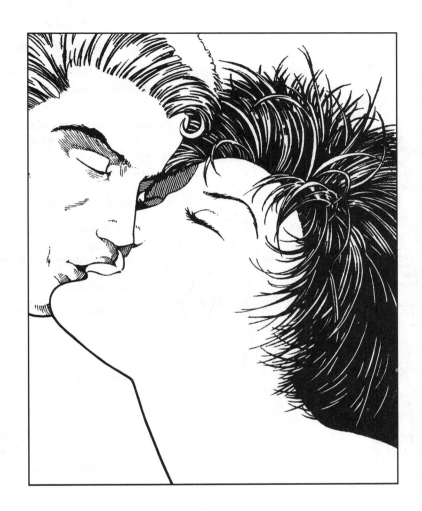

Welcome!

www.Guide2Getting.com

Guide To Getting It On!
Ninth Edition

V. 9.0 (9th ed, 1st printing)

Publisher's Cataloging-In-Publication
Joannides, Paul N.
Guide to getting it on! / Paul Joannides, author;
Daerick Gross, illustrator.--9th ed.
p. cm.
Includes bibliographical references
and index.
ISBN: 978-1-885535-17-7
1. Sex instruction. 2. Sex.
3. Man-woman relationships.

1. Joannides, Paul. 11. Title.

HQ31.J63 2017   613.9'6

Goofy Foot Press
Oregon, U.S.A.
www.Guide2Getting.com

printed in
Saline, Michigan
McNaughton & Gunn
Made in the U.S.A.

Guide To Getting It On

Unzipped!

author & publisher
Paul Joannides, Psy.D.

illustrator
Dærick Gröss Sr.

editor
Toni Johnson

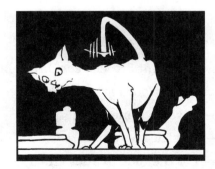

Goofy Foot Press
Oregon, U.S.A.

Bed of Contents

Warning & Disclaimer

Hard as I've tried, this Guide isn't perfect and it's not a final authority on sex. There will be times when it is better to consult with your best friend or TEDx. You might also speak to a physician or licensed sex therapist. Ultimately, it 's your body and your sexuality—venture beyond the bounds of common sense at your own peril.

This book talks about sex acts which are illegal in some parts of the world. Know the laws about sex and break them at your own risk; prison sentences, public stonings or beheadings could result.

The people who have contributed ideas to this book are psychologists, social workers, lawyers, teachers, writers, a couple of surfers, some prostitutes, a priest and 10,000 survey takers. Just because some of these people have college degrees doesn't mean they know any more about sex or relationships than you do. They all struggle at times. Still, their perspective might be helpful.

While the techniques mentioned in this book work well for some people, they might not be good for you. Check with a healthcare provider before attempting any sexual act that you are unfamiliar with, or do so at your own risk and with the understanding that bad things might happen. Consult with a physician if you have any condition which precludes strenuous exercise or erotic activity.

All readers, except those who are trying to get pregnant, are encouraged to use the most effective method of birth control, such as an IUD, and to adopt a medically-sound strategy for avoiding sexually transmitted infections. However, no form of birth control is foolproof, and diseases have been known to outsmart the finest of barriers. These are normal consequences of having sex and are this book's fault.

This book was written to help expand the consciousness of its readers. Neither Goofy Foot Press nor any of its minions shall be liable or responsible to any person or entity for any loss, damage, injury or ailment caused, or alleged to be caused, directly or indirectly, by the information or lack of information contained in this book.

This book contains anatomical illustrations which are at best simple approximations. If your anatomy differs from what is shown, take heart, everyone is unique. Hopefully there is at least some similarity with what's beneath your clothes and what's between these covers.

If you do not wish to be bound by this disclaimer, please return this book with a copy of the sales receipt to the publisher for a full refund.

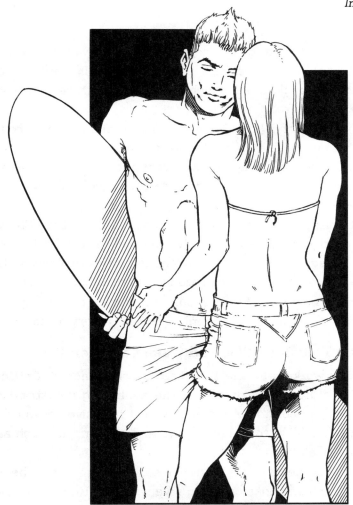

Introduction

When I started writing this book, the men who made Snapchat weren't even born and the founders of Facebook were six years old. There was no texting, Google, Grindr, YouTube, or Amazon. Porn was mostly in magazines that you hid under your bed, and phones were wired to the wall.

Scientists still clung to the notion that men wanted sex more than women and that women wanted to be married so they could have more children. We should be thankful that I began writing *The Guide* while sitting on the warm sands of Topanga Beach in Southern California. You couldn't help but look at the women on that beach and know that science had it all wrong.

Many things have changed since the 1st edition went to press. Yet humans still have the same genitals and a lot of us still want sex to be special. Hopefully, you'll have as much fun with this 9th edition as your parents did with the first.

I never expected this book would be used in more than 50 college sex education courses. Then students started telling me the book was the best sex-magnet ever. They would leave it out for others to see, and sex would often follow. (Why it's used in medical schools I'll never know. Medical students don't have time for sex.)

The first college to assign *The Guide* was Santa Barbara City College. I used to drive to Santa Barbara to hand deliver the books. Santa Barbara City College will be the first college to receive this new edition. East Carolina University will be the second, and then Miami of Ohio.

The Guide is now in its 9th edition. That wouldn't have happened without the help of many of you. Thank you so very, very much.

Who This Book Was and Wasn't Written For

When I was working on the 1st edition of the *Guide To Getting It On,* I met with a group of gay men in the publishing industry. I told them I wanted this book to be one of the most inclusive books on sex ever written. I wanted it to speak to gays and lesbians as much as to people who are straight.

The first thing they did was point to a sad looking shelf in the back of the gay and lesbian bookstore where we were meeting. They said it was the one shelf in the entire bookstore that had to be dusted the most often. It was the shelf where the inclusive books on sex were placed.

They explained that gay men don't want to read books on sex with chapters about vaginas and breasts. Did I really think a gay guy would want to buy a book with illustrations of a man with his face between a woman's legs like on pages 249 and 254? As for lesbians wanting a book that shows women teabagging men's balls like on pages 263 and 267...

Their advice was, "If you write it for everyone, it will speak to no one." They also asked if I woke up each morning with a hardon for other men. When I said no, they replied "Why would you think you can write about our experience when it isn't your experience?" They encouraged me to write what I know.

If you know about the politics of sex eduction, you would understand how shocking their response was. They were saying I need to make this book for people who are straight and mostly straight, as opposed to having a political agenda to make everybody love everyone. But their advice made sense, and that's what I did, with a twist—I made respect for sexual differences a cornerstone of this book. This has apparently worked, considering how many of the college instructors who have assigned the book are gay and lesbian.

I've also given up trying to please people who insist that every word of every sentence must not offend a single person on the entire planet. During this past year, I've been told I'm not supposed to say "a woman's clitoris" because it might offend people who are transgender. So instead of using words like "woman" or "man," I should say "a person with a clitoris and vagina" or "a person with a penis."

The same goes for menstruation. I'm not supposed to refer to women as having periods. They want me to use the gender-neutral term "menstruators" for persons who menstruate. Otherwise, according to the Society for Menstrual Cycle Research, I would be reinforcing "the rigid gender binary that perpetuates privilege and oppression." As for the dude who drives across town in the middle of the night to buy a box of tampons for his menstruating girlfriend, I guess I'm supposed to call him a "non-menstruator."

It used to be the biggest enemy of this book were movies of childbirth they show in high school health classes in an attempt to scare girls from having sex. Instead of teaching about consent and the importance of learning about your body and talking to your partner about what feels good, they show close-up videos of 9-lb blood-covered babies forcing their way out of the vaginas of screaming women. From the time I started writing this book until now, our country has spent $2 billion promoting *Abstinence-Only Sex Education* and its message of shame. Based on the recent elections, there may be even more abstinence-only sex education, purity balls and virginity pledges.

And now, anything and everything having to do with sexuality has been landmined by academic types who see micro-aggressions and plots from the patriarchy lurking in every corner. When these people aren't saying mean things to anyone who doesn't agree with them, they are often dismissive and act superior.

So each prior edition of this book has had to weather whatever storm our sex-confused culture could throw at it. This edition is no different. It's totally up for the task.

As for the buyer at the Babeland sex toy stores who refuses to carry *The Guide* unless I re-write it in a way that she approves of, I'd like to say there's way more to diversity than using impossible pronouns and espousing only those beliefs that mirror your own. I've spent a lifetime fighting for the rights of people who are gay, lesbian and transgender. I've also written a book for men and women who like to have sex with each other. I'm proud of both, and will not be changing a thing.

Paul Joannides, Psy.D.

Page Layout Software : Adobe InDesign CC
Hardware : MacBook Pro
Prepress/Press : McNaughton & Gunn
Queen of Copy Editing : Susanne Schunter
eBook Guru : Ron Bilodeau

for Toni Johnson

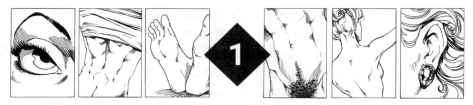

The Beginning

Each of the lovers you have in life will want something different from you. Some will want you to touch between their legs, others will want you to touch their soul. This book tries to help you with both. It encourages you to explore dimensions of sexuality that people usually aren't told about—from the emotional part of getting naked together to why a guy who takes his penis too seriously might have trouble pleasing his partner. It covers subjects like hand jobs and heart throbs, kisses above and below the waist, friendship, and sex in different kinds of relationships.

Whether you have lots of experience or have yet to be with your first lover, a good place to start is with our Goofy Foot Philosophy:

It doesn't matter what you've got in your pants
if there is nothing in your brain to connect it to.

Do With It What You Want

Since this is a book about sex, it makes sense to begin with a definition of what sex is. But trying to define sex is like chasing a rainbow. The closer you get, the farther it goes. Here are a few things to consider:

😎 People think of intercourse as the ultimate sex act, the real thing–*ipsum fuctum.* But if intercourse is the ultimate act, then why can making out or holding hands be sweeter and more meaningful?

😎 Almost all sex acts can be painful, obnoxious, or boring if you aren't doing them with someone who turns you on. Does this mean that the mental part of sex is more important than the physical part?

😎 Why does one couple find a particular sex act to be highly erotic while another couple finds the same act to be disgusting?

😎 A person has sex and an orgasm with a partner of many years, but the sex doesn't feel particularly exciting. The next afternoon he or she nearly bursts with excitement after catching the brief but intense gaze of a sexy stranger. How can a glance from a stranger take your breath away more than sex with a long-term lover?

😎 You are getting a physical exam. You are naked and your genitals are being touched. You feel no sexual excitement. However, if you were naked and being touched in this way after a fun night out, it might be incredibly sexual. How much do we rely on the context of a situation to tell us what's sexual and what isn't?

😎 How can a song, car, or piece of clothing be sexy?

Needless to say, we have given up on trying to pin a tail of definition on the big donkey of sex. It seems that any definition of sex needs to fit who you are as an individual as well as your particular situation. Instead of pretending to know what that might be, consider this:

> *Learning about sex and intimacy is a lifelong adventure. Even with years of experience, we still blow it on occasion. The best any of us can do is to tell you what we wish we had known about sex when we were young. That's what this book is about. Do with it what you want.*

Morality & What's in Your Pants

In much of America we still try to equate morality with whether you keep your pants on. We also associate morality with religion. But there are Christians, atheists, Jews, and Muslims who are moral people and there are Christians, atheists, Jews, and Muslims who are immoral people. The same is true for people who are sexually active and for those who aren't. Morality is about respecting and caring for your fellow human beings. It has little to do with how you enjoy your sexuality, unless what you do breaks a special trust or is not consensual.

Hmmm. A Book on Sex

Consider the books on sex that were written between 1830 and today. Many of these books gave a woman a psychiatric diagnosis if she liked sex as much as men. And men were told they would go insane if they masturbated. Today's books on sex make all sorts of claims as well. So keep two things in mind: that books on sex don't often pass the test of time, and this is a book on sex.

Sex books are merely a reflection of the time and culture that spawn them. Sexual fashion will change many times during your life.

How It Fits In

When your mom was in school, she couldn't sneak a phone between her legs and send a Snap of her pre-mom crotch to one of your potential fathers. You, however, are no longer constrained by the limitations of ancient technology.

But still, the reasons why people have sex are pretty much the same as they always were. Love and infatuation can be a driving force, but feeling horny and having fun are frequent motivators. People also have sex to make babies, to feel more grounded, to make money, to help them feel more desirable and less lonely, and the list goes on.

Sex with the same person can mean different things at different times. Early in a relationship, it might excite you and rev you up; later it might be a source of comfort and calm. In most relationships, there will be times when the sex is boring or when it makes you feel more distant than close. Just be aware that there's usually more to a good carnal experience than the hydraulics of sticking hard into wet. For some people, what separates good sex from bad are intangibles like fun, friendship, love, and caring.

As you get older, your expectations about sex may change. If you are 15, getting laid in and of itself can be a huge thing. But by the time you are 30, you'll have more experience under your belt. By then you might want your sex life to take you someplace different than when you were younger. Perhaps you will be searching for different qualities in a partner as well. Hopefully, you will want sex to be special no matter what your age.

A Red Flag—Matters of the Heart

Some sexual relationships are mostly physical. Others are emotional. Keeping it just physical is not an ability that everyone has or wants. Sometimes it depends on your situation and where you are in life, other times it's a matter of chemistry.

The emotions that accompany sexual relationships can be magical, enchanting, and wonderful. Then again, they can be awful. A cherished relationship can fizzle and go flat, leaving you with so much heartache you might wish you were dead. The tears can pour from a place so deep that you'll wonder if they will ever stop.

Lovemaking can be a way of working through fears and uncertainty, as well as a place for growth, fun, and friendship. Sex can help you be more honest, and alive with yourself and your partner.

No Assumptions Here

Most of us make assumptions about the sex lives and relationships of other people. Consider Tim, a computer geek, and Jake, a well-liked shortstop on his company's baseball team. Tim is bicep-challenged while Jake looks like he just leapt from the pages of *Men's Health.* Yet Tim-the-geek has a creative and fulfilling sex life with his partner, while Jake-the-hunk lives in fear that someone will discover his sex life consists of porn and and his right hand.

This book is just as much for Tim and his girlfriend as it is for Jake. It makes no assumptions other than you are curious about sex and might want to enjoy it even more. It also tries to accommodate a full range of sexual tastes and beliefs.

Smart vs. Dumb

Just about anything in this world that's worth doing will kill you if you're stupid about it. Having sex can be far less risky than driving on the freeway or even driving across town. It just depends on how smart you are about sex and how badly you drive.

You know the drill about condoms. And given that 50% of pregnancies are unplanned. IUDs are a great no hassle way to prevent pregnancy.

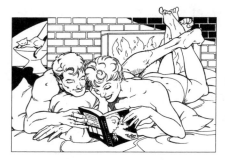

Dear Paul,

In my intro psych class, they wanted us to take a detailed survey about sex. My boyfriend and I really like sex, but I didn't feel comfortable doing the survey and left most of it blank. Does this mean I'm weird?

Athena from Mt. Holyoke

Dear Athena,

My own suspicion about sex surveys began two days before I took my first intro-to-anything class in college. I had spent my first 18 years in a small town that didn't have a lot of stop lights or two-story buildings. It did have as many bars as churches, and it wasn't unusual for girls to get knocked-up before the end of high school.

So I had spent the totality of my life in the nape of America's red neck. Then, I suddenly found myself as a freshman at UC Berkeley, where there were Krishnas instead of cows, and "weed" was no longer the hallmark of poor pasture management.

Back then, I had no idea that the nice, neanderthal-looking guy who lived upstairs in my dorm would become a co-founder of Apple, or that I would someday write a book on sex that people like yourself would have on their shelves or in their phones.

What I did know is that I had to show up at the student health center to take a physical exam. That's when I became one of hundreds of guys in their boxers or briefs, waiting in a mile-long line to pee on command. Then we got to stand in front of a row of doctors who pulled our briefs down and reported what they saw to the young nursing students who were sitting next to them with charts in their laps. Not being ones to take it on faith, the nursing students looked up and checked as well.

Then, when I got back to the dorm, there was a thick survey sitting on my desk. It wanted to know about my personal sexual habits. Being barely a man and just two days in the big city, I wasn't ready to confess "how many times I masturbated during the past week." But I did know that no matter how far from home you are and no matter how fast of a lane you have fallen into, what's personal is personal and nobody has a right to take that away from you. So, like you, I left the survey blank.

As I think back over the sex survey from my first few days in college, I am reminded of how complex and personal sex is for some of us, as it seems to be for you. At the same time, I appreciate that your roommate might be uploading videos of herself having sex on sites where everyone can see them. And what about all of the people who post intimate details of their private lives on social media?

Are you "weird?" Perhaps. But I suspect that's true for many of us.

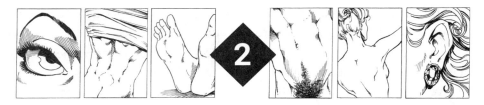

Romance

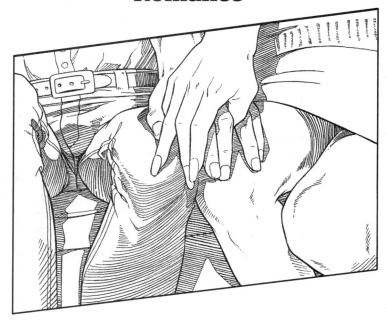

Romance is something thoughtful you do for someone you love. It's the Gorilla Glue that holds relationships together. It's lube for above the belt instead of below.

Romance can be as simple as leaving a note on the refrigerator that says "I love you," sending a thoughtful text, or giving an unexpected hug. It can include heroic gestures like helping your partner do a project or scouring the tile in her skanky-looking shower or taking a whole day to organize his or her *Nightmare-on-Elm-Street* closet.

Contrary to what the ads on TV show, romance does not need to cost a thing. It should not require an increase in your credit limit. You are deluding yourself if you think the only way you can be wildly romantic is by single-handedly jump-starting the economy.

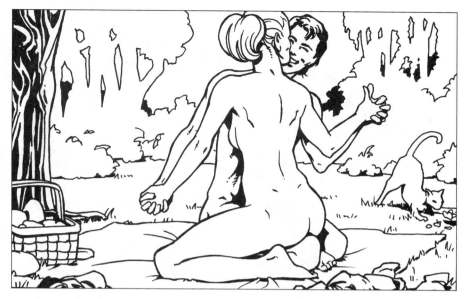

Romance vs. Sex

Try not to assume that romance will result in sex. Romance resides in a special universe somewhere between Platonic love and carnal lust. It can evolve into sex, and the sex can be incredibly romantic, but it's possible to have a romantic evening and end up in bed alone. When that happens, you do what the rest of us have done since the beginning of time: you romance your penis or clitoris yourself.

Romance When Dating as Opposed to When You Are Married

Getting the oil on your partner's car changed and having it washed can be a romantic thing if you are dating. However, if you are married, it's probably one of those things that's migrated from the romance column to being just another job on your to-do list. Hopefully it's something your partner appreciates, but it's unlikely to get you a night of oral sex because "you're so darned wonderful."

But when you were dating, going to a movie might not have been particularly romantic, given how you would do it at the drop of a hat. But once you have kids, going to a movie involves hiring a babysitter and maybe picking her up, getting dinner made for your children, and finding some way to defy the laws of parenting and get to the theater on time. By virtue of the wedding ring and your most excellent breeding skills, going out to see a movie goes from routine to romantic.

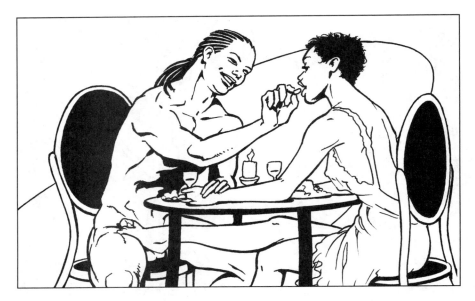

Likewise, your partner may have loved receiving stuffed animals before marriage, but after having children, the population of stuffed animals in your household may have reached critical mass. She's thinking, "How do I sneak this bag of stuffed animals to Goodwill without little Sophia having a meltdown?"

Married or not, getting a lover her favorite chocolate is almost always romantic regardless of the number of notches on the side of her uterus. Chocolate works on the same part of the brain as cocaine and heroin.

Getting Your Romance Meters in Sync

If the person you are lusting over feels like a keeper, try to figure out what is romantic to him or her. This might be different from what's romantic to you.

While things that make a big splash could be what catches your romantic eye, your partner might prefer the understated. Just because his or her style is different from yours doesn't mean you can't be wonderfully romantic in each other's eyes. Over time, you should make a mental list of things your partner goes "Wow!" over. That way you won't panic when the need for romance arises.

Romance during stressful times can require a different approach, such as turning into a rock your partner can lean on or quietly taking up the slack in other ways. If your partner has a huge project coming up or is dealing with serious drama, plan ahead for things you can do to help make it better, although being supportive doesn't always require "doing" something. Sometimes it just means listening.

Reliability vs. Excitability: Romance in Long-Term Relationships

In long-term relationships, all the romantic gestures in the world are meaningless if you aren't trustworthy and don't do your share of the work. Romantic gestures won't get you far if you didn't do the things your partner was counting on you to do.

On the other hand, when you hear people in long-term relationships say the sparkle has gone in their relationship, maybe they have worked so hard at being reliable that they have forgotten about the special touches that help make a relationship hot. Maybe they used to be more playful or daring. Maybe they made their partner feel incredibly attractive and alluring, but not so much any more.

There is a balancing act in long-term relationships, given how "reliability" means going to work and keeping your commitments, while "erotic" is more about dropping everything and surrendering to the moment. Doing fun things together becomes an important equalizer. It is as important as your best moves in bed.

When a Relationship Is New

It seems that during the first six months to a year in a new relationship, we process our lovers in the wild'n'crazy part of the brain. Our good judgment is mostly shot to hell and even a lover's most annoying habits seem endearing. We pine over them, obsess about them, and want to have lots of sex with them.

Then, after a year or so, we start to process our long-term partners with the "long-term relationship" part of the brain. We become more aware of the warts in a relationship. It can also be a time when partners sometimes stop trying as hard to be romantic. To protect your sex life from being lost in the kids-and-a-mortgage part of your brain, it helps to add novelty. Novelty is a way of lobbing your relationship back into the sexually-exciting parts of the brain. Maybe you can visit new and different places, have fun together, or try snuggling and making out when you are watching a movie.

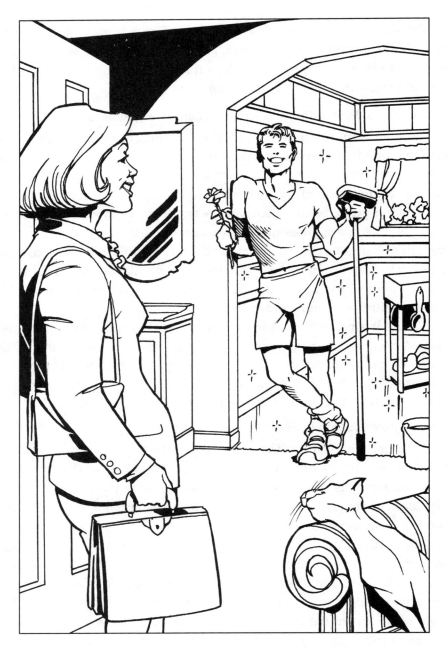

Men who help around the house get laid more often than dudes who don't, causing speculation that cleaning products in a man's hands are sexier than oysters and fast cars.

What Readers Have to Say about Romance

"Romance is being kind, gentle, and thoughtful. Sometimes intense as when making love, sometimes only on pilot light, but never off." *male age 70*

"Romance is when she and I can absolutely forget that the rest of the world exists. Just today we both had a million things to do to prepare for the coming work week, but I found a great Spanish song about a bull that falls in love with the moon. Soon we had dropped our work and were spinning each other around the living room like two people who had no idea how to dance flamenco." *male age 25*

"What is romance? Stroking my hair, holding my hand, helping me with the housework, cooking, talking, sharing the day with me." *female age 43*

"Romance is waking up in my partner's arms and being told that he loves me." *female age 27*

"Romance is sitting on a hammock together reading our books. It's when we go Rollerblading at the beach." *female 27 & male 32*

"For romance, I enjoy a great bubble bath together with candles and wine, lots of great smelling scents whether it's perfume, incense, or just the smell of my man." *female age 36*

"It's bringing home a single rose or a little something to say I was thinking of you today." *female age 34*

"Doing things that show he values me as a life partner and not just a bed partner." *female age 45*

"If he brings you flowers or jewelry and he's not there in any other way, it's not romance." *female age 45*

Dear Paul,

There's a really cool single mom at work who I'm thinking about asking out. I've never dated a woman with kids. Do you have any advice?

Mitch in Miami

Dear Mitch,

There is an amazing pool of women to date that some guys don't realize exist. They're called single moms. While plenty of single moms are only interested in long-term relationships, that's the last thing others will want. Having a trustworthy friend to meet once a week for sex and conversation or even just sex could more than fill the bill.

But let's say she is interested in something that's more traditional than casual. A man who dates a single mom needs to know about babysitters. No babysitter, no date, unless it's a family date or the kids are at their dad's. So the first words out of your mouth should be, "Can I help pay for the sitter?" and "It's too early in our relationship for me to be meeting your kids, but I can pick up a pizza for them?" This may not sound romantic to you, but few guys will be this considerate.

The next thing to know when dating a single mom is how kids can suddenly spike temperatures or start throwing up, especially when they don't want their mom to go out. And you won't believe the nasty array of colds, coughs and flus that kids bring home from school. So you will need to have patience and a willingness to masturbate when mom is suddenly hijacked by family matters. No matter how important you might be in a woman's life, you are not going to come between she and her kid's viruses, or hopefully not, anyway.

Until you've been dating for a while, think twice about getting super-expensive tickets for events. It will just make her feel bad if she has to cancel at the last minute, and it won't bother you nearly as much if the casualty is only dinner and a movie. If she suddenly has to cancel because of Junior's croop, you won't be anybody's chump if you leave a bouquet of flowers at the door with a note saying how much you look forward to seeing her soon. Yes, some parents are flakes and will use their children as an excuse, but you'll be onto that soon enough.

Do not try or expect to meet a single mom's kids for a long time. It's not fair to them if they become attached to you and you suddenly end up out of the picture. But you can still help. Ask about the things her kids like to eat. The 12-box carton of Mac'n'Cheese and frozen chicken tenders and chicken-pot-pies from Costco might be calling. At the end of a date, ask if she needs to stop by the grocery store on the way home. If that's the last thing she wants to be reminded of when she's out with you, she'll let you know. If you do meet her kids, don't go sticking your tongue down their mom's throat when they are around. Don't try to buy them off with gifts. Your friendship and concern about them is enough.

If you and their mom start having sex, you'll need to become logistical wizards like other parents do when kids are around.

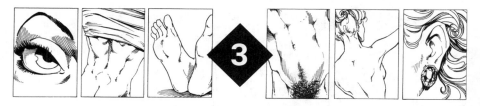

Kissing

It's funny how guys will worry about the size of their penises when they should be worrying about how well they kiss. Kissing usually says more about you and is more likely to be a deal breaker.

Kissing a partner on the lips makes more of an emotional statement than kissing him or her on the genitals, even if being kissed below the belt often feels better. One of this book's advisors, who makes her

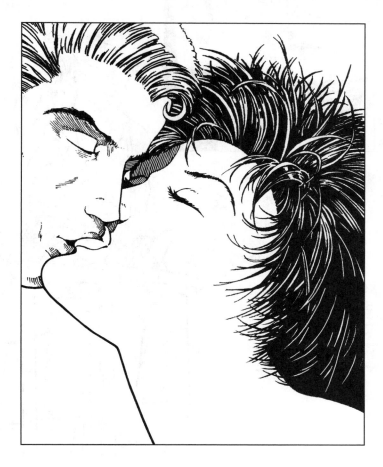

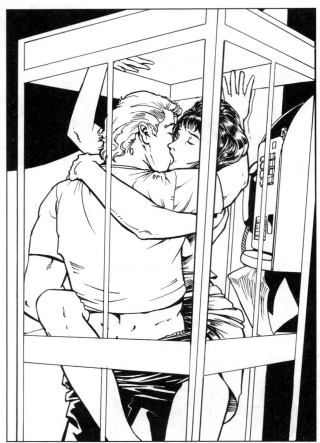

Then...

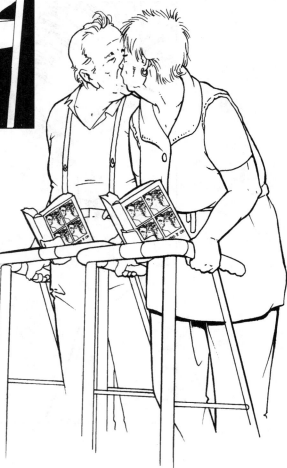

And now.
Same couple
50 years later.
Same Kiss?

living by having sex with different men, won't let anyone but her husband kiss her on the lips. And when a relationship starts to go sour, couples usually stop kissing on the lips long before they stop having intercourse.

There are reasons why kissing can be more intimate than getting into a partner's pants. From the moment we are born, most of us are kissed by moms, dads, aunts, uncles, grandparents, and anyone else whose approaching lips we can't successfully dodge. Being kissed symbolizes a love that we hopefully come into the world experiencing.

Another reason for the added power of kissing is so many of the major senses—vision, smell, hearing, and taste—have their outlets on the face. The face is so full of sensory centers that we have terms such as "You're in my face" or "Get out of my face" to express annoyance or social discomfort. The lips are also exquisitely sensitive to touch.

Look at the importance of lips in style and fashion. You can buy a zillion different colors of lip gloss and lipstick, with some that sparkle and others that make your lips look wet.

When Kissing Is the Main Course

Kissing on the lips often leads to other things, but there are plenty of times when kissing is all you get. Like when you are fifteen and necking all night long. Or when you are older but want to feel like you are fifteen. Or when a woman has started her period and she hasn't yet read this book's most excellent chapter on period sex, Chapter 27: *Surfing the Crimson Wave.*

Don't for a moment think that monster make-out sessions are kids' stuff. Some people experience these as hotter than much of the intercourse they've had.

If all you plan on doing is making out, be sure to put your gum in a safe place where you can find it afterward. It will help take the edge off until you can go home and masturbate.

Great Kissing Advice

"The best thing you can do is to ask your partner to kiss you the way he or she likes to be kissed. It really works. Just sit back and let him or her take over; you'll learn all kinds of things."

male age 26

We seldom take the time to ask a partner how he or she likes to be kissed. Maybe delicate butterfly kisses are what get your partner going rather than dramatic lip-lock action. You'll never know unless you ask.

Maybe you are too shy to ask a lover how she or he wants to be kissed. Why not do a search for "best movie kisses" and make a list of cinematic spectaculars to download? You and your partner can have fun trying to imitate some of the kissing scenes. Hopefully, your partner's favorite kissing scene isn't from *Lady and the Tramp.*

Readers' Smooch Advice: The Basics

"Please don't eat my mouth. A good kiss can make me wet with desire, with only the softest touch." *female age 23*

"Start really light. Barely brush your lips against hers. Be very aware of her response. Increase the pressure ever so slightly when she begins to meet your lips. Eventually, touch the tip of your tongue to her lips. If she opens her mouth, you can let your tongue enter just the smallest bit, but try not to force her mouth open." *male age 25*

"Kissing is not just a preliminary to fucking. Gently explore with your tongue, lightly suck on her lips and tongue. If she is into it as much as you, kiss with good suction, not lazily."

female age 45

"When you're kissing, be gentle; don't swallow a woman's entire face or dig your teeth into her cheeks." *female age 36*

Breathe or Die, and Don't Forget to Swallow

People who are new to kissing sometimes ask if they should kiss with their eyes open or closed. There is no right or wrong way. Experiment and see what works best for you.

Another question is what to do with your nose. When you are kissing, your mouth is often busy, while your nose is mostly in the way. Breathing through your nose gives it a purpose and keeps your partner from feeling like you are attempting mouth-to-mouth resuscitation. Tilting your head to the side can help avoid a collision of oncoming beaks.

You might find it helpful to take an occasional pause in the make-out action. Maybe you need to catch your breath; if you're a guy, maybe you need to adjust your erection. You can keep the momentum going during these intermissions by gently stroking the side of your partner's face with the back of your fingers, or you can tell them how much they turn you on or how lucky you are to be with them.

As for swallowing often, take these comments to heart:

"Try not to slobber!" *female age 25*

"Turn off the water works! There is nothing worse than a big slobbery wet kiss." *female age 27*

"An overly wet mouth is a turn-off." *female age 32*

"Girls love slobber. At least that's what they tell me. Maybe that's 'cause I slobber. Hey, wait a second!" *male age 22*

French Kissing

French kissing is spelunking with your tongues. However, it is not a tongue-to-tonsils regatta. Try swallowing first, and go gently. Pretend your tongue is Baryshnikov instead of Vin Diesel or The Rock, and you will do just fine. There is always time for tonsil-sucking later.

Don't occupy your partner's mouth like it's a parking space in New York City. Bring your tongue out for air. Try changing the pace by kissing your partner's neck before re-probing the deep.

Some people think their tongues should act like a penis when they are French kissing. A penis gets hard and likes to thrust in and out of anything that will have it. It can't help itself. But a tongue shouldn't thrust in and out like a penis and you shouldn't try to deep throat a partner with it.

"Take it slow and easy, but not too easy." *female age 26*

"Don't jam your tongue down someone's throat until she invites you in." *female age 38*

"Getting deep throated for fifteen minutes at a whack is no fun."
female age 48

First Time French Kissing Advice

You don't need to leap from closed-lip kissing to tonsil hockey in one fell swoop. If your partner is into kissing you and you've been at it for awhile, you might try opening your mouth a bit so there's a space

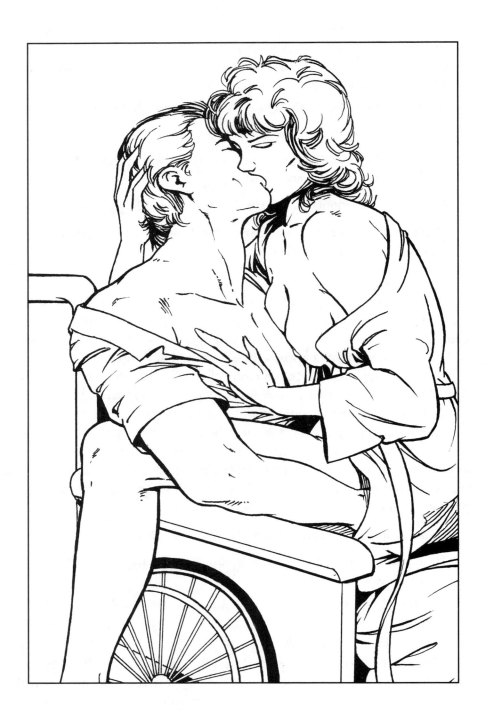

between your lips. You can then gently run the tip of your tongue around the edge of your partner's lips. That way, you're not invading their open-mouth space, but you're not being a weenie either. See how your partner responds. If they want your tongue, they'll let you know. They might even put their tongue in your mouth. Or maybe it will feel nice to gently suck on an upper or lower lip without anyone's tongue leaving its bullpen. Sooner or later, you might want to explore a partner's mouth with your tongue, but don't make them feel like they are at the dentist. Forge ahead in small steps, seeing how your partner responds before exploring further.

Tongue Sucking

When sucking tongue, you are basically doing the same thing to your partner's tongue that you would to a lollipop. Sometimes you can suck your partner's tongue into your mouth, which can be kind of cool. Be gentle and brief your first few times; see if your partner likes it.

Your Hands on a Partner's Breasts, Butt and In Their Hair

What you do with your hands when you are kissing can put a kiss into hyper drive or it can mess everything up.

Once the situation is warming up, a partner might enjoy it if you run your fingers through their hair while you are kissing. But if a woman has a head full of hair extensions or has done serious moussing, she might grab your hand and pull it away. Respect this. Run your fingers through a partner's hair once and see what their reaction is. Also, hair follicles contain nerves. Some partners will want you to run your fingers gently through their hair; others enjoy a firm grip on their hair.

Never assume it's okay to put a hand on a partner's breasts just because you are locking lips. Just because she might have her tongue down your throat doesn't mean you have a free pass to grope her breasts. If a woman wants a man's hands on her breasts, she should grab them and put them there. Unfortunately, not all women realize that if they want something they need to speak up and ask for it.

If it seems like a woman's breasts are calling to you for attention but she won't put your hand there, you might try sensuously running your hand up and down her side. Don't move your hands to her breasts until you get a loud and clear signal to do so.

It can feel really good when a partner runs a hand up and down your back while you are kissing. The same is true with a hand on the butt if your partner is cool with it.

Body Contact When Kissing vs. Dry Humping

It's hard to ignore that your chests and crotches are speaking to each other when you are making out. But you don't want your partners to feel like they're being dry humped if all they want is to be kissed. There will be times when making out turns into dry humping, but kissing passionately and dry humping are not the same. The safest and smartest route is to let it be a mutual decision, with plenty of feedback.

Flossing, Brushing and Death Breath

It is raunchy to kiss with pieces of food stuck in your teeth. Flossing and brushing can make you far more attractive than wearing cologne or sucking on breath mints. If you are concerned about bad breath, check with your dentist. Dentists know all about bad breath, as many of them have it themselves.

If you are eating food with garlic or onions, make sure the person you plan to smooch has some too. Flossing and brushing won't put a dent in breath that is laced with garlic. Your only defense is to share the offense.

Kissing When You Are Wearing Lip Gloss

Some people will refuse to kiss a woman who is wearing lipstick or lip gloss. They don't like the feel. Others enjoy it when a woman is wearing a particular flavor. You usually can't go wrong with a natural hydrating coating, but greasy glosses can feel gross.

Plenty of women will pull out a tissue and do a quick lipstick wipeoff when they're about to start kissing. This can be a wise maneuver if you are kissing someone for the first time. Once you get to know them better, you might try out your favorite flavors and see if they bite. As for glitter gloss, be sure to ask.

Out Damn Gum!

Even if you just popped in a new piece of gum, do not try to hide it in the back of your mouth when you are making out. There are couples who have no problem passing gum back and forth, but until you and your partner are that kind of couple, take the gum out.

If You Are Wearing Braces

If you have braces with rubber bands, consider taking the rubber bands out ahead of time. One reader barely escaped mid-smooch tragedy when a rubber band on his sweetheart's braces came unhooked and nearly shot him in the uvula. A direct hit would have triggered the same reflex that causes vomiting.

Also, an incoming tongue might get scratched or caught on metal edges that don't pose a problem for the wearer of the braces. Talk to your partner about this, so he or she can map out any danger spots.

Putting the "Neck" in Necking

In hundreds of sex surveys that male and female readers of *The Guide* have taken, a large majority say they wished their partner would spend more time kissing them on the neck. Lots more time. So don't forget the neck!

Hickeys and How To Hide Them

Hickeys are what happen when a lover sucks on your neck or other body parts with enough force to cause internal bleeding. The hickey is the resulting bruise. Some people love the feel of getting hickeys, it's how it looks the next day that can be the problem.

Hickeys go through stages, so you will need to change your cover-up makeup as the hickey goes from three-alarm to one-alarm.

If the hickey is blue-black-purple, use a yellow-based concealer. If it's reddish, try a green concealer.

If the hickey is greenish-yellow, use a pink-based concealer. Be sure to blend out the edges.

If your hickey is blue-black-purple at the epicenter and reddish around the perimeter, dab on yellow in the center and green over the reddish part. After the concealer is on, dab on your normal foundation. Do not rub. Then use your normal powder. If not being found out is of the utmost importance, try a translucent powder on top to help set it.

If you don't have green, use an oil-based concealer that is lighter than your natural skin color. That's because the hickey color will cause the lighter concealer to look darker. Focus the concealer only on the hickey area and not on the skin beyond it. Otherwise, the unbruised skin around the hickey will look like a big smudge, and people will know.

Teeth on Skin

Teeth on skin can feel really nice or really ugly. Lube your lover's skin with oil or saliva so your teeth glide along the surface. Then run your teeth back and forth. You might try a bit of biting action on large muscle groups such as the shoulders or buns. Be sure to get feedback and try not to violate your local cannibalism statutes.

Kissing in Other Cultures

Instead of kissing on the lips, Eskimos allegedly rub noses. What's closer to the truth is that Eskimos put their noses in close proximity to inhale the breath of a loved one. Perhaps they do this to keep their lips from freezing together.

Eskimos find that inhaling the breath of a lover is erotic; those of us from more temperate climates prefer exchanging wads of saliva.

Passion Pits Then, Netflix and Chill Now

Drive-in theaters used to be called passion pits. They were where younger couples kissed, groped, and petted themselves into a frenzy. Drive in theaters were so popular fifty years ago that your parents or grandparents might have been conceived at one.

It never hurts to have a "Drive-In Night" in your living room or back yard if you have a projector. Don't forget the popcorn and condoms.

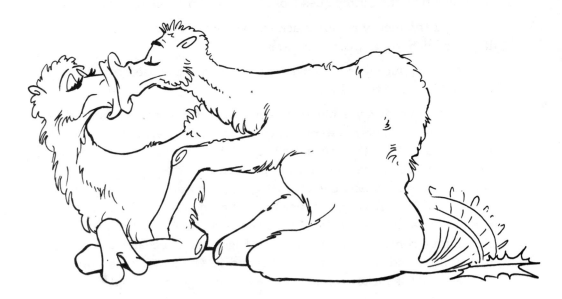

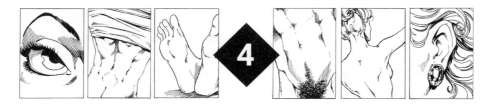

The Importance of Getting Naked

In relationships, there are different kinds of nakedness. Sometimes, we just get physically naked. Other times, we get emotionally naked as well. For some people, getting naked in front of a lover is easy and natural. Some sext naked pictures of themselves. For others, getting naked can be stressful or embarrassing. They might engineer situations where they can get it on without taking their clothes off in front of a partner. (High school athletes are so uptight about getting naked in front of each other that a lot of them won't shower before an after game dance.) This should give you an idea of how powerful getting naked can be, and how vulnerable we can feel about our bodies.

As a culture, we are so uptight about nakedness that we don't have street-corner fountains with cherubs peeing into pools of water or public paintings of naked Botticelli babes. A bare crotch on primetime TV is about as common as a snowstorm in Siam. We've relegated naked genitals to porn.

Don't Sell Near-Nakedness Short

Many of us are more aroused by near-naked images than by actual nakedness. That's because near-nakedness allows more space for our fantasies to imagine what's under a thong, bikini, Speedos, or whatever. The suggestion of impending nakedness can bring all sorts of intrigue.

The Naked-Nipple Rule

In North America, we believe that a woman isn't really naked unless her nipples are showing. In Europe, they still don't understand the big fuss over nursing babies and naked nipples. We have the naked-nipple rule on most beaches in North America. Hopefully, you can violate this rule with a lover at home as often as you both like.

Getting Naked—Hidden Possibilities

A lot of honesty and trust can be generated when you are naked together, something that rarely develops if the sole purpose of taking your clothes off is to have sex. It's how a guy can learn to have his penis resting on a woman's soft, warm skin without feeling like he has to perform with it, and how her vagina and breasts can be pushing against him while she dozes off.

Some couples enjoy undressing each other, while others make a game out of taking their clothes off, from playing strip poker to light-hearted wrestling. Getting naked happens naturally if you shower together or go skinny-dipping. Sometimes it happens when you are hot-tubbing, and some couples like undress each other while dancing.

It can sometimes be helpful for partners to tell each other some of the things they do and don't like about their bodies. Some women worry about their butts being too big or their breasts being too small or mismatched, or that their labia are not porn perfect. Some guys worry they aren't hung well enough, or they might be hung too well, or they don't have six-pack abs like the dudes do in Daerick's illustrations. Getting your fears out in the open with a partner will usually help you feel more comfortable.

One way for the shy to share their nakedness is by getting a fun top or T-shirt to wear with nothing on underneath. Or maybe you'd like to try a pair of cool boxers or boardshorts.

Guys Worry: Is Wood Good or Not So Good?

When it comes to getting naked, men sometimes worry whether they should or shouldn't have a hard-on. It's fine either way. The point is learning to associate nakedness with something other than just sex or taking a shower. And some people don't have the slightest hesitation to get naked for sex, but if it's getting naked just to talk or hold each other, good luck. They may become fidgety and fire off a rapidly dismissive, "Sure, we'll have to try that sometime...." Perhaps that kind of nakedness feels too intimate.

As for what to do after you've made love and are still naked, it might be nice to spend extra time holding and touching each other. Having orgasms clears the senses in a way that allows some of us to share a special kind of warmth and tenderness. (One reader comments, "Good

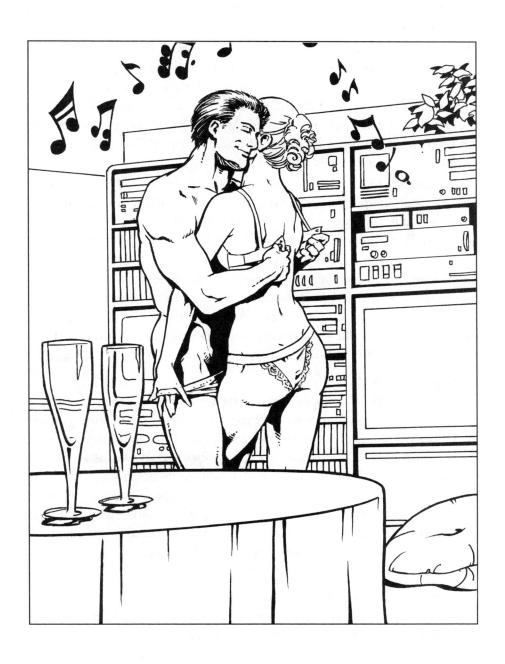

luck on this one. I've spent a lot of lonely time while my partner sleeps immediately after orgasm.")

Stripping

Getting naked for an audience is called stripping. Until a few decades ago, stripping was something that only women did. Then male strip shows became popular. (Contrary to what you might think, it's the women at the male strip shows who go wild and get aggressive, while the male audience members at female strip shows are expected to totally behave themselves and quietly pay for lap dances.)

According to *The Stripper's Guide to Looking Great Naked* by Jennifer Axen and Leigh Phillips (Chronicle Books), a stripper's appeal is all about attitude and having her own style rather than sporting the perfect body. Forget going on strange diets, and spending hours at the gym.

The Stripper's Guide says that when comes to trimming your pubic hair, women with a voluptuous or well-endowed body might try a landing strip. The vertical line balances the curves and draws the eyes downward. A woman with an I-shaped body might go for a more natural-looking pubic bush which helps make her hips look more round and curvy, assuming she still has a bush.

Playing Strip Poker

A fun and time-honored way of getting naked together is to play strip poker. For a woman who unexpectedly finds herself in a game of strip poker but hasn't trimmed her pubic hair in a month and is wearing a granny bra, *The Stripper's Guide* suggests that she head for the bathroom for her three minutes of ABT "allowable bathroom time." She should stuff the granny bra into her purse or into a drawer (better to be totally topless than shirtless with an ugly bra). She should run her fingers under cold water and tweak her nipples. And if the cards aren't running her way and she loses her pants, she should make a show of taking them off, but sit with her legs crossed.

Cam Girls — Nakedness Makes Online History

Until the invention of the webcam in the late 1990s, if you wanted to see a stripper strip, you went to a club that featured strippers. But then came huge leaps in technology followed by JenniCam which featured the Internet's first cam girl.

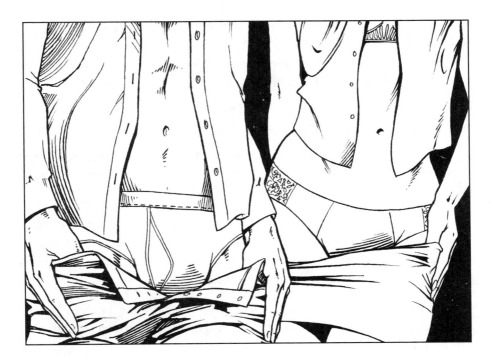

JenniCam was broadcast live from 19-year-old Jennifer's Ringley's dorm room in Dickinson College in 1996. There was only dialup back then, so the early webcams would only refresh once every three to five minutes. Live streaming wouldn't happen for years.

Early cam girls like Jenni were referred to as "lifecasters." They were the forerunners of reality TV shows like *Big Brother.*

The webcam was on in Jenni's dorm room 24/7. Much of the time, viewers would see nothing but an empty room, or they would see Jenni eating or reading. Jennicam viewership skyrocketed when her webcam started showing Jenni having sex with her boyfriend. It wasn't long before 3 to 4 million people a day were watching Jenni mostly do boring things, with a few minutes of sex thrown in every now and then. This was the magic of the early cam shows. Viewers could be the ultimate voyeurs.

A key part of the early cam girl experience was the blog or website where the cam girl would keep her diary or post her daily journal, answer viewer questions, and provide an archive of images. The early cam girl blogs were the Facebook pages of their day. But only a handful of cam girls would ever experience the level of celebrity and social net-working fame that Jenni Ringley did.

JenniCam was live for seven years. It was the perfect intersection of technology, exhibitionism, and voyeurism. People would spend hours waiting to see not much of anything.

Naked and Getting Naked Underwear Tips

😎 When going out, a woman might let a man know that she is not wearing underwear or reach into her purse and pull out a pair of pant-ies while saying, "Oops, I forgot to put these on!"

😎 Go down on your partner while she or he is still wearing under-wear. You can reach under the material with your tongue or pull a part-ner's underwear down with your teeth. If you are having a quickie, keep your underwear on and try working around it.

😎 Dry humping with only your underwear on can be fun. Taking a shower or bath while one or both of you are wearing your underwear can be fun.

😎 For men, the next time you are in a department store with your lover, nudge her into the men's underwear department and ask her what style and colors she thinks might look best on you.

😎 Some guys get very turned on when a partner is wearing panty-hose. If that's the case, a woman might try cutting out the cotton crotch on a pair of pantyhose. (She should cut out the crotch on the inside of the seam so they don't unravel.) Her lover can then go down on her or they can have intercourse while she is wearing the pantyhose with the new ventilation system. She can also purchase crotchless underwear, but probably not at Walmart or Target.

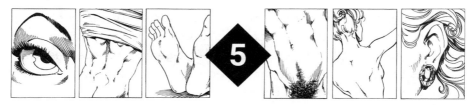

On the Penis

This chapter was written for women readers, although the men who have seen it claim to be amused. The topic is boys and their toys. Hopefully the following pages provide some insight into the relationship between a man and his weenie.

Toys, Pain & Pleasure

As a woman, the first thing you will find out about penises and testicles is that most guys take them way too seriously. There are reasons for this:

😎 The penis is the only childhood toy that a guy gets to keep and play with throughout his entire life. It is the only toy he will ever own that feels good when he tugs on it, that changes size and shape, and is activated by the realm of the senses. You won't find that at Amazon.

😎 One of the first things a man does when he wakes up in the morning and the last thing he does at night is to grab his penis and testicles. It's a ritual of self-affirmation that has little to do with sexual stimulation. A daytime extension of this is known as pocket pool.

😎 The average male pees between five and seven times a day. Each time he pees he has a ritual, from the way he pulls his penis out to how he wags it when he's done. When he is peeing alone a guy will often invent imaginary targets in the toilet to gun for. An especially fine time is had when a cigarette butt has been left behind. Gunning for floating cigarette butts is the male urinary equivalent of playing video games. While this may be a difficult concept for a woman to fully grasp, it makes for a certain amount of familiarity, friendship, and bonding between a man and his penis.

😎 How many women look down when they are peeing to see what's coming out of their bodies? Guys look down often. As a result, we males get visual reinforcement for the feelings we have in our genitals when we pee. Between erections, pocket pool, package adjustments and peeing, guys have more sensory experience with the penis than most women have with their vaginas. This must be why women sometimes call us "Dicks!" (Women have hand-eye-genital experiences when they use tampons and shave, but that doesn't start until after puberty and it's often associated with blood, cramps and razor burn.)

👓 You wouldn't believe how often the human male experiences a jolt of pain in his testicles. It is a discomfort that gives a guy the kind of extra-personal relationship with his reproductive equipment that menstruating women have with theirs. The source of agony can be anything from an elbow during a game of basketball to simply bending over and having your pants crimp the life force out of you. One of the great culprits in male testicular angst is the horizontal bar on the bicycle frame. It's where boys' balls land when a foot slips off the pedal. Why is it that girls' bicycle frames are V-shaped when it's guys who need the V?

👓 This may be difficult to fully appreciate, but there is the matter of the unwanted hard-on. The unwanted hard-on usually strikes with ferociousness first thing in the morning. Not only does it interfere with the ability to relieve a full bladder, but it provides logistical problems for a guy who has walk down shared hallways to get to the bathroom. The unwanted hard-on can actually feel painful for its most frequent victim, the adolescent male. The unwanted hard-on is much less of a problem after a man turns thirty, and by the time he's forty it is an event accompanied by a sigh of relief and a moment of thanks.

👓 Porn teaches us that sexual pleasure between a man and a woman depends on the man's ability to get hard and stay hard. What a demented view of sex. This puts a lot of pressure on guys to be consummate cocksmen. It makes us more dick-centered than necessary, at the expense of everyone.

👓 When life is full of despair, the one thing a man can usually count on for a good feeling is his penis, unless matters are totally out of hand, in which case he needs to consider something stronger like tequila or prayer.

These items aside, the most important thing for a woman to know about a penis is how it figures into a man's concept of his own manliness. Ridiculous, but important.

Weirdness in Locker Rooms

You might think that a man's primary concern about penis size has to do with what a sexual partner might think. But how he stacks up among his bros is just as important. When we asked men if they feel comfortable about being naked in the locker room, the majority answered the question as if they'd been asked about penis size, even if the words *penis* and *size* were never part of the question. These are the exact answers men gave:

"How do you feel about being naked in the locker room?"

"I used to feel uncomfortable back in my freshman year of high school. Then I realized that I was really a little bigger than average." *male age 21*

"I used to think that my penis was really small, and so I was shy about it. As it turns out, I'm on the high end of average when erect: I'm just not a hanger." *male age 32*

"I have an inferiority complex about the size of my penis. I don't care how many studies tell me that I am right in the middle of the curve, I will always feel small." *male age 25*

"I was raised in strict religious environment, so nudity of any kind was a no-no. My equipment is pretty small and I was a late bloomer. All this adds up to being very shy about my own appearance. In junior high and high school, when 'naked locker time' was mandatory, I would arrive as early as possible and change quickly so others wouldn't see me. If others were around me without clothes on, I gave myself tunnel vision or imaginary blinders so I wouldn't see other guys' equipment. I didn't want to be perceived as gay, and glancing around was a good way to get yourself taunted at least, beat up at worst."

male age 41

The men who said they were comfortable in the locker room often made reference to their penis size, indicating they were well hung. You can almost predict how a man feels about being naked by asking how he feels about the size of his penis. Hopefully, the following from a Marine who has been in combat helps provide perspective:

"The tradition of group showers is still strong in the Marine Corps. It makes us more comfortable with each other, and if you are trusting a guy to save your life, do you really think penis size is that big a deal? Before the military though, I worried I didn't 'measure up.'" *male age 27*

As for guys checking out other guys, you would think this curiosity would decrease as they get to be adults. Not so, according to researchers who hung out in rest rooms at a San Diego Padres game and covertly studied a hundred different men who were peeing.

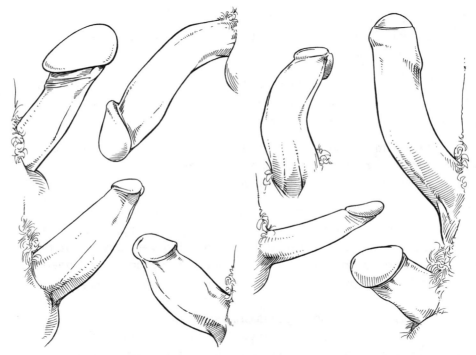

From these drawings of real-life erections, you can see that terms like "6 inches" or "normal" are meaningless. All of these erect penises are normal, yet very different from each other. In studies that included 15,521 penises, the average length of an erect penis was about 5.25 to 5.5 inches. The average circumference was close to 4.5 inches. The average length when not erect was about 3.5 inches. A penis that is 7 inches long when erect is in the upper 97th percentile of all penises. It's reasonable to assume that guys who are in porn or who upload videos of themselves have the largest 1% to 10% of all penises.

What's Inside a Guy

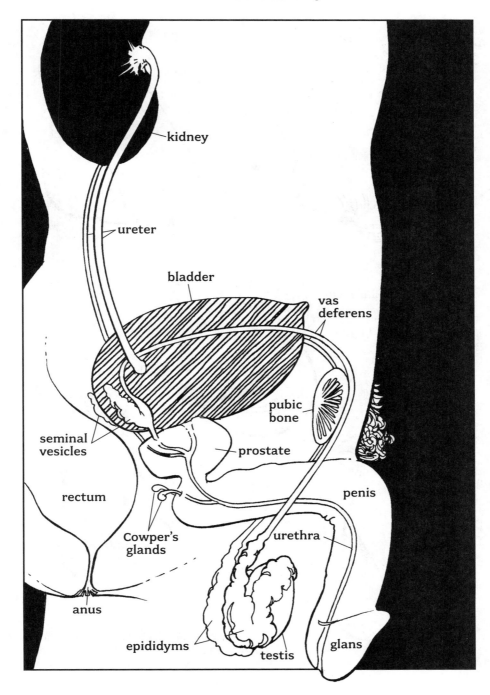

kidney

ureter

bladder

vas
deferens

pubic
bone

seminal
vesicles

prostate

rectum

penis

Cowper's
glands

urethra

anus

epididyms

testis

glans

THE GOOFY DICK GAME
Real Penises of Real Guys

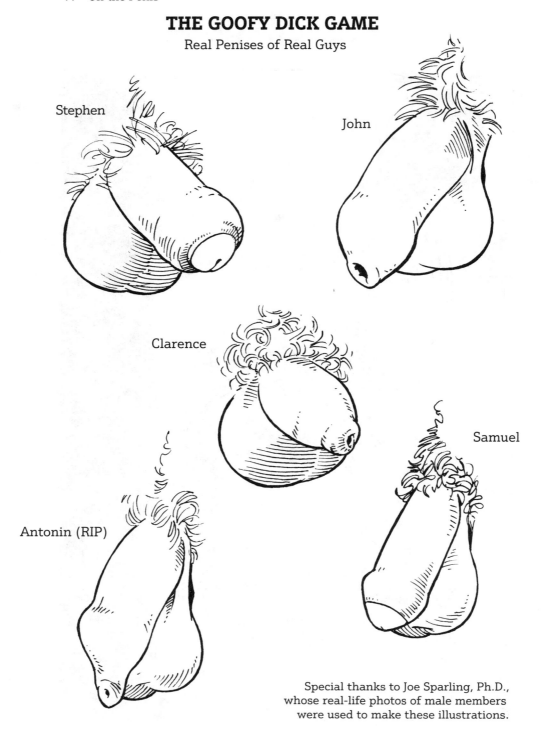

Stephen

John

Clarence

Samuel

Antonin (RIP)

Special thanks to Joe Sparling, Ph.D.,
whose real-life photos of male members
were used to make these illustrations.

YOU BE THE JUDGE!

Match Each Soft Penis On The Other Page
With Its Erection On This Page

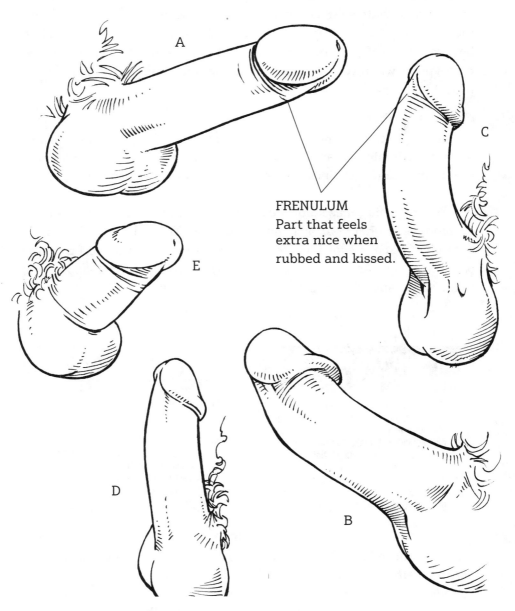

FRENULUM
Part that feels
extra nice when
rubbed and kissed.

Stephen-A   Antonin-C   Clarence-E   Samuel-D   John-B

Many of the men who were using the urinals made an attempt to check out the equipment of whomever was peeing next to them. Also, men who were well-endowed went out of their way to show their bigger units to the other men who were peeing. These tendencies might be more true of Padres fans than, say, Diamondbacks fans, who are usually too busy weeping in the men's room to check out the size of the other boys' bats. But if you are a man who has ever glanced down at another man's penis when you are peeing, take comfort in knowing that you are probably normal.

Manliness—What Is It?

In our culture, being manly means you don't act gay. It also means if you have feminine parts to your character, you keep them hidden. But that's an attempt to define masculinity by saying what it supposedly isn't.

What is being masculine? Is it a physical way of being? Is it a state of mind? Is it what your dick gets hard over? This Guide's definition of masculinity keeps evolving. Here it is in its current state (on the next page, anyway). As you will notice, it says nothing about being gay or straight, because that has nothing to do with masculinity.

Male Enhancement?

Ads like these have flooded the backs of newspapers and magazines since the 1800s. We now have TV infomercials and e-mails promoting products for "natural male enhancement." The products don't work. They never have, but the scams still do.

Masculinity Defined

Masculinity is mostly an invention of modern culture. It doesn't have a huge foundation in science or nature, yet it remains a powerful force in the way we view ourselves and each other.

To be manly or masculine, a guy should be a responsible person who can be independent when the occasion demands. He should try to be caring, comforting, and kind. He should be able to give and receive physical and emotional tenderness without being too controlling. He should have values and a good work ethic, and he shouldn't need to prove his masculinity by trying to scare or intimidate others.

He should have a presence that's greater than the Nike symbol on his shoes or the UnderArmour logo on his shirt. If there's a tough job to be done, he should volunteer to do it no matter how much he doesn't want to.

He should rarely whine or blame others for his own screw ups. He doesn't need to have a vagina-seeking sensor at the end of his penis, and his physical appearance can range from geek to movie star. Showering to prevent smelly balls and pits should be a priority.

Some men have none of these qualities, but appear to be studs nonetheless. These are guys who usually take their penises too seriously. That is because the only way they can convince themselves they are real men is by performing manly activities or drinking lots of beer or doing drugs, and then having a vagina nearby they can stick themselves into. They are more show than substance.

The man who doesn't take his penis too seriously doesn't flake out when it comes to doing the dishes. He may have his passions in life, often sports, music, gaming, work, or trying to fix things (sometimes successfully), but these usually help to center rather than isolate him. Sex with him is a natural extension of your friendship. It makes all the sense in the world.

As for "curing" the kind of man who takes his penis too seriously, you can't. No human being has ever changed because someone else wanted him or her to. It's something that has to come from within.

Friends and lovers can sometimes help if they are willing to call the guy on his nonsense, but they can't make the changes for him.

Why It's Difficult to Be Satisfied
By a Guy Who Takes His Penis Too Seriously

A penis is sometimes used to camouflage what's missing inside a man, as well as what's missing in a relationship. If a guy demands that his penis has a disproportionate amount of attention, then it gets in the way of his being at one with a lover.

Unfortunately, a lot of women grew up thinking that a distant, self-involved, dick-centered type of guy is what manhood is all about. Or they hook up with whiney dudes who they need to take care of. As a result, they end up with men whom they can never really get close to and spend the rest of their lives complaining about what duds men are.

Dumbed Down Dudes?

Researchers have been trying to figure out why the ratio of women to men on college campuses is approaching 2 to 1, given how it used to be the other way around not long ago. One of the things they are finding is that a lot of young men don't think it looks good to be smart. They think it's cool to be dumb.

Seriously?

The parents of girls often tell them "If you work hard, you can be whatever you want to be when you grow up." The "whatever you want to be" part might be a little extreme, but it could be that more parents should be providing their sons with more guidance and expecting more from them than is currently the case. And women should think twice about having sex with men who think it's cool to be dumb. What if the condom breaks and you end up having a kid with the guy?

The Penile-Pumping Regatta

Some men lose emotional connection once intercourse begins. Sex becomes a penile pumping regatta in order to prove dick-worthiness. This can be really boring for both partners.

To give you an idea of how much insecurity is involved, consider the words of a 29-year-old man who is starting to question why he takes his penis so seriously:

"It's like, I attack sex. I'm afraid of slowing it down. If I'm gonna be fucking, I'll fuck like crazy, gotta have a huge dick and fuck like crazy to avoid dealing with whatever's making me anxious. Women have always said to me, 'God, you can't get enough.' But I think the reason I can't get enough is that if I slow down, the fears start to crowd in on me. Does this woman really want to be with me? Is she going to leave? Is my cock good enough? It's hard for me not to use sex as a seal of approval."

—From Harry Maurer's *Sex: An Oral History*, Viking Press

Porn merely reinforces paranoia about dick worthiness. The fact that most porn actors consume nearly fatal amounts of Viagr to stay hard is lost on most men and women. And there are plenty of women who have their own insecurities. (Is getting breast implants or wearing a padded bra all that different from this guy's need for a perfect penis?)

Sexual Awareness: Hood Ornaments vs. Wet Triangles

When it comes to sexual awareness, the penis is positioned like the hood ornament on a car. It's difficult to ignore what your hood ornament is telling you. Sometimes we guys aren't even aware we are sexually aroused until we feel ourselves starting to get hard.

Women are not conditioned from early childhood to associate sexual arousal with specific body cues in the way that men are. While their genitals often swell and lubricate, the flags that get waved are sometimes more subtle. Most of the changes happen on the inside and can be chalked-up to a tingly sensation between their legs. Besides, "good" girls are usually taught to ignore their body's sexual cues.

While the penis can be a reliable indicator of sexual excitement, it does have its share of false positives and occasional negatives.

How a Penis Gets Hard

The penis contains three chambers inside that run the length of it. Two of the chambers are responsible for making it hard or rigid. They are called the corpus cavernosa. They run parallel to each other up the shaft of the penis. Think of a double-barrel shotgun, and that's how they sit next to each other. These two chambers are made of spongy material and are covered by a thin but extremely tough exterior. To make a penis erect, they fill up with blood. This makes them inflate. It puts pressure on the exterior covering and causes each of the chambers to feel hard. As a result, the blood pressure in an erect penis is way higher than the blood pressure in the rest of a man's body.

These chambers run beneath a man's testicles and are anchored inside of his pelvis. That way, he can't pull his penis off of his body when he's masturbating.

The third chamber that is inside of the penis is made of a similar spongy tissue as the corpus cavernosa. It is called the corpus spongiosum. It encircles the urethra, or the tube that a man pees and ejaculates through. While this tube expands during erection, it doesn't have a tough exterior covering like the other two tubes in the penis, so the surface doesn't become hard or rigid. If it did, it would crimp shut the urethra and there's no way a guy could ejaculate through it.

The corpus spongiosum also forms the head of the penis. While the head of the penis expands or mushrooms during erection, it stays relatively soft.

Unwanted Wood

"For some reason, out of nowhere, your penis starts to get hard, and it is extremely difficult to stop." *male age 25*

"It's totally embarrassing. You just want to get up and go, but you can't. So you start pulling on your shirt or sweater to try to cover up the bulge. You become very self-conscious; you think everyone is looking at your crotch." *male age 43*

"It's like being in an elevator with an umbrella that will not go down." *male age 42*

"It can physically hurt when your penis is trapped in your jeans pointing downward and it suddenly gets hard for no reason whatsoever." *male age 26*

"Most of my memories of unwanted erections were at school, generally during class, and I was terrified that someone would notice." *male age 24*

"I travel a lot for business and sometimes wake up erect after a flight. It's terribly embarrassing. If I can't think the damn

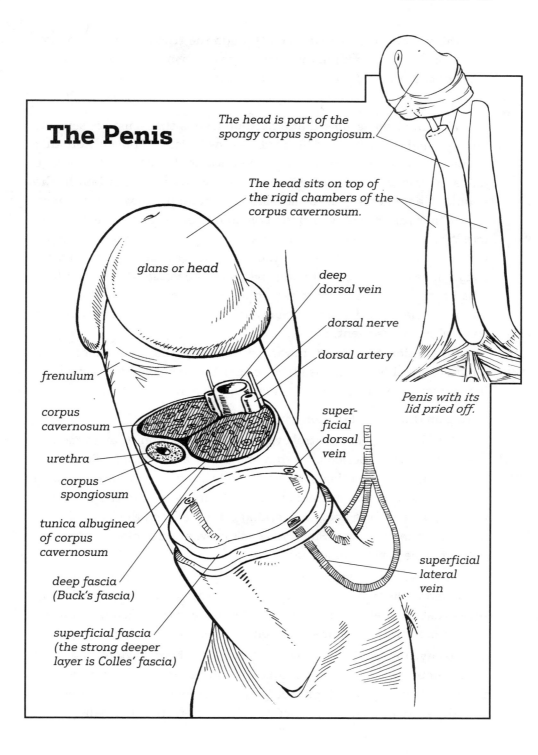

The Penis

The head is part of the spongy corpus spongiosum.

The head sits on top of the rigid chambers of the corpus cavernosum.

glans or head

deep dorsal vein

dorsal nerve

dorsal artery

Penis with its lid pried off.

frenulum

corpus cavernosum

superficial dorsal vein

urethra

corpus spongiosum

tunica albuginea of corpus cavernosum

deep fascia (Buck's fascia)

superficial lateral vein

superficial fascia (the strong deeper layer is Colles' fascia) thing down, then I have to go through the tricky maneuver of flipping it up, trapping it under my waistband without being noticed, and keeping my briefcase in front of me when I stand."

male age 25

Women often assume that a hard-on means that a man is sexually aroused, and that no rise in his pants means he isn't. If only it were that simple. Consider the occurrence of the unwanted hard-on: The average teenage male is capable of getting a totally unwanted hard-on in the middle of an algebra test for absolutely no reason, unless he is a member of that rare breed who finds polynomial equations sexually arousing. When you are a young man, hard-ons just happen; nobody is more befuddled than the possessor of the penis. To say that all hard-ons are a sign of sexual excitement badly overstates the case. One reader took a bad grade in an early-morning high school class because he couldn't go to the chalkboard due to his unwanted erections. His only thoughts were of embarrassment, not sex.

In addition to getting unwanted hard-ons, there are times when a man can feel highly aroused, yet either fail to get hard or have it go limp when he needs it the most (floppus erectus).

Hiding an Unwanted Erection

Guys have no more control over unwanted erections than women do over getting their periods. So thinking about awful things like french-kissing your grandmother isn't going to bring a raging hard-on down because it's probably not about sex to begin with. Pinching yourself until you bleed won't help, and jerking off more often than you already do won't change a thing. Since you can't prevent unwanted erections, it helps to have ways to hide them.

Avoid wearing sweat pants in public places. The sweat pant material is more likely to drape around your erection and show it off. Wear pants that are made of more rigid material like denim. You might avoid skinny jeans until unwanted hard-ons are less of a problem..

Baggy untucked Ts or sweat shirts have been saving men from boner embarrassment since the beginning of time. The same is true for a briefcase, backpack or laptop bag with long straps that you can casually shift in front of your crotch. If your erection normally points upward, put your hands in your pockets and nudge it under the waist-band of your briefs or boxers. This maneuver is called a 'waistband tuck.'

False Negatives: When Gravity Dings the Dong

Confucius says, If limp dick is worst thing that happens to your relationship, you live charmed life.

Hopefully, your lovemaking isn't solely dependent on the man's ability to get hard. If it is, your sexual relationship might be somewhat limited. It's also disconcerting to think that your entire sex life would be centered on the whims of the average penis, hard or soft.

Regarding the biology of erections, it is perfectly normal for a hard penis to partly deflate every fifteen minutes or so. As for the psychology of erections, hard-ons have been known to fly south for varying periods of time, from a single day to who knows how long.

The most unhelpful thing a woman can do when a guy can't get it up is to become defensive. Women often assume that erection failures mean the man doesn't find them attractive or that he might be gay. These are possibilities. But there are a billion other reasons for not being able to get an erection, from fearing you won't be good in bed to what just happened on Wall Street. Physical problems like diabetes can also be a factor. Given the stress of living in the modern world, it's a wonder we men are able to get it up as often as we do.

While most of us have been raised to think of a limp penis as a sign of failure, it's more productive to view it as an opportunity to bring a man and woman closer together. At the very least, it will force him to become better at pleasing a partner with his lips, tongue, fingers and imagination.

Betty on Dick

The following passage is from Betty Dodson's classic *Sex for One* from Harmony Books. In addressing the issue of misbehaving penises, Ms. Dodson speaks with welcome concern:

"Although I ran only a dozen men's groups, the experience helped me to let go of my old conviction that men got a better deal when it came to sex.... I thought they could always have easy orgasms even with casual sex, and I envied their never having to worry about the biological realities of periods or pregnancies. But the truth is that not all men are able to be assertive studs who make out all the time.... The most consistent sex problem for many men in the workshops was owning a penis that seemed to have a will of its own. An unpredictable sex organ that got hard when no one was around and then refused to become erect when a man was holding the woman of his dreams in his arms...."

If this sounds familiar, tell your partner there probably isn't a woman alive who wouldn't be happy to receive a long, lingering back rub and oral sex in the place of intercourse. Or what about a go at an orgasm from Chapter 19: *The Zen of Finger Fucking?* If his woody won't work, let him know there are plenty of other ways to please you sexually.

This Guide's Philosophy

Never, ever let a recalcitrant penis ruin sex for either of you!

When Young Men Use Boner Drugs Recreationally

There is an increasing number of young men who don't have erection problems but take erection drugs for recreational purposes. This might be due to unreal expectations that their penis needs to be like that of porn stars, many of whom are taking erection drugs themselves.

Young men who don't need erection drugs but start taking them can become psychologically dependent on boner drugs. They can also expect themselves to have erections that are harder than normal and are quicker to rebound.

Nature didn't create erections to be like baseball bats. Normal is not porn perfect. So no matter what your age, if you don't need erection pills, don't take them. The money would be better spent on romance. The following personal account from a reader echoes this concern:

> I was dealing with a pretty complicated personal life, along with stress and mild depression. So my erections weren't as consistent as I would have liked. My doc prescribed Viagra, at my request. I was able to take it and get a good effect from very small doses, which means it was probably just working as a mental crutch. Later I found myself with an interesting feeling of psychological dependence on the Viagra pills. They made me lazy. I didn't have to worry about relaxing, clearing my head, being present, the pills did all the work. Plus, I would

psych myself into problems, by worrying about not taking the Viagra, then worry myself into having problems, and then feeling shitty if I had problems and hadn't taken it. It was a very interesting dog-chasing-its tail syndrome.

So when they describe folks as addicted to Viagra, I get it. Even for young men, it can serve as a psychological crutch, taking off a lot of the very significant pressure we feel to get hard at a moment's notice. Even now, after not taking them for months, if I have the slightest twinge of low response, I can start to panic, and this can create a cascade effect where I keep thinking about how that little pill would solve everything..."

In case you are concerned about your erections not being perfect, take solace in knowing that after receiving 5,000 sex surveys from women over the past ten years, there have been very few complaints about a lover's ability to get an erection.

Penis Perceptions Driven By Porn

Dr. Stephanie Buehler, a therapist with years of experience, has been seeing an increasing number of normal young men who she says:

"Believe they should be studs who are able to perform any time, anywhere, with anyone at a moment's notice."

Physically, these young men are perfectly normal, but they think there is something wrong with them because they can't perform like the men in porn. This is especially unfortunate because one of the things women want most in a potential partner is a good personality. (Men in porn aren't defined by their personalities.) Porn is also helping drive unreal expectations in some women about the sexual abilities of men.

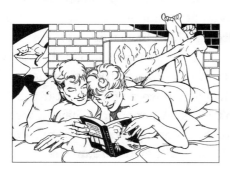

Dear Paul,

My boyfriend always wakes up in the morning with an erection. But when we start having intercourse, it goes down. He doesn't have this problem any other time. What's up?

Gretta in Marietta

Dear Gretta,

The erection your boyfriend has when he first wakes up is little more than a limp penis trapped inside of a raging hard-on. It happens because he wakes up while dreaming. Men usually have three or four erections during a normal night of sleep. These are caused by the changes in the body that happen during REM or dream sleep. They are triggered by a different part of the brain than normal erections. So your boyfriend is waking up with a leftover sleep erection. Men get them whether they're dreaming about being chased by wolves or being kissed by the love of their life.

Although his penis looks and feels hard, it's not the kind of erection he gets when he's been thinking about you. Even if it seems like it's ready for action, treat his penis like it's a floppy one that needs to be aroused. Try kissing or playing with it before jumping his bone(s). This might help turn it into a waking-state erection that's sex worthy.

Since his erection was not born from sexual desire, don't assume that your boyfriend feels like having intercourse. He might feel better if he could pee and brush his teeth. Or he may be just fine having sex with a full bladder and dragon breath.

Do a search for "morning wood" at www.Guide2Getting.com to see how men from our sex survey describe how their waking erections feel versus the erections they get when they are awake and sexually aroused.

Wet Dreams & Dry Dreams

A wet dream is when a guy has ejaculated in his sleep and managed to leave a sticky mess in his underwear, pajamas or on the sheets. However, plenty of orgasms when dreaming are dry, so the term "wet dream" a misnomer. And men will sometimes ejaculate in their sleep and not remember having had an orgasm or even dreaming about sex.

Both men and women have sex dreams. Men have them more often as teenagers, with the frequency decreasing as they get older. Most women don't start having sex dreams until they are in their twenties.

Some guys think they are more likely to have a wet dream if they don't masturbate. This usually doesn't work. A person can have a wet dream the same night he or she masturbates or has sex. So not masturbating probably won't increase your chances of having dream sex.

Amber Streams

Every once in a while a girlfriend will ask a guy if she can stand behind him and hold his penis while he pees. This is a completely normal request born of normal curiosity. But be forewarned that you are sometimes giggling so hard that the entire bathroom becomes a target. On the other hand, women sometimes do a better job of aiming the thing than we men do. One reader says she loves grabbing her husband's penis and writing their names in the snow with its amber stream.

Cramped Penis Alert

When a guy is wearing pants and he gets an erection, his penis will often be trapped in a downward or horizontal position. While it might be presumptuous for a woman to lend a helping hand if you are making out on a first date and his penis gets hard, it can be a nice gesture when you've been dating for awhile to reach inside his pants and pull his penis up so its head is pointing up unless it naturally bends down.

Getting Older

As things get older, they start to petrify or harden. This is true for logs, fossils and the human brain. Unfortunately, it is not true for the penis. As a penis approaches its fifth decade, it tends to petrify less fully than it did earlier in life. It can also squirt less fluid during ejaculation. Some women will cling to this information like a ray of hope, while others will be disappointed. As man gets older, he can compensate with wit and wisdom for what he loses in hardness and volume.

First Ejaculation

Before puberty, a young dude can stroke his pecker until it nearly falls off, but his orgasms will be dry except for a few drops of precum. This will change during puberty. Puberty kicks the prostate gland, seminal vesicles and testicles into semen-making mode. It creates semen and an adult ejaculation.

The process of going from a few drops to a full wad can be wonderful if you know what to expect. It can be disturbing if a guy hasn't been told about ejaculation and he masturbates for the first time after entering puberty. Here's how boys used to react to their first ejaculation before porn was so easy to access:

"I was eleven and discovered this new feeling when I rubbed this silky part of my blanket over my penis, so I kept doing it. Eventually, I got this intense feeling in my groin and then there was this goop everywhere. I was completely freaked and grossed out. I thought that I broke myself, but was too afraid to tell my parents." *male age 34*

"I was sure anything that felt THAT good had to be sinful and that my ejaculate was evidence that I was damaging my insides. Each time I'd masturbate (almost daily) I would feel horrible guilt afterward and swear to God that I would never do it again." *male age 44*

"I had heard about masturbation while sitting in the back of the school bus. When I tried it just the way the kids told me, it was almost like pain. For weeks I would stop short of actual orgasm for fear that I would do some sort of internal damage to myself. Finally, one day I kept rubbing through my fear and found that I enjoyed the hurting tremendously." *male age 35*

Today, most boys watch porn before puberty and know it's normal for men to produce a wad of semen.

Men Who Have Multiple Orgasms before They Shoot Semen

Most males experience orgasm as an overlapping two-part process—sensation and ejaculation. But some guys have learned to separate the two events and have a couple of orgasms before they ejaculate. According to Dr. Marian Dunn, who interviewed a number of men with this ability, a common thread was that their partner remained in a state of high sexual excitement after the man's first feeling of orgasm. This seemed to provide a path of feedback that the man could feel in his penis as it remained inside her vagina. It's also likely that the men had really good control to begin with.

Some of the men had small ejaculations with each orgasm, while others didn't ejaculate until the end. Some had been able to do this all of their lives; others had learned it recently. The men who had always been able to do it assumed that all men could and were surprised when a sexual partner pointed out the difference. This should not be confused with delayed ejaculation, where the man wants to have an orgasm but is unable to.

Hormone Advisory: The Impact of Testosterone

The bulk of men's testosterone is produced by the testicles. Men with higher levels of testosterone are more likely to be on the football or rugby team than men with lower levels of testosterone. They're more likely to be aggressive, to want to show off more to women, to want to pump iron, and they'll probably want to have sex more often than men with lower testosterone. Men with high levels of testosterone are also more likely to be in prison and they are more likely to be unemployed.

Men with lower or more moderate levels of testosterone tend to be more agreeable and less reactive than men with high testosterone. So a general or a diplomat whose effectiveness depends on consensus building rather than impulsivity is more likely to have a lower level of testosterone than a soldier who loves the rush of battle. And a prosecuting attorney is more likely to have a higher level of testosterone than a patent attorney.

A male with lower testosterone is more likely to be introverted, is less likely to perform extreme skateboard tricks and do dangerous and otherwise stupid things. However, there is no association with testosterone and courage or bravery. So the terms "he's got balls" or "grow a pair" aren't accurate. Nor does having low testosterone have anything to do with cowardly behavior or with being wimpy.

More important than the absolute levels of hormones is how a man has been socialized to behave. Also, we shouldn't assume it's testosterone that causes horniness. Sometimes the level of testosterone goes up because a guy is already feeling horny.

Men and Estrogen

Contrary to what you might think, testosterone in men is converted into estrogen. The estrogen is very important for how a man feels. So if a healthy twenty-year-old male were to suddenly lose his testicles and not produce testosterone, he would suffer negative effects from having no estrogen in addition to having no testosterone. He'd essentially go through menopause. He would have hot flashes and his bones would become brittle. These are things that estrogen protects men from experiencing—in addition to feeling depressed and having little sex drive which would result from his having so little testosterone.

Men who have prostate cancer and are being given drugs to stop their testosterone production should talk to their doctors about taking an estrogen supplement. That's because the men suddenly have no estrogen as a result of producing no testosterone, and they can feel like they are going through menopause as a result.

The Great Testosterone Sham

Drug companies make millions of dollars selling testosterone to men who may not need it. They have created ads that make men over the age of forty think they'll get their twenty-year old selves back by taking testosterone. This is dumb and probably dangerous, but good luck talking sense to a middle-aged man who is being promised a pharmaceutical miracle.

Performance Enhancing Drugs, Shrinking Testicles and Man Boobs

Performance enhancing drugs often contain testosterone. When the brain detects the level of testosterone is higher than normal, it will throttle down activity in the testicles in order to decrease testosterone production. This can cause the testicles to shrink.

Extra testosterone in the male body is converted into estrogen. This results in such a large increase in estrogen that it can cause a guy to grow man boobs. So athletes who are taking performance enhancing drugs will then take drugs that women are given for breast cancer. These cancer drugs will help lower estrogen and hopefully make man boobs smaller. Do you really want to do this to your body? Also, some of the muscle building supplements that you can buy anywhere are suspected of causing up to a 65% increase in a young man's chances of getting cancer of the testicles.

Guys & Horniness

It is assumed that the average male wants to have sex every hour of the day as long as the opportunity presents itself. There are plenty of men for whom this axiom does not apply. It could be the man has a nervous system that's sensitive enough to be impacted by some of the really disturbing things that happen in the world. Or maybe he is tired and needs a good night's sleep. It is sometimes difficult to drop everything and have sex. There are plenty of times when it's just as nice to cuddle up close to a lover and enjoy falling asleep in each other's arms.

How Often Do Men Think about Sex?

Two of the more common urban myths about sexuality are that men think about sex every minute, and that men think about sex way more than women do. Researchers have found that on average, young men think about sex once an hour and women think about sex once every two hours. This can vary greatly from person to person and from hour to hour.

To help put it into perspective: *College students think about sleep and food as often, if not more often, than they think about sex.* Also, not all sexual thoughts are created equal. Sexual thoughts can range from a brief and fleeting stirring that lasts a millisecond, to an elaborate fantasy that can cause a tent in your pants or a flood between your legs.

Something that can influence a woman's sexual thoughts more than men's is if she feels discomfort about her sexuality or if she worries that others will think badly of her for being interested in sex. If that's the case, she'll be less likely to have sexual thoughts, or less likely to admit to others that she has sexual thoughts.

Mercy Sex Basics—Making a Man Come Sooner

Let's say you are okay with getting a man off as an act of kindness but you aren't particularly into it, or you need a good night's sleep. Here are some suggestions to help a man come sooner.

Tighten the Foreskin: Pulling the foreskin taut around the base of the penis can cause a man to feel more sensation when it's is stimulated.

Focus on the Frenulum: The frenulum is the most sensitive part of the penis. It's just below the head of the penis, on the side where the seam runs up the shaft. During oral sex, you might focus on this area. If doing him by hand, make sure that your fingers run over this part of the penis during each stroke. Pumping too quickly may numb out the penis and be counterproductive. Also, if a guy is circumcised, using a well-lubricated hand rather than doing him dry might help speed things up.

Adding a Squeeze or Twist: Try giving a well-lubricated hand job where your entire hand wraps around the penis and twists up and down it as though it were following the red stripe on a barber's pole. Try a similar twisting motion with your head during oral sex. A slight turn of the neck is all that's needed, nothing to give you whiplash. At the same time, work the area between his testicles with one of your hands.

Visuals: If the man is turned on by your naked body, crank up the lights and park the parts he enjoys most in full view. If you have a particular bra or panties that get him going, suit up.

Play with yourself: Never hesitate to play with your nipples or vagina. Some men will be so turned on by watching you play with yourself that they will begin to masturbate and finish themselves off.

More nerve bundles: Some men have a spot on the part of the penis that is buried beneath their testicles which can deepen the sensation when pressed upon (see page 222). Keeping a finger on this spot may help move up launch time. When giving blow jobs, some women will work this area with one hand while pulling the skin on the shaft taut with the other.

Nipples: Some guys' nipples are quite sensitive; others aren't. Tweaking a man's nipples with your fingertips or caressing them with your lips and tongue might speed up arrival time.

On or Up His Rear: The human anus is probably the second-most sensitive part of the body. A wet finger on it, swirling around it, or pushed into it can speed some men up considerably.

Extras: If he gets turned on when you talk dirty to him, do it if you are in the mood. If he likes porn, put his laptop or iPad where he can see it. If you are having intercourse, try slowing down the thrusting rather than speeding up, or change the pace. If he is thrusting shallow, have him thrust deep. And don't let him pause, which is what a lot of guys will do to keep from coming. If you usually have sex in the bedroom, switch to the kitchen or living room if you can. A change in routine can help increase the level of excitement and speed of launch time.

If His Penis Goes Pop

A penis should never make a cracking sound or go "POP." Although rare, the pop might be from a fracture of the penis, which has nothing to do with what most of us consider a fracture to be. Unlike an arm or a leg, there is no bone in the penis to break. So a penis needs to be erect for a fracture to happen, which is when one of the chambers or cylinders in the penis tears. The way they fix a penis fracture is by sewing up the tear in the side of the chamber.

A penis fracture can also be related to a snapping of the ligament in the penis. If it breaks and is not cared for soon, internal bleeding might permanently damage the penis. A fractured penis will often make a cracking sound, followed by rapid loss of erection, pain, swelling, and hemorrhage. The outcome is excellent if the penis is surgically repaired within a couple of hours. If you wait longer, the damage could be permanent, including a penis that's shaped like a deflated circus balloon, or an Allen wrench.

Any kind of genital pain that lasts more than ten minutes needs to be tended to by a physician. Long-term damage can often be averted if you get medical help right away.

Two Strange Causes of Penis Fractures

Penis fractures are rare. I a study of sixteen men who had fractured their penis, half of the men were having extra marital affairs when the injury occurred. Only three of the men were having sex with their own spouse in their own bedroom. So the sex was often rushed, aggressive, awkward, and it happened in unusual places like cars, elevators, offices and public rest rooms, where the men were unable to protect their penis from the sudden downward thrust of their partner.

Another cause of penile fracture can be an extremely aggressive form of masturbation. There is an area in Iran where this kind of penis bravado is practiced and it results in several fractured penises each year. It would be an awful thing for men in other cultures to start imitating.

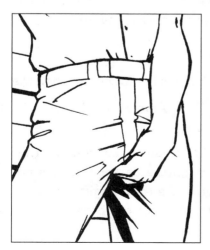

Dear Paul,

Why are guys always touching and grabbing at their genitals?"

Eva from Evanston

Dear Eva,

When the skin on the balls sticks to the thighs, or the skin on the penis sticks to the skin on the balls, you get a claustrophobic feeling. It's like if you had to keep your arms pressed against your sides all the time. Try it for just five minutes. When this happens with a guy's penis and scrotum, he's gotta dig to lift and separate or it starts to feel like he's going to go nuts. Body powder can sometimes help as long as it doesn't contain talc. Underwear that doesn't fit right can make matters worse.

———————

Dear Paul,

When guys are peeing, why can't they aim it right? Would it kill them to get all of it in the bowl?
                                                                    Nancy in Niagara Falls

Dear Nancy,

The problem is not with the aim, but with the unpredictable nature of the stream. It breaks up about as often as the signal on a cell phone. Sometimes a rebel tributary appears and shoots off to the side, a healthy stream will suddenly turn into a spray, or it goes where you aim it, but the toilet water splashes up and makes a mess on the rim.

Another cause can be when a guy has a foreskin that extends past the glans of his penis and he doesn't retract it when he pees. Whatever the cause, there is no reason why a guy shouldn't grab a wad of toilet paper and clean up after himself (bowl, floor, walls, shoes, ceiling). This is something that parents should teach their sons. Also, I don't know if you are aware of the first law of fluid dynamics, but a man never pees on his pants leg unless it is one minute before an important meeting, first date, or job interview.

I'm told that women can be wickedly messy when they pee in public rest rooms. But that's a different story for a different chapter.

———————

Dear Paul,

The skin on the shaft of my husband's penis is a lot darker than the skin on the rest of his body. Is this normal?
                                                                    Amber from Brownsville

Dear Amber,

It's perfectly normal. Penises vary as much in skin tone as they do in size and shape. One man's penis might be darker than his normal skin color, another's might be lighter, and a third might even have freckles or blotches. You can't predict the tone of the bone until the pants are down.

Dear Paul,

When my husband's penis is erect, it almost points down instead of up. Is this normal?

Diane in Bend

Dear Diane,

Penises often point up, at approximately a 30-degree angle from the stomach. But plenty of erect penises stick straight out, and others point down. You might try an intercourse position where you are on top but facing his feet. His penis may be able to tickle parts of you that a man with an "uppie" would miss. Most important is that you and he experiment with positions that feel good for both of you.

———————

Dear Paul,

My penis has a curve in it, but it only shows when I'm hard. Did I cause the curve by the way I masturbate?

Curly in Canton

Dear Curly,

It's perfectly normal for guys to have a curve in their penis which only shows up when they have an erection. Contrary to the urban myth that curves are caused by the way men masturbate, most curves happen before boys are born—when they are still fetuses in their mother's wombs and their penises are first forming.

In a very small minority of men, the curve can be so extreme that intercourse is not possible. But for most men, this is not a problem. A curve can be a strength if there are special spots in a lover's vagina that can benefit from the focused attention that a curve can offer.

———————

Dear Paul,

When it comes to pleasing guys, why are they so focused on their penises? There's so much of the body that feels good when it's kissed and touched, yet they seem to want everything to focus on the penis.

Flabbergasted in Frankfurt

Dear Flabby,

Let's say you've ordered the best takeout and have a romantic, candlelit dinner for your lover. You've gone to the gym, shaved, and are wearing killer jeggins and your sexiest thong. You want him to want you more than he wants his car, his phone or Halo. But when the lights finally go down, there's no party in his pants. No matter what you try, he's not able to have an erection. So tell me, what's going through your mind? Are you worried he doesn't find you attractive? Do you wonder if he'd rather be with someone else?

The truth is, you are probably just as focused on his penis as he is. It's the ultimate indicator that you are attractive and that he is excited about you. So once a penis gets hard, a guy figures he'd better start doing something with it ASAP. If the thing suddenly goes down, especially when your legs are wrapped tight around his waist and you've just cried out, "Fuck me harder," he'll be a big disappointment to you and an even bigger disappointment to himself.

Also, a man sometimes feels a strong need to ejaculate once he becomes aroused. This need is more pronounced in the teens or twenties than later in life. It makes us focus on having to do something with the penis rather than being able to enjoy what's going on around us.

In Praise of Geeks!

What better way to end a chapter like this than with the following sentiment from a female reader:

> "I don't know about other women, but I have discovered that the *geek* crowd which doesn't often get laid in high school has a great deal of time to contemplate what they'd do if they ever got their hands on a woman. They are far better lovers because they've taken the time to contemplate something other than *scoring*. As a friend of mine used to say, 'Nine-tenths of sex happens in your mind; the rest is all in your head.' Geeks think, while jocks avoid it at all costs because in high school, thinking is not cool. Besides, geeks know how to be passionate rather than just *stoked*. Give me a geek any time."

A reader asks "Help, my new boyfriend's penis is HUGE."
The response is on pages 326 - 328.

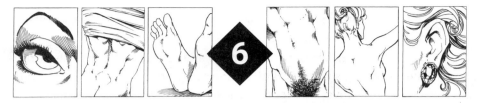

Semen Confidential

A woman from Utah asked, "Why does male ejaculate smell vaguely of cleaning products?" This one question has lead to an entire chapter—about semen, not cleaning products. It's all here: why semen can cause stains, what semen allergies are, why you might get an upset stomach after swallowing semen, why semen gets clumpy in water and sticks to hair on the shower drain cover, and an answer to the mother of all semen questions: "Why does my boyfriend's semen burn when it gets in my eyes?"

Semen doesn't pour out of a penis homogenized like milk from a carton, even if a guy has been bouncing on a trampoline. The first squirt of each ejaculation has secretions from the Cowper (bulbourethral) glands and the Littre glands. The prostate gland manufactures the next squirt, which makes up 15% to 30% of the total volume of each ejaculation. This is followed by the relatively small but potent contribution of sperm from the testicles. The seminal vesicles hold up the rear of each ejaculation with a blast of liquid that produces up to 80% of the entire wad.

Why Semen Smells Like Bleach

When Ms. Utah asked why male ejaculate smells "vaguely of cleaning products," she is referring to a bleach-like smell, unless the semen of men in Utah smells like Windex, 409, or Janitor in a Drum.

Contrary to what you might think, the testicles make less than 5% of semen. The lion's share of semen comes from two other sources: the seminal vesicles and the prostate gland.

Urologists know that when you cut open a testicle, there is no odor. So we can rule out testicles as the source of the bleach-like smell. The seminal vesicles aren't the culprit, either. That leaves the prostate gland, which produces a chemical called spermine. This is what gives semen its characteristic cleaning-product smell. Semen can also smell like fresh bean sprouts, which makes good sense because bean sprouts contain the chemical spermine.

The reason why some men's semen smells more bleachy than others is due to changes in the pH of semen and variations in how the body buffers it. The pH level impacts how spermine behaves. This is also why a man's semen might smell more like bleach one day and less the next.

For science and history buffs, spermine phosphate crystals were first found in semen in 1678 by Anton von Leeuwenhoek, father of the modern microscope. Semen was one of the first things Leeuwenhoek looked at under his new microscope (big surprise...). Two hundred years later, German chemists gave spermine its name, although women have known about the cleaning-product smell of semen since the time of Aristotle.

As a man is about to ejaculate, the components that make up semen collect in the part of the urethra that's at the base of the penis. To create an ejaculation, the muscle fibers surrounding this part of the urethra squeeze it like you might the bulb of a turkey baster. During this process, the phosphate in the spermine-phosphate molecules gets pried off. This allows the free base of spermine to be released which creates the bleach-like smell. Semen stops smelling like bleach after it's been in the air for a while because the free bases in spermine start linking together to form an odorless compound.

Why Semen Makes a Partner's Eyes Burn

A reader asked why her boyfriend's ejaculate burns when it gets in her eye. Spermine appears to be the culprit for that, as well. Pure spermine carries harsh warnings. The material safety data sheet for commercially produced spermine says:

> **Danger!** Corrosive. Causes eye and skin burns. May cause severe respiratory-tract irritation with possible burns. May cause severe digestive-tract irritation with possible burns. May cause central- nervous-system effects. May cause cardiac disturbances. *Causes eye burns.* May cause chemical conjunctivitis and corneal damage. Causes skin burns.

Fortunately, the concentration of spermine in semen is quite low when compared to pure spermine. While there might be other chemicals in semen that cause your eyes to burn, the number one culprit is sperm-ine. Also, semen can be a bit alkaline, which could possibly cause eye-ball irritation.

Why an Upset Stomach?

Some women report getting a stomach ache after swallowing semen. This is usually blamed on the prostaglandins that are in semen, which might make it similar to the kind of stomach upset that some people get after taking aspirin. However, after reading spermine's material safety data sheet, you can't help but wonder if spermine is also involved.

Why Semen Tastes Like It Does

When looking at why semen tastes the way it does, the amount of citrate ions stands out. These ions help semen to be a strong buffering agent, which makes it more friendly for sperm. They also create calcium citrate, which tastes salty and sour.

Semen also contains zinc ions. There's a taste test where people who are suspected of having low levels of zinc in their bodies are given a solution of zinc to drink. If their body has an acceptable level of zinc, the zinc solution tastes strong and unpleasant. However, if they can't taste anything, it's because their body has a zinc deficiency. This means that semen may taste better to people who have a zinc deficiency, although it's probably not wise to phone your healthcare provider and say, "My boyfriend's cum tastes really good to me. Does this mean I'm zinc-deficient?"

Bottom line: for most people, the zinc in semen is not going to help it taste any better. The same is true for the magnesium and sodium that's in semen. On the bright side, semen does contain fructose and glucose. However, the amount of fructose and glucose can vary by as much as four-fold from man to man.

When Semen Smells Bad Rather than Just Bleachy

Most women who've had sex with men have a baseline sense of what semen smells like. However, semen can occasionally have a pun-gent odor that can be the result of a hidden prostate infection. This might be a combined bleach-like odor and fishy smell. The fishy part comes from the polyamines that are released from decaying white

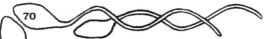

blood cells that end up in the semen due to the infection in the prostate.

Semen normally contains some white blood cells, but at a very low level. When a man has a prostate infection, the white blood cell count in his semen increases, which results in more of the smelly polyamines being liberated: As our consulting andrologist says:

"Since I do a lot of semen analysis in my office, I can tell the semen that has lots of white blood cells when we open the container. It has a really strong, bad odor—to the point that my research assistant is able to suspect that men have an infection just from the odor of semen when we are preparing slides."

Men who have prostatitis might notice yellowish, jellylike globs in their semen. Suspicions also rise when semen has a honey-like sweet smell. This can be the result of a staph infection. Healthy semen tends to be mostly white and has the smell of clean, fresh bleach.

Semen Stains

Ever notice that some mens' semen stains are worse than others? Semen contains a lot of protein, much of which is albumin. This is the same kind of protein that is in egg whites. As protein dries it changes optical qualities and color. The yellowish staining quality of semen is related to the concentration of protein in it. The sperm concentration can also have an impact. The higher the sperm count, the more opaque or yellowish semen will be. These factors determine why one guy's semen may have a greater tendency to leave yellowish stains in underwear, sheets and socks (a lot of guys use their socks for clean up when they jerk off).

How Thick Is Semen?

Viscosity is a measure of how fast or slow a liquid flows from a container. The viscosity of water is around 1.0 cP. The viscosity of semen that's fresh from the penis can vary from 1.3 cP to 23.3 cP. This means some men's semen is almost as thin as water, while other guys almost need a grease gun to squirt it out. (Some women cite the texture of semen as being the reason they don't like to swallow when giving blow jobs. So with one partner, it might be a problem, but not so with the next.)

The viscosity of semen starts to change as soon as it is ejaculated. That's because during ejaculation, prostate-specific antigen (PSA) mixes with the rest of the semen. This starts a reaction that makes semen become more watery so sperm can swim in it. Due to the liquefying power of PSA, semen becomes almost as thin as water within 5 to 30 minutes, regardless of how thick it may have been when it first shot out. If you doubt this, have a guy ejaculate in a clear glass and watch it for the next 30 minutes. The change happens even faster when semen is in the vagina. It's why semen drips out of a woman's vagina after intercourse.

Average Volume

The average volume of an ejaculation is between 2.3 ml and 4.99 ml, which is from half a teaspoon to a full teaspoon. For an inter species comparison, the average bull weighs between 1,000 and 2,000 lbs. He ejaculates between 4 ml and 8 ml, which is not much more than the average human male.

Semen Allergies

A semen allergy is caused by an allergic reaction to a protein in semen. The protein is made by the prostate gland. A woman could have been just fine with a partner's semen for years, and then suddenly start having an allergic reaction to it. Or she may have had a semen allergy from her first contact with semen. As with food allergies, a semen allergy might go away as fast as it arrived.

Semen allergies are very uncommon. Only 40,000 women in the United States are thought to have them. The symptoms can include pain, redness, burning, swelling, and itching. And once a woman develops a semen allergy, it's not just to semen in her vagina. The burning and itching can occur anywhere semen touches her skin, including in her mouth or up her bum. One way to decide if a woman's symptoms are due to semen allergy or chronic vaginitis is to use a condom during intercourse. It's best to use a polyurethane condom, given how her symptoms might also be from a latex allergy. If the symptoms stop when the couple is using a condom but begin again when they are not using a condom, it's time to consider a semen allergy.

Aside from a complete gynecologic exam, a woman will need to get intradermal testing to see if she has an allergy to semen. This is where a small amount of semen is injected under the skin. If this were done on the Syfy Channel, an alien child would start incubating at the injection site. But in real life, it simply determines if there's an allergic reaction.

Fortunately, there is a desensitization treatment for semen allergy that is safe and effective. You need to do it under the supervision of an allergist or immunologist. It is called a "graded challenge" where diluted solutions of semen are placed in the vagina every twenty minutes until the woman is able to tolerate undiluted semen. The couple has to have intercourse at least two to three times a week from that day forward to maintain the desensitization.

Also, a woman doesn't get a bad reaction to the semen of just one guy. If she did, switching partners would be a treatment option, although not always a practical one. If she gets a semen allergy, it's usually to all semen from all men.

Theoretically, a woman's semen allergy might go away if her partner had to have his prostate gland removed, that the prostate is what makes the offending protein. No studies have been done.

Why Semen Gets Clumpy in the Shower or Bath

You may have noticed that semen gets clumpy, stringy and sticky when it's in water, like when a guy masturbates in the bath and the semen clumps up and sticks to his skin and body hair, or when he masturbates in the shower and clumps of semen stick to hair that's on the drain cover.

When semen first comes out of the penis, it's hydrophobic which means it hates water. Even though it's a liquid, when fresh semen makes contact with water, it will form clumps, like the bubbles in Lava lamps. These clumps are semen's way of protecting as much of itself as possible from water. You'll see this occur if a guy will ejaculate into a glass of water. Everyone will be amazed.

Given semen's propensity to stick to shower floors and hair on the shower drain, it's only right for a guy to clean up the shower if he has roommates. (Dorm shower floors and drain covers—GROSS!) Semen will only clump up if it makes contact with water as a man is ejaculating.

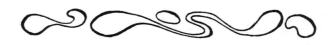

Otherwise, semen will liquefy or get watery in ten to fifteen minutes. This is why you should tie off the end of a condom, to keep the liquefied semen from dripping out.

Spying on Sperm

It can be very cool to look at your own or a partner's semen under a microscope. What you thought was a gob of goo is actually a metropolis of biological activity. It's like looking down at New York during rush hour, only there are sperm instead of Taxi cabs. Here's how you do it:

You'll need access to a microscope that has 100x and 400x magnifications, a microscope slide, coverslips, and a human male with a hard-on. Make sure the microscope has a good light and that you can focus on the edge of a coverslip that's on a glass slide.

If you don't know how to produce semen, there are chapters in this book that can help. If you need lube, only use saliva. Most commercial lubricants do evil to sperm. You'll want to have the semen under the microscope within 60 to 90 minutes after it is produced.

As you might recall from the start of this chapter, semen doesn't squirt out pre-mixed. So you'll need to collect the entire ejaculation in the same container. If you don't, you might not be collecting the squirts that have sperm. Do not collect the specimen in a condom unless it's a condom made from polyurethane and has no lube inside. The materials in most condoms are not sperm friendly.

While it tends to come out thick, semen will liquefy within 15 to 20 minutes—so much that it will become almost as thin as water. After it has liquefied, give it a close look with your naked eyes. According to our sperm consultant:

"If it is clear (transparent), the sperm count is probably low. If it is cloudy but you can see through it (translucent), it is a medium sperm count. If it is creamy white or yellowish and you cannot see through it, it is probably a fairly high sperm count. This is not a measure of fertility, just something interesting. Besides, it only takes one sperm for paternity, and the number of sperm depends on many things, including how often you ejaculate, if you've been in hot tubs or hot baths, what medications you are taking, etc."

Keep the sperm specimen between body temperature and room temperature. Any colder or hotter, and sperm start dropping like flies. If you're taking the semen from your dorm to the biology lab, keep it warm and safe.

Once you are ready to make the slide, lightly swirl the semen in the container to mix it. Put a drop or two on the slide, and then place

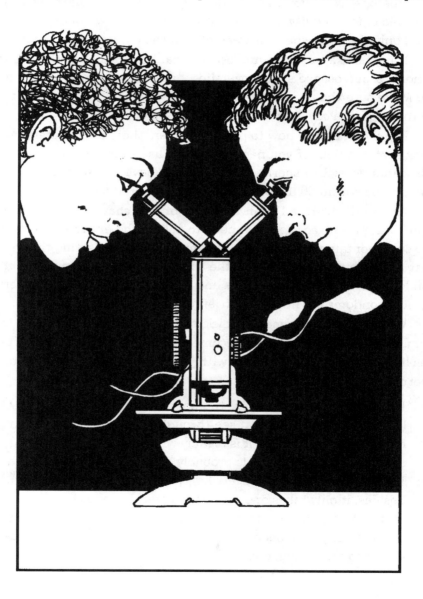

a cover slip over it. Place the slide on the microscope's platform and observe it with the 10x objective (at hopefully a 100x magnification). The sperm are going to be very small and difficult to see. Once you spy sperm, change to the 40x objective, but don't make any significant changes in focus or you risk breaking the slide with the lens. If you need to make changes in the focus, go back to the 10x objective and do it that way.

Semen has more than 300 constituents, including proteins, fats, immature sperm cells, dead parts of old sperm, and occasionally blood cells. Given the less-than optimal conditions you are probably working under, it wouldn't be surprising if 50% or more of the sperm are dead as doornails before you look through the microscope. Only about 15% of sperm are the beautiful type with flowing tails.

Precum

Precum is a clear slippery fluid that begins to ooze out of the penis when a man becomes sexually aroused. It's made by two small glands at the base of the penis called the Cowper's glands. Some men produce almost no precum, while others make more precum than they do semen.

Since precum is made at the base of the penis, it bypasses the part of the male reproductive system that causes semen to spurt or ejaculate. So it oozes or drips instead. You can tell precum from urine by touching it with a fingertip and then pulling your finger away. Precum will stay connected to your finger, making a clear cool-looking spindle.

Because it's so slippery, precum is nature's sex lube for the penis. It helps the foreskin slide more easily over the head of the penis, and it helps the head of the penis slide more easily into a vagina. Precum also makes the walls of the urethra more slick so ejaculate has less resistance, and it helps to neutralize or deacidify the urethra to make conception more likely.

As for the popular idea that precum has no sperm in it, up to 40% of men have precum that contains low amounts of sperm, regardless of when they last peed or ejaculated. Whether this is enough to get a woman pregnant remains a matter of debate. Precum definitely carries sexually transmitted infections, including HIV. So if you are concerned about getting a sexually transmitted infection, make sure a condom goes on as soon as a man gets an erection.

Readers' Comments

What did you think the first time you saw a guy ejaculate?

"I was a little shocked. I was young, 15, and I don't think I understood exactly what was going on. It's also when I realized that tissues weren't just for noses anymore." *female age 27*

"I did it right! Good job! I was proud of me. Then I thought, 'Geez, I hope my mom doesn't come home early.' " *female age 22*

"I remember being disgusted and oddly fascinated at the same time, and I couldn't believe how far that stuff could shoot out!" *female age 32*

"It just kind of oozed out. For some reason I thought there was supposed to be more of a stream." *female age 37*

"I was jealous he could actually project it from his body and I couldn't." *female age 23*

"I was kinda grossed out by the whole thing." *female age 45*

"I was proud that I made him ejaculate, but I couldn't believe that people actually would let that go in their mouths. I was a senior in high school." *female age 25*

"I wondered what it felt like. I wondered what it tasted like. Also, I wondered what it would feel like to have that happen inside of me." *female age 25*

"I vaguely remember thinking, it's amazing how their bodily process is. Also, there is what is needed to help form a human being." *female age 36*

A Very Special Thanks: to Steven "Dr. Sperm" Schrader, Ph.D., Darius A. Paduch, MD., PhD, Urology & Reproductive Medicine, Weill Cornell Medical College, and Jennifer Collins, MD, Albert Einstein School of Medicine.

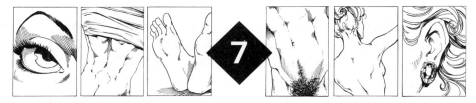

Fun With a Foreskin

Dear Paul: Cut to the chase: I am an RN and have seen hundreds of uncircumcised males. No turn on. But when my most recent lover happened to be such it was so totally unexpected that my sexual arousal rate went up 200%. I am very turned on by stroking him to expose the head, kissing and licking it and then covering it again by pulling the foreskin back up. Sucking ever so gently with the skin covering the head gives him pleasure, but pulling it down near the base of his penis completely exposes him and his reaction is amazing. All it takes is tender gentle swirls to drive him crazy.... The wanton horny bitch that resides within myself has been released and owes the author of *The Guide* the best blowjob ever!

Dear RN: Drive south on I-5 until you reach the Corvallis exit...

What Foreskins Do

Foreskins protect the head of the penis. They have nerves that can feel touch and warmth. They make it easier to masturbate and give

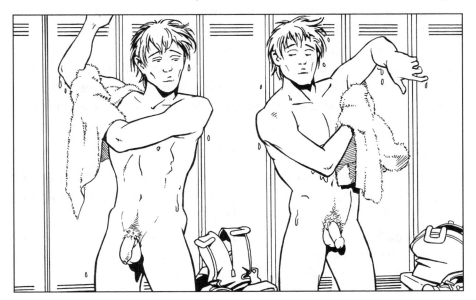

handjobs. And during intercourse, the head of the penis spends part of each stroke sliding inside the foreskin. Then it pops out and slides along the walls of the vagina before it pops back into the foreskin. This can make intercourse feel better for some women. Some have described this as feeling like a subtle "bump." It can also help keep more of a woman's natural lubrication inside of her vagina during intercourse.

For Parents—Foreskin Care

The average age of a boy when his foreskin retracts is 10.4 years. Not 10.4 days, weeks or months. Yet physicians in American still tell parents to forcibly retract the foreskins of their infant sons to wash around them. This can cause trauma.

During infancy and childhood, the inner surface of the foreskin is attached to the head of the penis. This protects the opening of the penis from irritation, infection and ulceration. Over time, the cells that attach these two surfaces start to dissolve on their own. Trying to retract the foreskin prematurely will rip apart these delicate tissues that nature has "glued" together. A number of males don't fully retract their foreskins until they are teenagers. This is normal and will usually happen as a boy starts to play with his penis. You don't need to encourage or coax him.

Parents do need to tell their teenage sons about cleanliness. They should explain that once a boy is able to comfortably retract his foreskin he should clean it every day in the shower. As for whether that daily cleaning should include soap, one of our urology-consultant physicians is himself uncircumcised. He is concerned that soaping the retracted foreskin daily might destroy the protective bacterial mantle and may result in foreskin odor. He suggests only soaping it a couple of times a week, while retracting it and washing it with water the other days of the week. Other healthcare providers might recommend differently.

Reader Comments

"I love the way his penis slides in and out of his foreskin when he's inside me. It not only stimulates me physically, but the thought of it also really turns me on while we are making love." *female age 30*

"The only Jewish guy I ever slept with was also the only uncircumcised guy I ever slept with. He seemed to have more stamina than any of the others, but that might just be a coincidence." *female age 21*

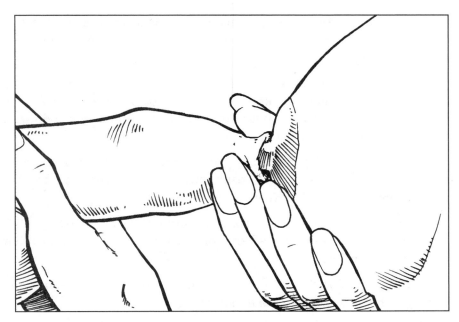

Our video "A Woman's Guide To Men's Foreskins" has several lovemaking tips. www.Guide2Getting.com/videos

"Just ask the guy how he likes it. Some like you to pull the foreskin tight; others say this hurts." *female age 20*

"I use my foreskin to massage her clitoris with." *male age 65*

"I'd never seen an uncircumcised penis until my current lover, but I've decided now that it's the best thing since sliced bread. The foreskin makes hand jobs 100 times better and easier because it slides over the penis so you don't need lube. I was kind of nervous about it at first but then I realized how stretchy the foreskin is even though it looks kinda fragile. For blow jobs, I pull the foreskin down and massage it there and go to town. *female age 18*

"For a blow job, pull the foreskin up over the head and stick your tongue down inside of the opening and swirl it around." *female age 38*

"Once my wife and I are ready for penetration, I roll my foreskin all the way shut. I press it gently against her labia while spreading them slightly, and push the glans in just a little. Then, I withdraw the glans back inside the foreskin, never exposing it to open air. What this does is spread her lubricant all over the first half of my penis. After several strokes like this, I am able to slip inside easily. Sometimes we find this so pleasurable that we continue a good long while before penetrating farther." *male age 38*

"The inside of a foreskin is where there is the most feeling, so gentle movement of it over a cockhead and down the shaft feels great. The best part of getting a blow job is what a tongue and mouth can do with that inside lining." *male age 59*

"One thing I find particularly stimulating is to lubricate a finger or thumb, slip it between the foreskin and the head, and massage the glans. It feels really, really great." *male age 19*

"When did I first retract it? I was around ten. I would slowly pull it back every day in the shower. After about two weeks I was able to pull it all the way down." *male age 22*

"Letting the foreskin balloon is quite nice both when peeing and when enjoying the pool jets." *male age 37*

"I like to clamp the end shut while peeing and making it swell up. Also, a similar and a more satisfying experience is to leave just a bit of the end open and put it under a strong flow of water so that the water flows in but has a place to get out." *male age 20*

"My fiancee does all the foreskin movement for me. It's such a turn-on when she pulls it back and then returns it to normal. She does this with her mouth constantly while she gives me a blow job." *male age 19*

"There is nothing worse than cracking an erection in your pants and not being able to make it go away because your foreskin is retracted and the head of your cock keeps on rubbing on your pants." *male age 18*

"The tip of the foreskin (like the rim of a volcano) can be very sensitive when you're soft. A light, caressing finger running around the edge can feel electric. If she's giving you a handjob and her ring isn't tight around her finger, the flesh of the foreskin can get caught in between and pinch like hell. On the flip side, there's something pretty erotic about handjobs while she's wearing your engagement ring." *male age 23*

A Special Thanks to Marilyn Milos who founded the National Organization of Circumcision Information Resource Center.

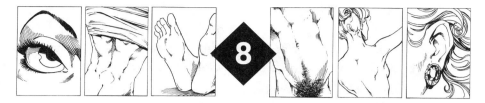

Hypospadias

Hypospadias is a condition where the urethra doesn't go to the end of the penis. The urethra is the tube inside the penis that urine and semen pass through. In mild cases of hypospadias, the urethra comes out near the end of the penis, but not quite. In more severe cases, it can come out anywhere from below the head of the penis to the area between the scrotum and anus which is called the anogential region.

Hypospadias is one of the most common birth anomalies there is. It occurs in 1 out of every 125 to 250 boys, although mild forms of hypospadias may be even more common than this.

Some of the known causes of hypospadias range from genetics and environmental pollutants called endocrine disrupters to maternal age, diet and drugs or hormones the mother may have taken before or during pregnancy. One study has shown that a vegetarian diet or a diet lacking in meat and fish may increase the risk of hypospadias. Maternal obesity might be a factor, as well as cocaine and drugs given as part of fertility treatments.

It makes sense that hypospadias occurs on the bottom side of the penis. This is where nature creates a seam as the penis is forming in the womb. The urethra goes just inside the seam and usually exits out the end of the penis. When there is hypospadias, the urethra exits before it reaches the head of the penis.

While hypospadias is sometimes very serious, about 85% of cases are classified as mild. A German study found that "All but 6 of the 225 men diagnosed with hypospadias were not aware of any penile anomaly... All patients participated in sexual intercourse without problems and were able to void in a standing position with a single stream."

Hypospadias can cause the head of the penis to be more mushroom shaped and it can also effect the part of the foreskin that's on the underside of the head of the penis. Chordee can also occur, which is when the head of the penis is bent downward more than usual. One study found that about half of the penises of young men with hypospadias were smaller than average either when flaccid, erect, or both.

When hypospadias is severe, it can result in shame and feelings of isolation. The boy's penis will often be handled by strange adults during numerous medical exams, and multiple surgeries are sometimes done. For many men, it's the medical exams and surgeries they endured as children rather than the hypospadias that have caused the most problems. (While medical intervention is sometimes helpful, there are plenty of guys who would have been far better off if their penis had been spared the surgeon's knife, and the repeated medical exams that resulted in feelings of shame and inferiority.)

With hypospadias, the most important issues to deal with are often psychological. Men with serious cases of hypospadias often grow up in fear that other males will find out and make fun of them. Fortunately, the Internet is making it possible for men with hypospadias to meet and talk to other men who have the same condition.

Men with hypospadias sometimes grow up fascinated by other guys' penises. This is perfectly logical when you consider how often their penis gets handled by parents and doctors, often without a helpful explanation. It also makes sense that a guy with hypospadias can be focused on how his penis is different from other penises. However, there is no evidence that hypospadias results in a different sexual orientation unless that's what was going to happen from the start, hypospadias or not.

As for sex and relationships, hypospadias can loom far more massively in the mind of the man who's got it than in mind of a potential partner. There is nothing about hypospadias that makes a man any less of a man, or any less of a lover. As one female reader said, "I can name you hundreds of other things women are more concerned about in a man than if his pee or cum shoots out straight or from the side–most women wouldn't give a rat's ass. Only guys worry about things like that."

There is no reason why a man with hypospadias can't become a father, so birth control is just as necessary as with any other guy. The urethral opening for men with hypospadias is sometimes bigger, which

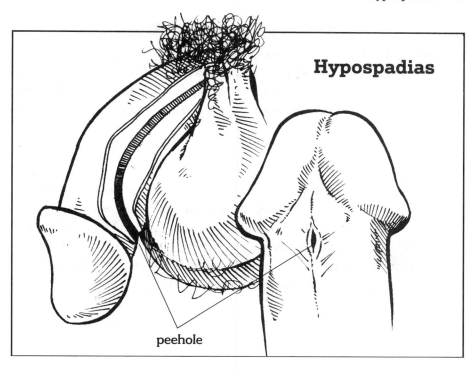

Hypospadias

peehole

can make a man more prone to urinary tract infections. So drinking extra water and peeing after sex might be a good habit to get into.

Men with hypospadias recommend that you tell a partner about your hypospadias sometime after you've gotten to know each other but before you've got your hands in each other's pants. You can always pull out this book and point to this page if you need an ice breaker.

Parents should discuss the condition with their sons who have it, offering reassurance and helpful information. Any parents who are considering surgery for a son with hypospadias should first read an article by Alice Dreger titled *Do You Have to Pee Standing Up to Be a Real Man?*

Epispadias

Epispadias is when the urethral opening opens on the top of the penis. The opening can be in one spot, or it can run the entire length of the penis. While it might seem that epispadias is simply a case of hypospadias turned on its ear, it is an entirely different anomaly than hypospadias. It is also very rare. Where approximately 1 in 125 to 500 boys has hypospadias, 1 in 117,000 boys are thought to have epispadias.

While they aren't sure what causes it, it is thought to result from a problem in the way the pubic bone develops.

Every once in a while, a girl will have epispadias, with it occurring in 1 out of 478,000 females. When this happens, the urethra will either exit higher than normal, between the clitoris and labia, or as high as the abdomen.

Resources: If you or your partner has hypospadias, an excellent resource is the Hypospadias and Epispadias Association: www.heainfo.org. The website of the Hypospadias UK Trust (www.hypospadiasuk.co.uk) is also a very helpful website. It covers everything from causes to emotional consequences, but their explanation of possible sexual side effects is wonky and appears to be from the early 1900s.

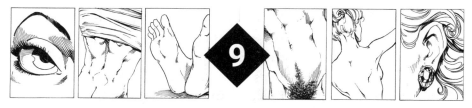

Balls, Balls, Balls

Balls usually take a back seat to the penis. That's because the pleasure a man gets from his testicles is more subtle. But that doesn't mean they should be ignored.

Testicles are far more rugged than you might think. You can squeeze or pull them with no problem. They can bang against a partner's thighs with impunity. But pop them with a simple flick of a finger and you might have to peel their owner off the ceiling. It's just the way the nerves are wired.

Testicles feel a bit like hard-boiled eggs without the shell, but they won't be that big unless the man is related to a racehorse.

When a guy is highly aroused or is just about to come, his scrotum and testicles will pull up to hug the shaft of the penis. In some men this is so extreme you'll wonder where his testicles went.

The Scrotum

The scrotum surrounds the testicles. It's a thin layer of skin that is lined with muscles. It is made from the same tissue as the outer lips or labia majora of the female genitals. This is why the skin on the scrotum has the same kind of sweat and oil-producing glands, hair follicles and nerve endings as the labia majora. The scrotum should produce the same kind of feelings when it is kissed and caressed as the outer lips of women's genitals.

Nature creates the scrotum by zipping up the two lips that would otherwise become the labia majora. This is why the scrotum has a seam up the middle. It's where the two labia fused together to make a scrotum. The scrotum remains empty until shortly before birth, when the testicles drop down into it from the abdomen where they were created.

People assume that if the scrotum were opened up, the testicles would fall out. This is not true. The testicles are held in place by the spermatic cords which suspend them from the lower abdomen where they originally descended from. Even without the scrotum, the spermatic cords will still hold the testicles in place like yoyos on a string.

The scrotum is lined with a layer of smooth muscles that allow its surface to pucker up. This helps move the testicles closer to the body when they are too cold, and farther from the body when they are too hot. However, it's the cremaster muscles that surround the spermatic cords that lift the testicles closer to the shaft of the penis when a man is about to ejaculate. The cremaster muscles can also reel the testicles against q man's body when he is frightened. So there's a lot more going on down there than most people imagine.

Sperm Go Into a Man's Body before They Come Out of His Penis

The testicles are glands or factories that produce testosterone and sperm. One testicle is often bigger than the other, and one hangs lower.

Sperm are produced in the testicles inside of small units called the seminiferous tubules. From there, the sperm are stored and aged in the epididymis, which sits above each testicle. Sperm are then pushed up into a man's abdomen through the vas deferens.

So contrary to what you might think, sperm don't go straight from the scrotum and squirt out of the the penis. Instead, they flow into a man's abdomen to an area that's behind his bladder. Then, as he's about to have an orgasm, the sperm move into a tube that runs through the prostate gland. They collect at the base of the penis, which is like a launching pad for semen. As soon as the man starts to ejaculate, out they go, squirt, squirt.

An Undescended Testicle

The medical term for undescended testicles is "cryptorchidism," which is Greek for "hidden gonad." One way to get a hidden gonad is to go surfing during the winter; another way is to be born with it.

Contrary to what seems logical, the testicles in the male fetus don't form in the scrotum. Instead, they develop inside the abdomen. They don't descend into the scrotum until shortly before birth.

Almost 3.5% of males are born with an undescended testicle. In most cases, it's just one of the testicles that is undescended. The testicle will often descend on its own without medical intervention, so that by a year of age, only 1% of males still have an undescended testicle.

The problem with a testicle remaining undescended past the first

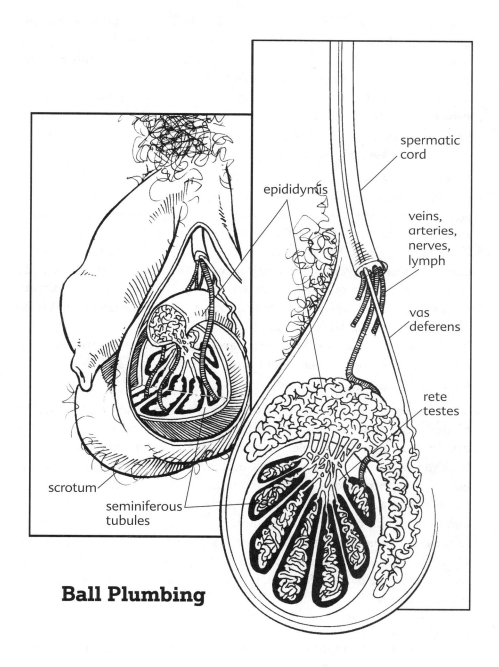

spermatic cord

veins, arteries, nerves, lymph

vas deferens

rete testes

epididymis

scrotum

seminiferous tubules

Ball Plumbing

year of life is that it tends to become infertile. So if the testicle remains undescended, the current practice is to treat it surgically. Attempts to coax the testicle down with hormone therapy have unacceptable side effects and any gains are usually short-lived.

If you are the parents of a child with an undescended testicle, be sure to get a second or third opinion from a pediatric urologist. As Dr. Joseph Dwoskin says, "There are as many opinions about testes as there are physicians who examine them."

Late-Breaking News

Physicians are beginning to find that some guys who are sterile as adults got that way because they were playing sports without a cup and took a significant knock in the nuts. Any man or boy who is involved in a contact sport should wear a cup. Ditto if he is playing catcher in baseball. The downside of wearing a cup is the discomfort. The upside is they can make a guy look really well hung. For links to some cutting edge cups, enter "cups" in the search box at Guide2Getting.com. These are not your grandfather's cups.

Performance enhancing drugs are also a leading cause of male infertility. They can do very bad things to your testicles.

What Is a Varicocele?

The testicles need a supply of fresh blood to function. It's not difficult for the heart to pump blood into the testicles, because the flow is usually downhill. The problem is how to get the blood from the testicles back to the heart when a man is standing. To accomplish this, the veins leading away from the testicles contain small one-way valves. When these valves aren't working correctly, the blood can pool in the veins and make them bulge like a small bag of worms. This creates a condition that's called a varicocele, which effects 1 out of 6 to 7 men under the age of 25. Approximately 35% of men with a varicocele are infertile. For photos and more information, enter "varicocele" in the search at Guide2Getting.com.

Testicle Pleasure

Ball Tending

If you are attempting to give your partner's testicles a satisfying caress, start by placing your fingertips on the sides of his scrotum and caressing lightly. Let his verbal feedback guide you. You might also try resting the palm of your hand over his penis with your fingertips pointing down. Experiment with lightly massaging the back part of the scrotum, where it attaches to his body. As your fingers move, the part of your wrist that's resting on his penis will move as well, which will double his pleasure.

You can handle a man's testicles during intercourse from positions like the reverse cowgirl where you are on top facing his feet. Different rear-entry positions may also allow you to reach between your legs and caress his testicles. Experiment and see what brings the most pleasure.

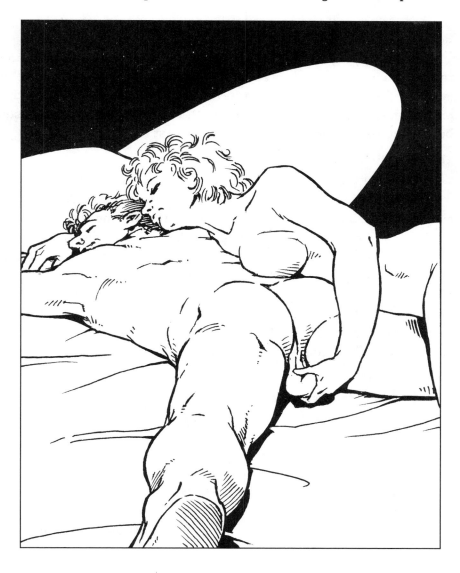

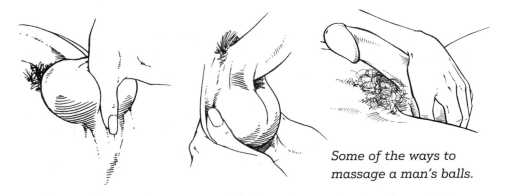

Some of the ways to massage a man's balls.

Perineum: Taint, Gooch or Grundle

There is a patch of anatomical real estate between the testicles and rectum which is often ignored but has the potential for sensation. It is called the perineum. (Women have one, too.) Place your fingertips on this area with enough pressure so the skin moves over the tissue beneath it. Experiment and see what feels best.

The Exquisite Brush-Off and More

Have your partner spread his legs and gently brush his inner thighs, testicles and whatever with a soft makeup brush or an artist's brush. Do circles around his scrotum. The sensation is subtle, somewhere between a feather and a fingertip. It can feel relaxing and exciting at the same time. If you enjoy taking control, you might tie your partner up first. If you're lucky, he'll grab the brush later and return the favor.

Also, don't hesitate to reach between your partner's legs and cup or cradle his genitals at nonsexual times, like when watching TV or while falling asleep. Some men will find this to be comforting and caring. For others it will be too arousing or unwelcome.

Cancer of the Testicles

The term "cancer of the testicles" is a misnomer. It should be cancer of the testicle (singular), given how it's usually only one testicle that gets the cancer. The good news is we only need one testicle to be fertile and to have a perfectly normal sex drive. The reason for having the other testicle is for back-up and pocket pool.

Anyone with testicles can get testicular cancer, but it is more likely to affect younger men between the ages of 15 and 35. It is curable 97% of the time if detected early. Considering the testicles are hanging out

and easily examined, you would think it is almost always detected early. But most guys between the ages of 15 and 35 assume that cancer is something that happens to people their parents' age, so it is beyond their consciousness to check every month.

Another problem is that a lot of men would rather sit naked on a fence post than call the doctor's office and say, "I'm concerned about my testicle, and I'd like you to check it out." So they wait until the cancer has spread before getting care. This isn't good, since some forms of testicular cancer can double in size in fewer than thirty days, and you won't feel a bit of pain as it is happening. It would be easier if cancer of the testicles always caused pain. Then most men would go to the doctor immediately. But cancer of the testicles usually doesn't hurt.

In spite of the way men feel about their own testicles, women are not necessarily enamored by them. So unless you've been caught cheating, most women would want you to be healthy with one testicle rather than dead with two. In fact, some guys who have lost a testicle to cancer play the cancer card quite effectively. Women are sometimes curious.

Partners and Symptoms

Cancer of the testicles is one of the few cancers where it is often a partner who discovers the problem. This can be a lifesaver. Hopefully, women readers will learn how to examine their partner's testicles in the name of health as well as pleasure.

The most common symptom to look for is a small lump or nodule on the side or sometimes the front of the testicle. It's usually not painful when you press on it. Another symptom is hardening of the testicle. While testicles can swell and shrink, it's time to get it checked when the entire testicle starts to lose its spongy texture. The same is true if there's unusual swelling in the scrotum. Less common symptoms include pain or discomfort in the testicles, back pain, swollen man breasts, or a feeling of heaviness or unusual discomfort deep in your pelvis.

Most of the things you will find in a scrotum besides balls aren't cancer and can often be treated with antibiotics. So don't assume your doctor is going to present you with bad news.

The mother of all ball-cancer websites is Doug Bank's incredible Testicular Cancer Resource Center: tcrc.acor.org.

BALL CHECK!

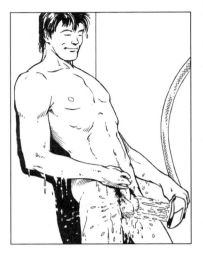

You need to do a ball check every 30 days or 10,000 strokes, whichever comes first.

The best time to check your testicles is after a warm shower, but not when you have an erection. An erection can raise your testicles and make them harder to examine.

One of the things you are looking for are changes since the last exam, so it's important to know what your testicles usually feel like.

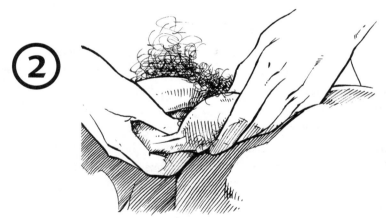

Use both hands. Grab a testicle. Roll it between your fingers. You are looking for any bumps or lumps. They can be smaller than a pea. Check the sides really well, and the top and bottom.

BALL NOTES If you ever get popped in the scrotum and the pain lasts for more than ten minutes, get it checked by a physician. If not treated quickly, testicle trauma can cause your huevos to become sterile. Also, one ball is often bigger than the other. Nature made them that way.

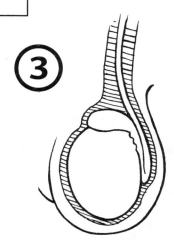

(3)

What You Are Feeling

When you feel your scrotum you may notice there is more inside than just two testicles. There are a couple of spaghetti-like cords that attach to each testicle at the back, toward the top. They are called the epididymis. They form a structure that is shaped like a comma. These might be fuller if you haven't ejaculated in a while. It may feel a little strange, but check out your comma for any small nodes, lumps or changes since the last time you checked.

(4)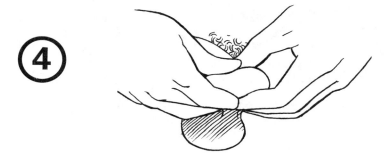

Squeeze that puppy. It should feel a bit spongy, although this can vary. Be aware if a testicle becomes extra firm or tender or starts to lose its spongy texture. Also note if the testicle is larger or smaller or heavier than it used to be.

(5) 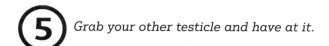 *Grab your other testicle and have at it.*

(6) 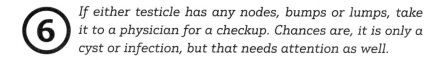 *If either testicle has any nodes, bumps or lumps, take it to a physician for a checkup. Chances are, it is only a cyst or infection, but that needs attention as well.*

(7) 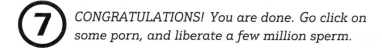 *CONGRATULATIONS! You are done. Go click on some porn, and liberate a few million sperm.*

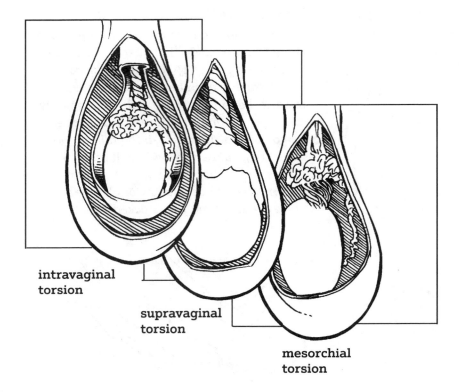

intravaginal
torsion

supravaginal
torsion

mesorchial
torsion

Testicular Torsion

Testicular torsion occurs when the testicle twists in the scrotum, causing the blood vessels in the spermatic cord to twist shut. It is very serious. If emergency surgery is not performed within four to six hours, it is quite possible that the testicle will be lost. This is why any sudden or acute pain in the testicles that lasts for more than ten minutes should result in an immediate trip to the emergency room. The same is true for an excruciating pain that appears for a few minutes and then suddenly stops. Don't take a wait and see attitude, as it might be too late if you gambled incorrectly.

Torsion happens more often in teeNagers, but adult males can get it as well. The potential for torsion is created when the testicle is not properly anchored in the scrotum. The three most common types of testicular torsion are illustrated above. *These testicles were modeled after the illustrations in the excellent book "Imaging of the Scrotum," by Hricak, Hamm & Kim, Raven Press.*

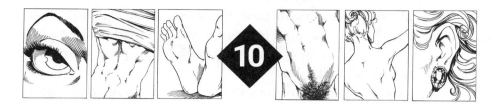

The Prostate & Male Pelvic Underground

This chapter is about the glands that produce more than 90% of semen—and they are not the testicles. When it comes to semen, the workhorse glands are the prostate and the seminal vesicles.

One of the truly cool things about the prostate gland is that it is completely hidden. It's the one sex organ a guy doesn't have to worry about the size of when he's naked at the gym or with a lover. Prostates are measured in grams instead of inches, and a man would have to be extremely neurotic before he'd worry about how his prostate stacks up against another guy's. Better yet, you will never hear one woman say to another, "You won't believe the size of Brandon's prostate!"

The other sex glands that are tucked inside a man's pelvis are the seminal vesicles, but you don't hear as much about them as the prostate gland because they rarely give a guy trouble. The seminal vesicles sit on top of the prostate like a pair of rabbit ears on an old time television set. They can make up to almost 80% of semen, depending on the man.

Without seminal vesicles and the prostate, tissue would only be for tears and runny noses, and porn actors would have nothing to do facials or creampies with. Ejaculation would be a non-event..

From Marbles to Golf

The prostate gland of a boy is about the size of a marble. If he jerks off, only a few drops of clear sticky fluid will come out. But his dad's prostate is the size of a walnut, small plum, or golf ball. That's because before puberty, the prostate and seminal vesicles are but a twinkle in the eye of their mature semen-producing selves. It will take a jolt of testosterone from a boy's teenage testicles to make his marble-sized prostate morph into a man-sized gland and to wake up his sleepy seminal vesicles.

The prostate is located at the bottom of the bladder. The urethra (tube you pee through) runs through the prostate like the Mississippi runs through the heartland. The prostate wraps around the urethra like a donut around a straw, or your hand around your penis when your spouse says, "Not tonight, dear."

The prostate is made up of smooth muscle fibers, connective tissue, small tubes, and clusters of glands that produce a clear fluid. It's a little like a miniature orange, with a tough skin and pulpy insides. To begin the process of ejaculation, the muscle fibers in the prostate squeeze the fluid from the tiny glands that are inside the prostate into the urethra.

The seminal vesicles are about two inches long. They sit above the prostate on the side of the bladder. They are a pair of puffy rabbit ears. The seminal vesicles have special cells that make a gelatin-type of juice that puts the "thick" in semen. The seminal vesicles manufacture most of the fluid that makes up semen.

While the testicles are the master glands of the male pelvis, they contribute less than 5% of each ejaculation. The testicles are hugely important when it comes to keeping a male looking like a man, but they don't produce much of his semen.

Why Women Drip after Intercourse without a Condom

Did you ever wonder why ejaculate shoots out of the penis thick, but drips out of a woman's vagina like it's water as she's tearing out of bed and trying to get to work or class on time? Blame it on the prostate.

Just before a guy ejaculates, the ingredients that make up semen collect in an area that's located near the base of his penis. These include a tiny squirt of sperm, a big squirt of thick fluid from the seminal vesicles, and a smaller squirt of prostate fluid that contains an enzyme called PSA. (Semen has more than 300 ingredients in total.)

The reason the fluid from seminal vesicles is thick is because this helps semen to collect near the woman's cervix once her partner's penis shoots it into her vagina. But then it needs to become more watery so the sperm can swim thru the opening of her cervix. PSA from the prostate gland is the catalyst that changes the semen from thick to thin, but it takes from 10 to 30 minutes to do its job. If you can't contain your excitement to learn more about this, see Chapter 6: *Semen Confidential.*

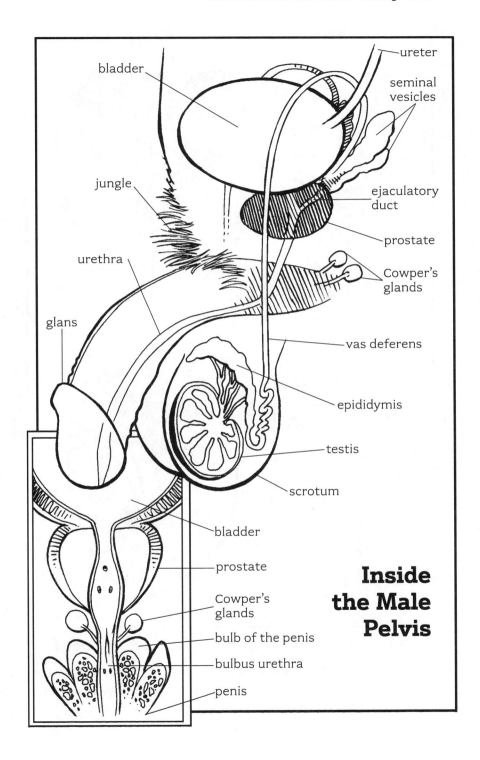

ureter

seminal vesicles

bladder

jungle

ejaculatory duct

prostate

urethra

Cowper's glands

glans

vas deferens

epididymis

testis

scrotum

bladder

prostate

Cowper's glands

bulb of the penis

bulbus urethra

penis

Inside the Male Pelvis

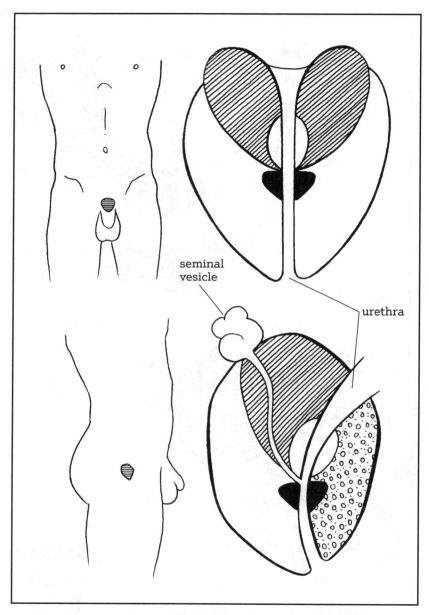

The Prostate Gland Cut in Half. Front and Side Views

*Some people think of the prostate as a lump. However, as you
can see from this diagram, the prostate is a complex organ
that has a number of different parts to it.*

The Prostate Was Named Correctly, But Not the Seminal Vesicles

The prostate was named in 300 B.C. by Herophilus. The word prostate meant "guard of the bladder." The prostate glands that Herophilus studied were fresh and in working condition, as he was allowed to dissect the bodies of criminals while they were being put to death.

The name "seminal vesicles" implies they are containers that hold the semen. But that's not correct. They manufacture several ingredients that go into semen, but the seminal vesicles never see fully-mixed semen any more than an ice-cream machine sees a hot-fudge sundae.

Curiosity Will Not Kill the Prostate

Some people can read about the prostate and that's that. Others will want to reach out and touch one.

There are two ways to feel a prostate: one is by doing the type of exam that a healthcare professional does. This is called a DRE (digital rectal exam). It will answer your curiosity, but not give a man pleasure. Be sure to trim and file the nail on the finger you are using. Put on latex exam gloves, and slather a generous amount of lube like KY Jelly on your finger. Have the man bend over.

You don't want your finger (or a sex toy, for that matter) to enter an anus at the same angle that an arrow does when you shoot it at a bull's eye. Instead, you want the pad of your finger to lay flat against his anus like it is when your are putting it against your lips and going "Shhhhh!" As you are pushing the pad of your finger against his anus it should eventually begin to relax. This is your opportunity to ease the pad of your well-lubed finger farther into the opening. Then flip the tip of your finger from vertical to horizontal as you are pushing your finger up his butt. As long as you are gentle but firm there shouldn't be any need to call an ambulance.

Slowly push your finger in a couple of inches and start to explore. The illustration on the next page should help. The surface of the prostate will probably feel a bit like the tip of your nose, only bigger, or like the padded part of your thumb where it meets your wrist.

If you explore the entire surface of the prostate from side to side, you might discover it has an indentation running down the center. Also, experiment with different levels of pressure. Be sure to get lots of feedback. If a man can contort himself, he should be able to feel his own prostate with his finger. But the angle is terrible and it won't be comfortable.

Prostate Play vs. Prostate Treatment

It's one thing when you are exploring a lover's prostate for fun. That's what the last part of this chapter is about. But it's quite another thing when a guy is having prostate problems and a health care professional tries to get fluid from it to study under a microscope.

One theory says that some types of prostate problems are caused by small pockets of infection that get trapped inside the gland. These pockets become surrounded with a hard material that encapsulates the infection. The purpose of a prostate massage as done for medical analysis and treatment is to push hard enough to burst these pockets of infection open. This requires a good deal of pressure that's not any more sexually arousing than having a mammogram done. But when you are stimulating a man's prostate in a sexually exciting way, you are pushing only as firmly as he tells you to. There is no medical agenda.

Getting a Good Prostate Exam

A lot of physicians who are too embarrassed to do a good prostate exam will stick a finger up a guy's rear with lightning speed, touch it long enough to say, "Tag, you're it," and yank their finger out. It's a wonder why they even bother. This would be the same thing as waving a wand over a woman's crotch and telling her she's had a pap smear.

One of the reasons why a "Tag, you're it" type of exam is useless is because all the examiner can feel is the surface of one-third of the entire prostate gland. He or she is trying to get a lot of information without being able to put a finger on most of it. Some of the things they are trying to determine are the size and symmetry of the gland, if there are lumps in it that might raise suspicions about cancer, and if it is spongy or hard.

Our medical consultant estimates he has done more than 35,000 prostate exams during his career in urology. He says a thorough prostate exam takes time and concentration. He tends to close his eyes once his finger reaches gland zero so he can focus better on the limited amount of information he is receiving. For him to feel like he's done a good job, he has the man stand or kneel square with his butt pointing up in the air.

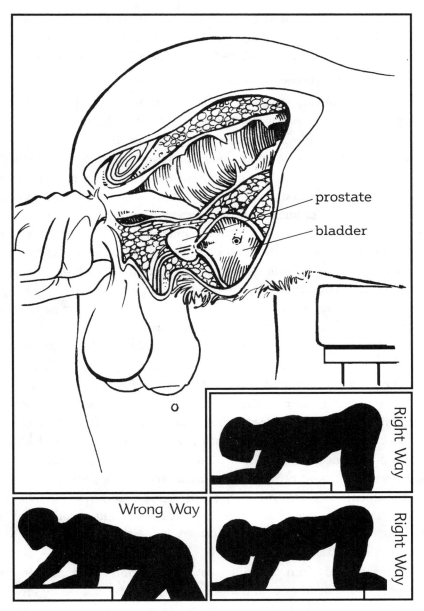

DRE—Digital Rectal Exam

*The examiner can reach only about a third of the entire pros-
tate. So she tries to check for symmetry in the lobes of the gland.
To do this correctly, a man needs to be standing or squatting
square, with his butt sticking up and out.*

While a DRE isn't going to provide any answers by itself, it is one piece of information that might be helpful in ruling out conditions like BPH, prostatitis, and cancer. Yikes — BPH, prostatitis and cancer?

Trouble in the Pelvic Underground

A gland that has to spend its entire life next to a guy's asshole is going to get uppity every now and then. We're talking a life sentence without parole inside a human porta-potty. So if the gland wants to revolt, what are its options? Its most immediate targets are the bladder and the urethra. With a little enlargement here and there, the prostate can nearly cripple a man's ability to pee normally and to fully empty his bladder. It can cause such an urgency to urinate that he can't hold it for long or it can make him wake up four times a night. It can also interfere with his ability to ejaculate or to even walk or sit without discomfort.

Most prostate glands get bigger as a man gets older. This is perfectly normal. The problem is there's no room in a man's pelvis for prostate expansion. As you can see from the illustration on the next page, if the gland grows one way it's into his bladder, the other way it's up his rectum. Or the growth might occur on the inside of the gland, where it can push against the urethra and clamp it shut.

The prostate is one of the most understudied parts of the human body. Scientifically valid studies on the prostate are few and far between. Although prostate cancer is the third-most-common kind of cancer men get, there isn't a huge amount of science to guide physicians. Half of all men will at sometime have BPH (Benign Prostatic Hyperplasia) or prostatitis, yet treatment remains more of an art than a science.

Prostatitis is a syndrome that can include pain in the pelvis, painful ejaculation, pain with erections, an array of urination problems, and pain with life in general. Some men say it feels like they've got a golf ball up their butt."

Prostatitis is often described as a young man's disease, yet it can pummel the pelvis of any man at any age. It can be caused by anything from an infection to chronic tension in the pelvis, although infection is found in less than 10% of all cases of prostatitis. To quote an article in the *Journal of Urology*, prostatitis is a syndrome that is "poorly defined, poorly understood, poorly treated, and bothersome." Or to quote our prostate expert, "Prostatitis is a young guy's disease that is not diagnosed properly and is not treated properly."

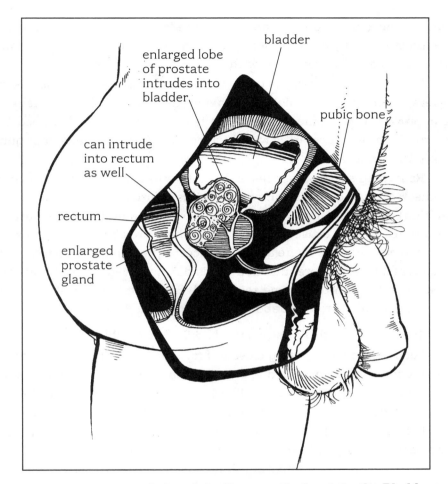

bladder

enlarged lobe
of prostate
intrudes into
bladder

pubic bone

can intrude
into rectum
as well

rectum

enlarged
prostate
gland

When the Posterior Lobe of the Prostate Pushes into the Bladder

*This is what it looks like when a lobe of the prostate swells and pushes
into the floor of the bladder. It can cause intense bladder discomfort.
When a man tries to urinate, this enlarged lobe can push against the
opening of the urethra and block the flow.*

If a man experiences a sudden, acute attack of pain in his pelvis,
he should see a physician as soon as possible. This kind of prostatitis can usually be treated successfully. But if he has chronic prostate
problems, heaven help the poor dude. He will need to educate himself
about prostatitis. An excellent source of information is www.prostati-
tis.org. After he has an idea of just how many theories there are and

how complex the problem can be, he needs to find a good urologist. The prostatitis.org website usually keeps a list of urologists who people have had positive experiences with.

Since chronic prostatitis tends to wax and wane, a lot of men take several courses of antibiotics, thinking that the antibiotics helped it improve the last time around. This is not a good idea. You need to approach chronic prostatitis with patience and intelligence. A shot gun approach is not wise.

Regarding sexual practices and prostate health, there aren't many studies to offer guidance. Having anal sex without a condom (bare-backing) makes the man who inserts his penis vulnerable to prostatitis because E. coli can cause prostatitis, and there are abundant legions of E. coli in our rectums. There are also concerns that a man can be leaving bacteria from a prostate infection in his partner's vagina, and this can be a route for him to become reinfected. So if you have prostate problems, talk to your urologist about your sexual practices.

BPH (Benign Prostatic Hyperplasia)—Middle-Age or Older

Let's say you are getting close to fifty and you notice that the wall doesn't shake anymore when you are peeing at a urinal. Or maybe you don't make it through the night like you used to without having to get up to urinate. This could be due to a prostate that is getting larger.

It is called BPH when your prostate gland is enlarged and physicians don't think you have cancer. The symptoms can range from mild to severe. One of the fascinating things about BPH is that the prostate can be greatly enlarged in a man who experiences no troubling symptoms, or it can be completely normal in size but the man is in agony. In the latter case, the swelling might be on the inside of the prostate, clamping the urethra shut.

Although BPH and prostatitis are supposed to be two different things, a man who is under 40 is likely to be given the diagnosis of prostatitis while a man who is over 50 is likely to be given the diagnosis of BPH, even if they have the exact same symptoms.

Prostate Cancer

At least one-third of all men over the age of fifty have an early form of prostate cancer, as well as 90% of men over the age of ninety. Most of these cancers stay where they are and the men never know it is

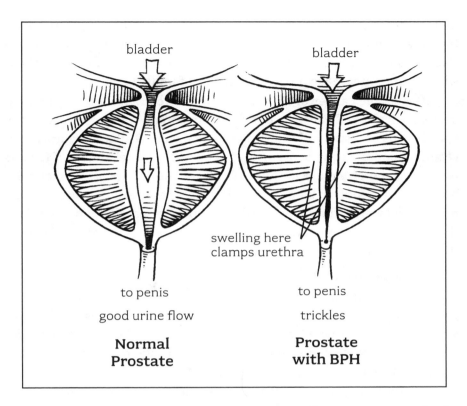

there. When this kind of cancer does grow, it often remains inside the prostate and is not aggressive. However, some forms of prostate cancer can be very aggressive. The challenge is in determining which is which.

Prostate cancer is sometimes diagnosed on a wing and a prayer. One of the big concerns with prostate cancer is deciding when to treat it aggressively and when to take a "wait and watch" attitude.

One test that can possibly indicate the presence of prostate cancer is called the PSA test. PSA is the enzyme that makes a guy's ejaculate go from thick to watery. When the level of PSA in the bloodstream starts to rise, it might be due to cancer of the prostate. On the other hand, BPH can also cause the PSA level to rise, and some men who have prostate cancer show no rise in their PSA level at all. Researchers are trying to find ways to improve these tests. Either way, if you have any concerns, please check with a healthcare provider.

According to Newton Malerman, author of *The Prostate Health Workbook*: "If you are diagnosed with prostate cancer or any other serious illness, take someone with you to your doctor's appointments. My wife was able to ask much clearer and tougher questions than I was. If you are single, or your spouse or partner is too emotional about what's happening, take a trusted friend or family member."

If you have cancer or BPH and if surgery or radiation is being suggested, ask if it will cause incontinence, impotence, a shorter penis, dry ejaculations or if you will squirt urine when you ejaculate. Inquire about vacuum pumping your penis after surgery. Search websites and forums because some of your best help will come from the posts of men who have been through it before you. However, be aware of which companies contribute funding to the websites you are searching. It is unlikely these companies will tolerate posts that question wisdom of taking their products.

Prostate Massage for Pleasure

Prostate play should never feel like a rectal exam. If a healthcare provider took the time to caress and massage your anus like a lover should before sticking a finger up it, he or she would probably lose their license. Or they would be so popular it would take months to schedule an appointment.

The following tips are from Charlie Glickman's *The Ultimate Guide to Prostate Pleasure: A Guide for Men and Their Partners* and from a video called *A Guide For Prostate Massage* from The Pleasure Mechanics.

😎 For prostate massage positions, there's face up and face down. See which one works best for both of you.

😎 Lube up your fingers with massage oil. Begin with external massage just below the testicles in the perineal area. Glide a well-lubricated finger around the outside of the anal opening, making circles around it. Don't try any penetration until the opening becomes relaxed.

😎 Don't push your finger into the anus. If you've massaged the outside for long enough, the anal sphincters will relax and allow easy insertion of the finger. Gradually increase the pressure, but don't push your finger farther in than feels comfortable for the man.

😎 Sometimes all that's necessary is putting your finger in a quarter or half of an inch. Massage there and call it a day if plumbing your man's depths is not pleasurable.

👓 The sphincter muscles are like two small donuts that sit above the anal opening. If your finger encounters resistance when it reaches the sphincters, stop there. It means the man is not relaxed enough to go farther.

👓 Once you reach the prostate, you might try a "come here" motion. Also try moving your finger in circles around the prostate. It should never feel painful or uncomfortable for your partner. Also try gliding your finger from the outer edge to the center of the prostate.

👓 Some men experience prostate stimulation as being midway between the sensation of needing to pee and having an orgasm. Men who enjoy prostate stimulation say it can create wavelike sensations through their entire pelvis and body. Orgasms that occur from stimulating the penis while the prostate is being massaged can sometimes last longer and result in more sensation.

👓 When you are ready to stop, let your finger glide out slowly; never pull it out quickly.

👓 The surface area of a dildo or anal sex toy is larger than that of a finger. This results in a different sensation on the prostate than a finger. Some men prefer the sensation of an anal sex toy on their prostate more than a finger, others like the greater precision that finger massage offers.

👓 You might try stimulating his penis at the same time you are stimulating his prostate with your other hand. You may need to go easy on the penis, as it might be more sensitive due to the simultaneous prostate stimulation.

👓 The prostate will swell as the man becomes more aroused. You'll be able to feel this with your finger, especially right before ejaculation. You should be able to feel ejaculation-related swelling with your finger.

👓 Some men find that direct prostate stimulation results in a super intense orgasm, while others find it's too much or it dulls the feeling of orgasm. They might prefer that you just push against the rim of the anus with a finger.

👓 For men who want to stimulate their own prostates, an S-shaped lucite sex toy like the Crystal Wand or a special butt plug might help. There are several different devices for prostate stimulation.

Resources for Prostate Massage and Pleasure:

The Ultimate Guide to Prostate Pleasure: A Guide for Men and Their Partners by Charlie Glickman, Clies Press, 2013. A thoughtful and well-written book for any man or couple who wants to explore the prostate and its potential for extra sexual pleasure.

A Guide For Prostate Massage from The Pleasure Mechanics. This is a brief video that couples will feel very comfortable watching together. www.PleasureMechanics.com.

Resources for Prostatitis and BHP

Be sure to visit the extremely thorough and competent website of the Prostatitis organization: www.prostatitis.org.

Thanks: A very special thanks to Dr. Joe Marzucco, formerly of the Portland Kaiser Urology Department and now a sex therapist in private practice in Portland, Oregon. Thanks also to John Schulman, a sex educator in Corvallis, Oregon, who helps students learn how to do prostate exams.

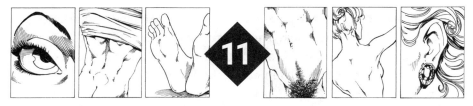

What's Inside a Girl?

What follows is an experience I had with women's genitals when I was 11-years-old. I had been in the city for a week visiting relatives and it was time to catch the Greyhound bus to return home.

Busses didn't always have bathrooms, so it was good to go before you boarded. The men's bathroom in the Greyhound bus depot was a palace of porcelain fixtures and horrible smells. At the end of a long row of sinks sat three vending machines.

One of the machines had men's colognes; you could spritz yourself with Old Spice or Brut for a dime. The next machine had a strange looking product from France that claimed to tickle women. And the third machine said *Instant Pussy—2 Quarters.*

To put this into perspective, candy bars weren't much more than a nickel, and two quarters amounted to a near fortune. But the front of the third machine promised a facsimile so exact that you couldn't tell the instant pussy from the real thing.

For the next fifteen minutes, I pondered the ultimate existential question: ten candy bars or instant pussy, ten candy bars or instant pussy, ten candy bars or instant pussy.

It was different for boys back then. There was no Internet and "porn" consisted of nudist magazines with women who had so much pubic hair that it looked like a Pomeranian dog was sitting on their laps. Beaches were no help either—bikinis as we know them were a dream of the future, and the bottoms of two-piece bathing suits were a cross between granny panties and Spanx. You learned more from reading the instructions in your sister's box of Tampax.

So you can understand why a boy might have left the men's bathroom with two fewer quarters and a sense of hope that a box of Instant Pussy would reveal something about one of life's greatest mysteries. The rest of the day was spent in quiet anticipation, with thoughts of instant pussy overwhelming whatever sights and sounds the long trip home had to offer. After hours on the bus, I arrived home and anxiously opened the small box. The instructions said, "Place capsule in a large glass of warm water." I took out a thermometer and made sure the water was a perfect 98.6. Then came the big moment. I crossed myself and revved up my courage. My trembling fingers dropped the capsule into the glass. Then I waited for the mystery to unfold. And I waited. And I waited.

Forty minutes went by before the gelatin capsule melted and revealed a thin piece of sponge in the shape of a cat.

A grown man would have known to go for the candy bars. But I was still clinging to the hope that there were answers to questions that were so much bigger than I was.

Porn vs. Reality

Porn has become the gateway for all things having to do with sex. In porn, a woman's vagina and rectum are pleading for a penis any time a guy gets hard. There is no discussion, preparation, or need for permission. If a man approaches a woman's genitals in the same way he does his own—or the way he sees it done in porn—he and his partner might be missing out on a lot of fun.

Women's Sexual Anatomy — The Nerve of It All

Years ago, a scientist named Kermit Krantz dissected the genital regions of eight dead women. He explored how women's genitals are wired. It is difficult to find a single research report on women's sexuality that is of more value than the one produced by Kermit Krantz.

Dr. Krantz found a great deal of variation in the way the nerve endings are distributed throughout the different women's genitals. While there tended to be a higher concentration of nerve endings in the clitoris, the amount varied significantly among the different women. Some had more nerve endings in the labia minora (inner lips) than in the clitoris, and some women's nerve endings were highly concentrated in one area while other women had nerve endings that were spread out over a larger area. To quote Dr. Krantz:

"The extent of innervation in different females varies greatly."

What this suggests is that no two women get off sexually in the exact same way. Each woman needs to explore her own unique sexual universe, from where to touch to the kinds of fantasies that get her off.

One woman might love oral sex and only be so-so about intercourse, while the next craves a penis between her legs. Another woman might prefer oral sex with Trevor, but intercourse with Isiah.

A man won't know what a woman likes in bed until she tells him. It's not the sort of awareness he is going to assimilate during a one-night stand or from watching porn. He needs to feel comfortable asking questions and taking direction. She needs to feel comfortable teaching him about her body. If she doesn't know, they can learn together.

Show & Tell

"While women speak to each other in graphic terms about things like menstruation, blow jobs, and the ratio of penis size to male ego, we usually don't talk to each other about what our crotches look like; not that we'd necessarily want to." *female 34*

Most guys know what their penises look like. That's because penises stick out. Guys often wag or squeeze them each time they pee. Not so for women. A lover often sees more of a woman's genitals than she does. Even when women do look at their genitals, much of the sexually reactive parts are hidden inside of their pelvis where they can't be seen. In this chapter, we'll try to even the score.

What to Call Women's Genitals

Men and women often refer to everything between a woman's legs as her vagina or "down there." Sex educators, (and I used to be among them), would come unglued about this. That's because what sits between a woman's legs is her vulva, not her vagina. You don't begin to see a woman's vagina until the lips of her vulva are spread.

I've gotten over this. Every time I say "vulva," someone will look at me strangely and say "You mean the car?" What concerns me far more than the name we use is that too many young women and men think that women's genitals are dirty or smelly. I'm also hearing from college instructors that a lot of young women feel "it's nasty" for them to masturbate. It's okay for men to masturbate, but not women. So I'm fine with whatever you want to call women's genitals, as long as you give them the awe and respect they deserve.

The Mons: Love-Making Ally

The mons pubis is a fleshy mound of tissue that sits on top of the pubic bone. It is made up of fat and is usually covered by pubic hair, unless a woman shaves.

The tissue inside the mons is sensitive to estrogen. So when a woman goes through puberty, the sudden ramp up in estrogen makes the tissue expand and turns the mons it into a mound.

The mons pushes the upper part of the larger labia out and forms the pudendal cleft, which is the top part of what some people call "the camel toe." Some mons are very prominent, others not so much.

The suspensory ligament of the clitoris has its base in the mons pubis, and the neck of the clitoris runs through part of the mons. This is why some women will push, pull, or make a circular motion with their fingers on their mons when they masturbate. A woman might also enjoy it if a partner pushes the mons up with his fingers when he's giving her oral sex. This can change the angle of the clitoris and could increase the sensation. A woman might also like it when her partner rubs the mons in a circular motion or gently tugs on her pubic hair.

Outer Lips

The ancient Romans got it wrong. They named the outer lips "labia majora" (big lips) and the inner lips "labia minora" (small lips). They should have called them "inner" and "outer," given how the inner lips are often more major than the outer lips. The outer lips or labia majora can vary greatly in size, shape and color.

The outer lips are made from the same tissue as the scrotum. This is why their skin is so similar to that of the scrotum. Both have similar sweat glands, nerve endings and hair follicles, and both produce the same nice sensations when they are kissed and caressed.

As a woman becomes sexually aroused, the blood flow into the outer lips increases. However, the increase is not as large as occurs in the inner lips and other parts of women's genitals during sexual arousal.

In terms of human development, if a fetus is going to be a boy, nature fuses the outer labia together to create the sack that will become the scrotum. The seam down the middle of the scrotum is where the outer labia were fused together. Otherwise, the lips don't fuse together.

Inner Lips

The labia minora or inner lips often give women's genitals their unique personalities. They start just beneath the clitoris and can run all

The Vulva

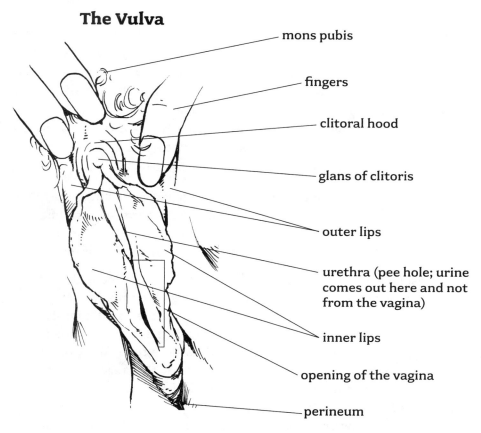

mons pubis

fingers

clitoral hood

glans of clitoris

outer lips

urethra (pee hole; urine comes out here and not from the vagina)

inner lips

opening of the vagina

perineum

the way to the bottom of the vagina. They fan out in different ways and when a woman is aroused, they perk up and deepen in color.

The inner labia come from the same tissue as the head of the penis, only they are thinner. They are sexually reactive, which means the tissue becomes engorged with blood and can double or triple in thickness when a woman is sexually aroused. The skin on the inner labia has no hair, and the edges of the labia minora are packed with nerves. This is why touching and caressing the inner labia can feel so good.

Since the inner labia attach to the bottom of the glans of the clitoris, some women enjoy it when a lover gently tugs on them or massages them. This is an indirect way of stimulating the clitoris. Some women will tug on their inner lips or stroke them when they are masturbating.

The inner lips can be from three-quarters of an inch long to four inches long, and they can be from one-quarter of an inch to two inches wide. They can stretch a bit when pulled on. They are often asymmetrical, and it's normal for one to be double the width of the other. In some parts of Africa the labia minora can be as large as eight inches because the women intentionally stretch them. Here in the States, women worry their inner labia are too big and some even consider having them surgically downsized with an operation called labiaplasty.

During intercourse, the inner lips are pushed and pulled with each stroke of the penis, which can tug and stimulate the glans of the clitoris.

Porn Is No Friend of the Inner Labia

Porn loves small inner labia. Some porn actresses have inner labia that are naturally petite, while others had theirs surgically trimmed. As for perspective on what labia of women really look like, one of the best people to ask would be a lesbian photographer and pornographer:

> "Lesbians are at an advantage in the vaginal knowledge department because we see our lovers' pussies all the time. We get up close and personal with real cunts in all of their real imperfection. But most straight women don't have the kind of access to vaginas that you get from licking box all the time. Many of my straight female friends have told me that the majority of up-close-and-personal views they've had of various vulvas have come from porn. Worse than that, some women feel insecure about their own coochies when they don't look like the ones in *Playboy*. Well, let me just set the record straight: Cunts don't really look like that. Trust me. I'm a pornographer."
>
> –From Diana Cage's *Box Lunch:*
> *The Layperson's Guide To Cunnilingus*

Perfection is no more common between a woman's legs than it is between a man's. A lack of symmetry is one of the wonderful things about being human.

Clitoris: Point Guard for Women's Genitals

Most people think a clitoris is the small tip you see at the top of a woman's labia when she spreads her legs. But there's much more to the clitoris than that.

The glans or tip is a small but potent part of the clitoris. The hood-like structure that drapes over the glans is just that—the hood. It's like the foreskin on a penis. When women masturbate, they often press a

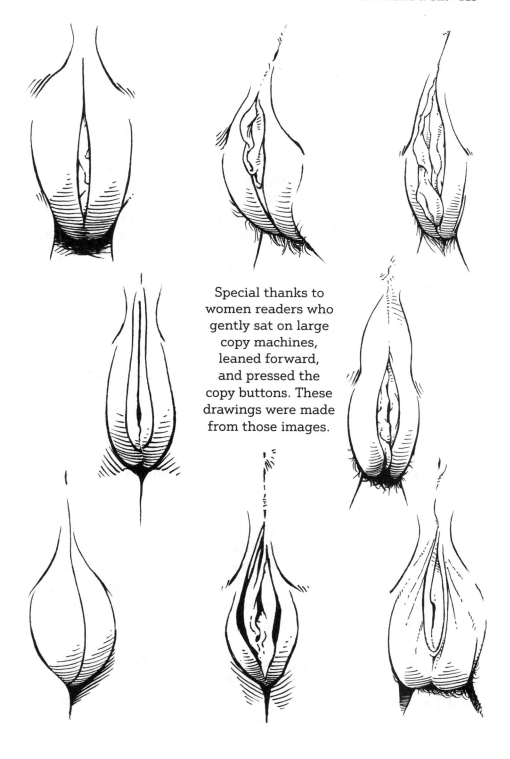

Special thanks to women readers who gently sat on large copy machines, leaned forward, and pressed the copy buttons. These drawings were made from those images.

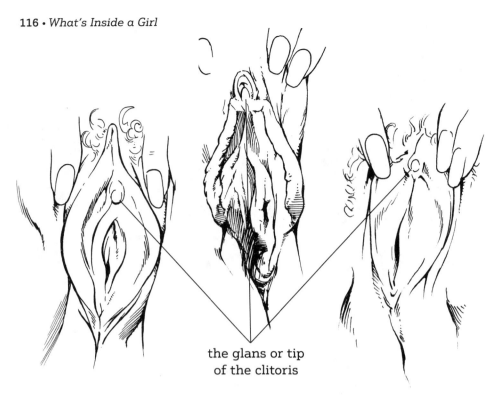

the glans or tip
of the clitoris

fingertip against the hood and rub it in a small circle or back and forth.

The hood of the clitoris can usually glide over the glans without it feeling abrasive. However, some hoods are bonded to the clitoris. This is perfectly okay and the sexual sensation usually feels fine. Surgery to separate the hood from the glans is seldom necessary or wise.

Some women find their clitoris changes sensitivity with the time of the month, in others it keeps an even keel.

As a woman approaches orgasm, it can seem like the tip of her clitoris disappears or retracts. This can be confusing for a partner who is trying to stimulate the clitoris by hand or mouth. Should he play Hercule Poirot and give chase, or wait until the clitoris returns? No one is sure why the clitoris seems to sometimes disappear at the height of sexual arousal. It could be due to pelvic muscle contractions that cause the shaft and glans to straighten out, or by a swelling of tissues around the glans of the clitoris, or by things we don't know about.

If you are stimulating the clitoris with your finger or tongue and it suddenly feels like it's starting to hide or retract, you are most likely doing something right. Don't change a thing unless the woman indicates otherwise. Let her clitoris play its game of cat and mouse.

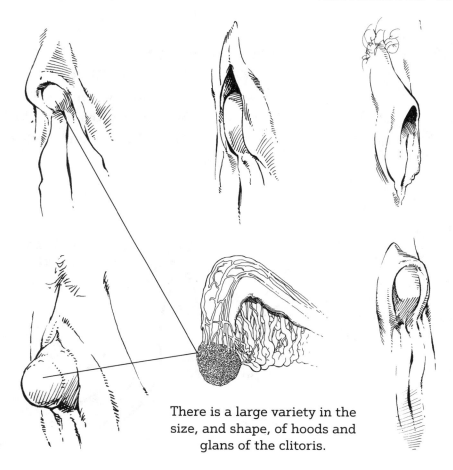

There is a large variety in the size, and shape, of hoods and glans of the clitoris.

Many women have a favorite side or place on their clitoris that they focus a finger or vibrator on. We used to believe that women who are right handed are more likely to focus on the right side of their clitoris, and women who are left handed go for the left side. Then we started asking women on our sex survey. As many right handed women said their favorite side of their clitoris is the left side as the right side. Oops!

The Size of the Clitoris

Guys aren't the only ones who worry about genital size. Some women worry that the tip or glans of their clitoris is too big, others wish theirs were bigger. The size of the tip or glans of the clitoris can vary greatly. In some women, it nearly pops out to shake your hand; in others it can hardly be seen. It is usually a little smaller than a pencil eraser, but can range from being barely noticeable to the size of a toe or

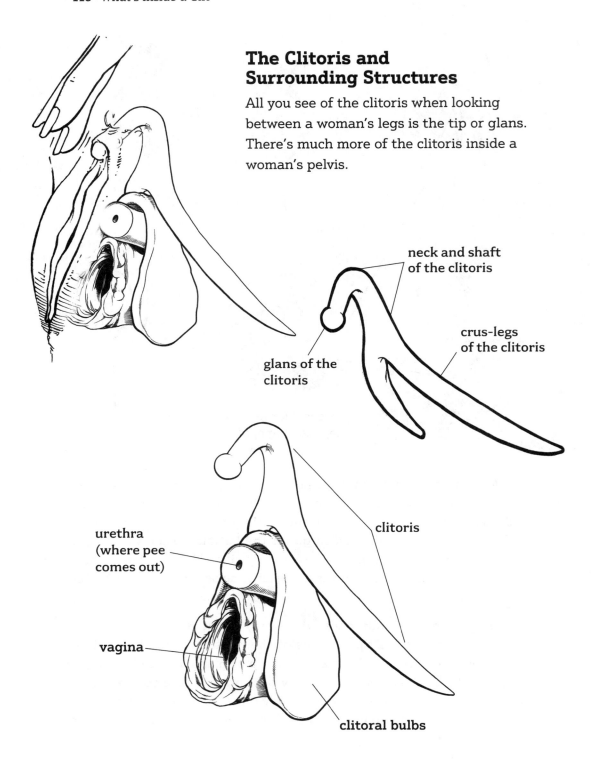

The Clitoris and Surrounding Structures

All you see of the clitoris when looking between a woman's legs is the tip or glans. There's much more of the clitoris inside a woman's pelvis.

neck and shaft of the clitoris

crus-legs of the clitoris

glans of the clitoris

clitoris

urethra (where pee comes out)

vagina

clitoral bulbs

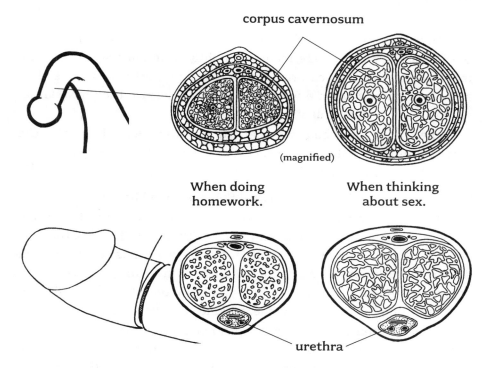

corpus cavernosum

(magnified)

When doing homework.

When thinking about sex.

urethra

Cross-Section of the Shaft of the Clitoris and a Penis

a small penis. Clitorises also enlarge from 50% to 300% when a woman is sexually aroused. It's unfortunate anyone worries about the size of a clitoris, because there is no limit to the enjoyment a woman can have with her clitoris regardless of how big or small it is. The size of the clitoris is impacted by hormones which rev up during puberty. By the time a woman is in her early thirties, the tip of her clitoris will be up to four times larger than it was when she began puberty.

The Crura of the Clitoris

The clitoris has three different parts: the glans or tip, the shaft, and the crura or legs. The crura look like the legs of a wishbone. They extend beneath the labia. The shaft and crura contain erectile tissue like the cylinders that are in the penis.

The Bulbs of the Clitoris or "Vestibular Bulbs"—Clitoris Adjacent

Mother Nature planted a pair of bulbs inside her favorite garden. They are called the bulbs of the clitoris, and they swell and blossom each time a woman is sexually aroused.

The bulbs are close to the clitoris and communicate with it through blood vessels, but they are made of slightly different tissue. They are more elastic than the clitoris. They expand proportionally more than a penis or clitoris when a woman is aroused because they have larger spaces that blood can rush into.

There is debate about whether the bulbs are actually part of the clitoris and if they should be called the bulbs of the clitoris or the vestibular bulbs. Either way, they appear to be sexually reactive.

The Axis of Arousal—Clitoris, Clitoral Bulbs & Labia Minora

When a woman becomes sexually aroused, her clitoris, clitoral bulbs and inner lips become engorged with blood. These structures seem to communicate with each other when a woman is becoming sexually excited. It's not like they text, but all three are highly involved when sexual excitement is in the air. Researcher Helen O'Connell might suggest including the urethral sponge, making the axis of arousal a quartet.

Some women enjoy it when a partner does a deep fingertip massage of the tissue that's beneath their labia. It might seem like it would be painful, but it may be stimulating rich vascular beds. With feedback and a willingness to explore, you'll learn what feels good and what doesn't. (For more, see Chapter 19: *The Zen of Finger Fucking.*)

The Clitoris during Intercourse

"I rub the heck out of my clitoris during intercourse. I do it to reach an orgasm when my partner is almost there." *female 25*

"I almost always rub on my clit during intercourse. I usually make small circular motions, which is not how I move my finger when I masturbate. I love when he does it too, although sometimes I have to move his hand into the correct spot."
female age 24

"I have tried rubbing my clit once or twice, but prefer to focus my attention on his dick inside of me." *female age 20*

The glans of the clitoris is seldom positioned to rub noses with an incoming penis. Many women enjoy the added stimulation of a finger or vibrator during intercourse, or they push the clitoris against the shaft of a lover's thrusting penis or grind it against his pubic bone.

More than 85% of the women who have taken our sex survey and who have orgasms during intercourse do not have orgasms from thrusting alone. Either they or their partner stimulate their clitoris with their fingers while the penis is thrusting, or they grind their clitoris into a partner's pubic bone. However, other women do just fine with thrusting alone. Research is beginning to suggest that a woman may be more likely to have orgasms from intercourse if the glans of her clitoris is located closer to the opening of her vagina, possibly allowing it to get more direct stimulation from the penis.

A Final Note on the Clitoris — How Do You Pronounce It?

If you are wondering how to pronounce the word *clitoris,* write *clitoris* on one piece of paper and *penis* on another. Ask friends of different sexes to say the words out loud. No one will hesitate in pronouncing *penis,* but good luck with *clitoris.* Both cli-TOR-is, and CLIT-or-is are correct, although many people punt and call the clitoris "it."

Urinary Meatus — Might Be More Fun Than It Sounds

The urinary or urethral meatus is a small circle of firm tissue that wraps around the end of the urethra, which is the tube that pee flows through. It is located in an area of women's genitals called the 'vestibule' which is between the inner lips and the tip of the clitoris and the mouth of the vagina. The urinary meatus is sensitive enough that some women rub it when they masturbate, while others avoid it.

The Vagina

The human body is made up of many different tubes. The favorite tube of many men and women is the vagina, which is a hollow canal with walls that contain four layers of tissue. The size and shape of vaginas differ as much as the size and shape of penises. The average length of a vagina when it is not aroused is 2.4 inches, with a range from 1.6 inches to 3.7 inches. The narrowest part of the vagina is around the opening, where the average is around 1 inch in diameter. The widest part averages 1.6 inches, which is in the back around the cervix.

The relatively short length of many vaginas might indicate that not all women want or can handle porn-sized penises.

When the vagina is not aroused, its walls lie flat against each other like a fire hose without water. When a woman is aroused, her vagina

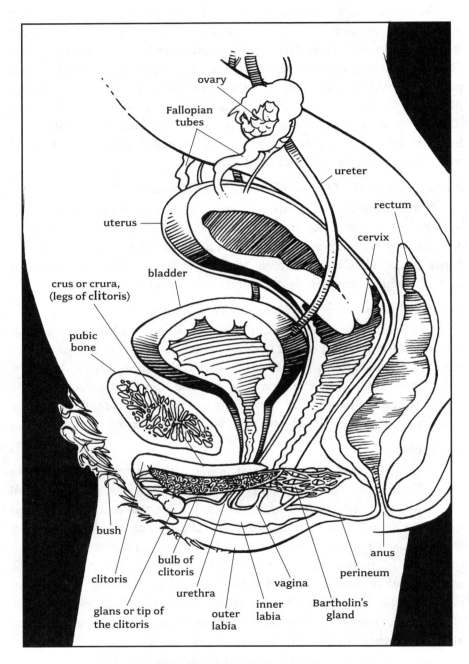

What's Inside a Girl

straightens out. The first third of the vagina becomes narrower, while the back part may balloon a bit. Some women especially enjoy stimulation at the opening of their vagina. That's because the opening of the vagina has touch receptors.

> "The main request I ask of my partner is to tease me with his cock. That's because most of the sensitivity in my vagina is at the opening." *female age 25*

While the first third of the vagina is often sensitive to touch, the back two-thirds are more sensitive to pressure. This is why some women find that having a thicker object such as a penis or dildo in the back of the vagina can feel extra good during masturbation or when her clitoris is being stimulated.

Keep in mind that women don't necessarily use dildos to mimic intercourse. A woman might not want a lover's fingers or a dildo thrusting in and out of her vagina when he is stimulating her clitoris. It could be the fullness that feels good, while the thrusting is an unwelcome distraction. Each woman is different so be sure to ask.

Vaginal Ruggae

During the years between puberty and menopause, the surface of the vagina has tiny folds or ridges that make it seem corrugated. These are called the vaginal ruggae. They help the vagina to expand during intercourse and childbirth. But before puberty and after menopause, the surface of the vagina is mostly smooth.

Vaginal Tenting

As a woman becomes more aroused, the back of her vagina will often expand or balloon open, and her cervix will raise up. This is called vaginal tenting. You can feel it with your fingers if you have them extended into the back part of a woman's vagina when she's highly aroused. Vaginal tenting might cause a woman to long for something inside her vagina which the rear walls can grasp.

pH and the Vaginal Microbiome

During the years between puberty and menopause, a woman's vagina becomes acidic. This is very important for vaginal health, and it happens as a result of microorganisms in the vagina that make up what's called a microbiome. This is so important to know about that a chapter on the vaginal biome follows this one.

Queefs aka Vaginal Farts

"My boyfriend was performing oral sex on me and fingering my vagina. When I sat up, all of the air in my vagina came rushing out and made a huge fartlike noise. I looked at my boyfriend with shock on my face. Then we both started laughing." *fem. 25*

Air that's trapped inside a vagina can make a fartlike noise when it comes out. It's just normal room air. Unlike real farts, it doesn't smell. It can happen when a woman is exercising or even when doing yoga.

Vaginal farts are more likely to happen after a woman has had an orgasm and the back of her vagina has ballooned open. The farting noise occurs when the vagina is returning to its resting state and the collected air rushes out. The Scottish utilized this principle to create the bagpipe.

A Tipped Uterus

The uterus is an upside-down pear-shaped organ that is located between a woman's bladder and her rectum. It is where human infants spend their first 40 weeks. Many people consider it to be the strongest muscle in the body.

In most women, the uterus tips toward the front of the body. But up to 30% of women have a uterus that is tipped, retroverted or tilted, meaning the uterus points up or more toward the back. This might be why some women with a tipped uterus experience period pain more as a backache than a pain in their abdomen, and why they tend to have more back pain and diarrhea when they are menstruating. (This is because prostaglandins are released that cause the muscles around the uterus to contract. This helps push out period flow. Unfortunately, the prostaglandins also activate the muscles in the walls of the bowels. This might be worse for women whose uterus is closer to their rectum.)

It's not unusual for a woman with a tipped uterus to prefer intercourse positions where she is face to face with her partner. Rear entry or doggie style positions can feel painful. So the missionary position might be her favorite, or she might enjoy a woman-on-top position where she's facing forward as opposed to a reverse cowgirl.

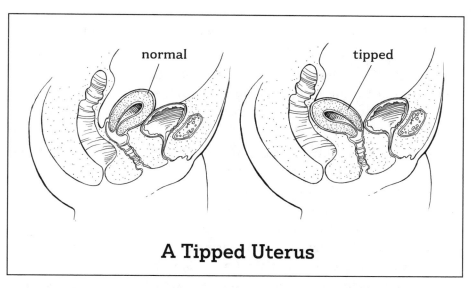

A Tipped Uterus

A tipped or tilted uterus points toward the back instead of the front or it can be aligned at any point in between.

The pain during rear entry intercourse might be due to the penis banging into the woman's uterus or ovaries—which would not usually be the case for a woman whose uterus is not tipped. The pain might also come from extra air that can accumulate during intercourse in the vagina. So the lover of a woman whose uterus is tipped needs to understand that while his former partner might have been the Reverse Cowgirl Queen, this position could cause a lot of pain for a woman with a tipped uterus. Here's what three women who took our sex survey say, but this isn't necessarily true for every woman who has a tipped uterus:

"My uterus is tilted. It makes doggy-style intercourse painful. I prefer to be on top of my boyfriend."

"I have a very tipped uterus. Unless I'm pregnant they can't pick it up on a regular ultrasound because it leans so far backward. Intercourse feels best with me on top or missionary. I've found that doggie style isn't very comfortable, nor is me being on top while facing his feet. As long as we are close to each other, belly touching belly, deep thrusting is fine. If we are separate, like if I'm laying down and he is in an upright position, deep thrusting can be uncomfortable. Where I'm at in my cycle also plays a role in how comfortable or uncomfortable things are."

"I have a tipped uterus, and this may be why it hurts when my partner thrusts too deep. It may also be why I don't like to be penetrated from the rear. Being on top is the most comfortable position for me and the one that provides the highest likelihood of orgasm."

Many women with a tipped uterus go their entire lives without knowing it's tipped. Poorly fitted bras will cause more inconvenience for most women than a tipped uterus. Also, there is a myth that women with tipped uteruses can't conceive easily. Don't believe it.

Some women with a tipped or tilted uterus refer to it as an "inverted uterus." However, an inverted uterus is a rare event that happens when a uterus turns inside out right after a woman has given birth. Also, the uterus can become tipped due to a problem such as endometriosis, so if you start having discomfort with intercourse, be sure to tell your doctor.

The Cervix and Fornix

The cervix is a small, fleshy dome in the rear of the vagina. It acts as a gatekeeper into and out of the uterus. The cervix can be as small as a cherry in a woman who has not delivered a baby through her vagina, or it can be much bigger. It has a dimple in the center called the os that menstrual fluids flow out of and male ejaculate flows into. Science doesn't yet understand the role of the cervix in sexual response.

The cervix sometimes feels softer during ovulation, when mucus passes through it to help bathe the vagina. This keeps the environment clean and more acidic, which are conditions that encourage conception. At mid-cycle, when conception is most likely to occur, the mucus becomes clear and slippery, like raw egg-whites.

The cervix has a space around it called the fornix. This is a delightful area to explore with a finger. When women are approaching orgasm, this part of the vagina will often balloon open. (See "Vaginal Tenting" on pages 203 - 204.) Some women find stimulation of the space around the fornix to be pleasing. It is also a good space to know about when a vagina isn't particularly deep or her lover has a long penis. Couples can experiment with intercourse positions that encourage the penis to slide under the cervix and into the fornix.

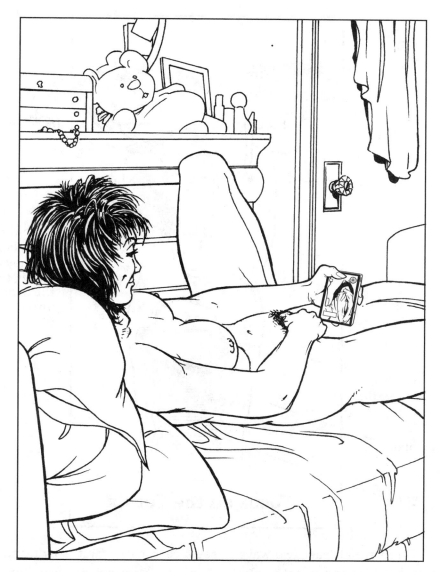

It's easy to use a phone or a mirror to check out your genitals.

From a sex therapist: Women often report feeling pain during sex that is deep in their vagina. What they may be feeling is the pain of their partner's penis hitting the cervix. Women are often surprised and don't realize what they are feeling is their cervix! In many cases it happens because they are not aroused so their vagina is not fully tilted. They should slow down and get more aroused or change position.

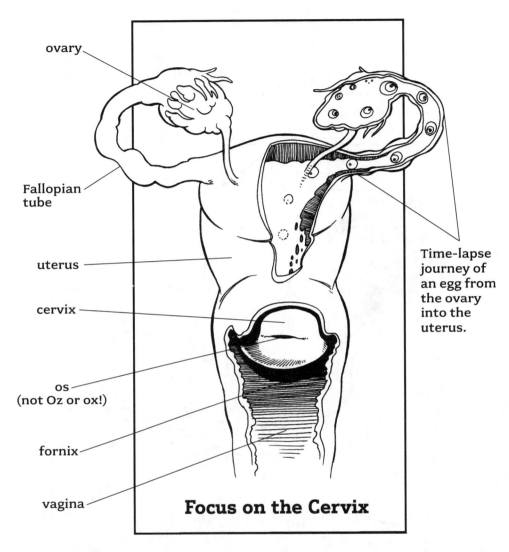

ovary

Fallopian
tube

uterus

cervix

os
(not Oz or ox!)

fornix

vagina

Time-lapse
journey of
an egg from
the ovary
into the
uterus.

Focus on the Cervix

There are at least two ways to see a cervix. The first is by using a
speculum. This is a metal or plastic device that physicians insert into a
vagina to help push the walls apart. It allows the physician to see parts
of a woman that few sexual partners ever do. If you have a healthy
curiosity, get a speculum from your physician or medical-supply store.
Put lube on it, gently insert it into the vagina and add the beam of your
favorite flashlight or phone. For a woman to see her own cervix, she will
need to incorporate a hand-held mirror or the camera from her phone.

Ovaries

A man's testicles announce themselves whenever he gets naked. Not so with a woman's ovaries. It's possible to have a long-term relationship with a woman and not even know her ovaries are there, except indirectly through events like periods and pregnancy.

The best time to feel a woman's ovaries is when she is lying on her back and is in an "It's okay if you feel my ovaries" mood. Rest one hand on her lower abdomen below her belly button. Gently slide a lubricated finger or two from your other hand deep into her vagina. When you encounter the rear wall of her vagina, veer to the left or right and push up while pushing down with your other hand that's on her abdomen. You will need to rely on her instructions from there. If a woman doesn't know where her ovaries are, she might ask her gynecologist to show her.

Sponges Around the Urethra

There is a spongy area above the walls of the vagina called the urethral sponge. The urethral sponge is tissue that surrounds the entire length of the urethra, which is the tube that takes urine from the bladder to the toilet. It runs along the roof of the vagina. If a woman is sexually aroused and you put your finger in her vagina and make a "come here" motion, you are pushing into the urethral sponge. Some women find this feels good. Others find it to be annoying. Even if she enjoys it, you should not do this until she is already highly aroused.

The tissue of the urethral sponge contains tiny periurethral glands that have an embryological and histological similarity to the male prostate. However, there is no prostate gland in the female pelvis. People who refer to the urethral sponge as "the female prostate" don't know what they are talking about. The prostate gland is an actual gland. It has specific functions and layers of organization. See pages 95-108.

G-Spot Area

Over the past few decades, the G-spot has become its own industry, complete with G-spot books, G-spot vibrators, G-spot toys, and videos.

While researchers don't question the orgasms that some women have with G-spot stimulation, there isn't any special wiring or trigger-tissue in the G-spot area that would make its stimulation universally wonderful for all women.

Until recently, we've mainly been limited to doing research on cadavers. While some of these dead women might still be orgasming in the afterlife, researchers can't see how different parts of a person's sexual anatomy interact when they're dead. With newer technology, we'll find more answers regarding the G-spot area. However, the debate will continue for a while longer.

One explanation of the G-spot has been proposed by one of our gynecology consultants. She says, "I always felt that the G-spot was actually a stimulation of the area that corresponded to the trigone of the bladder and that was why many women felt even greater sensations when their bladders were slightly full during sex. I have some patients who intentionally drink fluids to fill their bladder prior to sexual play because it 'feels better.' I think this causes the trigone to press down more on the anterior vaginal wall and is more easily stimulated." This corresponds with the experience of many women who find that G-spot area stimulation causes a feeling of bladder fullness:

> "When my partner is going down on me and inserts his finger,
> placing pressure upwards on the top wall of my vaginal canal,
> it feels really really good if I ignore that it also feels like I need
> to pee." *female age 24*

One of the world's top sex researchers was kind enough to weigh in the G-spot controversy for readers of *The Guide.* His take on the G-spot area is that when you are stimulating the anterior wall of the vagina you are stimulating parts of the urethra, the urethrovaginal 'space,' the clitoris via the ligaments connecting to it, the vaginal wall, and possibly Kobelt's plexus. He believes that all of these structures participate in arousing the brain. But he also says that where and how you fit the G-spot into an 'anterior vaginal wall complex' is a challenge.

The G-Spot Bottom Line

With all of the media hype and sex-store attention about G-spot stimulation, some readers might be thinking, "Why spend so much time with a woman's clitoris when I could be stimulating her G-spot?" The answer should depend totally on what your partner wants rather than on what someone else tells you.

Mercifully, Claire Yang, M.D., a neurophysiologist and researcher in the Department of Urology at the University of Washington, has the following to say:

> "I think that because the sexual response is so closely linked to emotions, the experience of pleasure, and in particular sexual pleasure, it is not going to be tied directly to anatomical structure, even during sexual arousal. For instance, why do women not feel sexual stimulation when those same areas that you describe are being examined during a gyn exam? The bottom line is: the entire genital area has nerves (as does the entire body), and in the context of sexual arousal, the processing of the messages is what makes the experience, not just the manual stimulation. I think the processing of sexual stimulation by the female brain is extremely variable, and to pin down a particular area (or situation) that is universally arousing is not possible at this time. That is why the concept of the G-spot has not gained universal acceptance. That is why the pursuit of a female sexual-arousal drug has been elusive. That is why the female sexual response will remain a mystery for a little while longer."

The writers at the major women's magazines routinely call me to ask about this spot or that spot, and what do I think is the mother of all intercourse positions. It's seldom enough if I say, "This might feel good for some women, but not for others. A woman should explore for herself and find what does and doesn't work for her."

Variations in Wetness

Some women's vaginas get so wet when they are sexually aroused that they need to wring out their underwear. Other women can be every bit as aroused but their vaginas remain dry. Wetness also varies during certain phases of a woman's menstrual cycle. And contrary to what you might think, some women need to add lube for period sex. That's because a woman's estrogen levels are at their lowest point during her period, and this can result in a decrease in natural lubrication.

Men shouldn't be so silly as to gauge a woman's level of sexual arousal on vaginal wetness alone. It's possible for a woman to be very aroused, but not be very wet. Also, thanks to porn, it is now popular to assume a woman's vagina is always ready for anything a guy wants to ram up it. Maybe this is one of the reasons why so many women in their teens and twenties are experiencing pain during intercourse.

Female Sexual Arousal

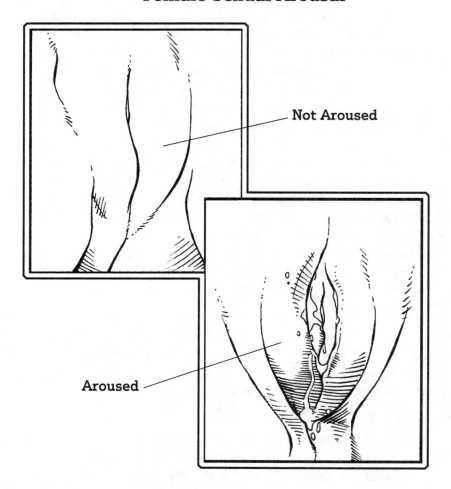

Not Aroused

Aroused

Not all vulvas show this degree of change with sexual arousal, but the changes inside a woman's pelvis during arousal can be extensive. While some women are quickly aroused and are ready for fingering, oral sex or intercourse as soon as the women in porn, most women require actual effort on the part of a partner in the form of kissing, caressing, and fun before they are ready to have sex. This doesn't mean women like sex any less than men. It's probably because sexual arousal occurs differently in women's brains than in men's, but no one knows for sure.

Sex educators used to say that most women require at least twenty minutes of making out and fooling around before a partner should reach between her legs. We stopped saying this because some women are raring to go before a guy can pull his penis out. But when I speak at colleges, the males seem surprised when I suggest a woman might want more than five or ten minutes of fooling around before having intercourse. And more women than you might think respond with "You mean it's not just me?" So I think we should go back to recommending the twenty-minute rule unless a woman indicates otherwise.

Female Ejaculation, Squirting or Gushing

Some women expel extra fluid at the time of orgasm. The biggest problem with this is that women who do it sometimes feel embarrassed and try to prevent it. As a result, they keep themselves from fully relaxing, and this can inhibit orgasms and pleasure.

The second problem is porn. A few years ago, a porn actress wrote a book on *female ejaculation.* She began giving workshops where she claimed that *female ejaculation* was nothing short of amazing, and that any woman could become a female ejaculator with the right training. Rather than just a few milliliters of "female ejaculate," women were being encouraged to ejaculate a cup or more of fluid.

Now, more than a decade later, we know that a woman's paraurethral glands can only produce 2 to 4 mls of fluid, or less than a teaspoon. Much more than that, and it's urine from the bladder. And some experts in female sexual health are starting to be concerned that women who have been forcing themselves to squirt during sex might be causing their bladders to prolapse. However, this has not put a dent into the *gusher, squirting* and *female ejaculation* categories of porn.

As for what we currently do and don't know about female ejaculation, some women release up to a teaspoon of fluid from their urethra at the time of orgasm. This is not urine. It is most likely produced by the paraurethral glands and it may often go into the bladder instead of squirting out of the body, so the woman is not aware of it. (More studies need to be done. For now, the best we can say is this is what seems to happen.)

We also know that when women release more than a teaspoon or two of fluid, it seems to be a dilute form of urine that comes from the woman's bladder.

For women who don't squirt or release fluid during orgasm, please do not attempt to train yourself or force yourself to do this. Forcing yourself to ejaculate might not be good for your bladder over time.

For women who do release fluid during orgasm, there is absolutely nothing wrong about it and hopefully you will not feel embarrassed by it. It could be a result of how your body is wired, combined with becoming extremely relaxed during sex and the way your partner is stimulating you. What's not to like about that?

If you release fluid during orgasm, why not put towels on the bed before making love? Also, they now make waterproof mattress pads and covers that don't crinkle or feel weird, but the manufacturer doesn't mention anything about squirting on the package.

Female ejaculation summary: There is nothing wrong with squirting and nothing wrong with not squirting. Squirting is not a sign of better sex. Not squirting is not a sign of inferior sex.

Being Wet When You Are Not Aroused & Not Being Wet When You Are

Our gyno consultant says that too many women think there's something wrong with their vaginas because they are moist during the day when they are not thinking about sex. She says this is perfectly normal, assuming a woman is in good gynecological health.

Also, a woman shouldn't feel there's something wrong with her if she gets really wet from thinking about sex when she's alone, but needs to add lube when she's with a partner or before intercourse–assuming she and her partner have spent enough time on the arousal part of sex before trying to have intercourse. Extra lube can especially help when a partner is wearing a condom, or if he is circumcised and the glans of his penis is pulling a woman's natural lubrication out of her vagina with each outbound thrust during intercourse.

Menopause

Menopause is what naturally happens to a woman's body when she is over 40 and stops having her monthly periods and no longer has to worry about getting pregnant. People have always believed that a

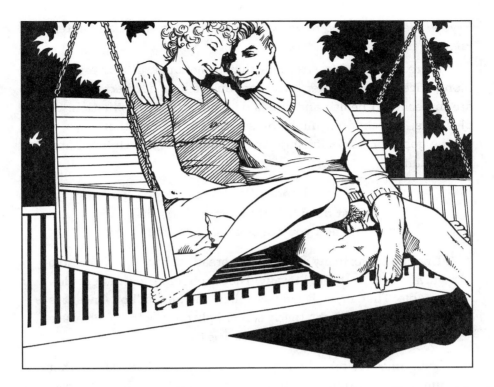

woman's sex drive goes down as she enters menopause. Yet researchers have discovered that when a menopausal woman gets into a new
relationship, she can be as horny as many 20-somethings. It could be
the excitement she is feeling toward her partner that determines how
much she wants sex, rather than the level of her hormones. Then again,
it can be difficult for any person, male or female, to feel sexual excitement if their hormones are below a certain threshold.

Some menopausal women become less wet when they are sexually aroused. The skin in their vagina may begin to feel less elastic or
more sensitive during menopause. While there are hormonal creams
that can help, the women from *Touch of a Woman* strongly recommend
that a woman or her partner massage her vulva and the opening of
her vagina every day with a moisturizer to help keep it more elastic. If
you are approaching menopause, please give this totally free, drug free
program a look. And keep in mind that the woman who has written this
protocol is an MD and is extremely knowledgable about women's sexual
health. The title is *Still Juicy: Maintaining Sexual Health Through and*

Beyond Menopause. Go to www.sexualityresources.com and enter "still juicy" in the search box.

There are also life stressors that a menopausal woman will commonly face, such as if her own mom and dad or her partner's parents are in declining health and she is dealing with their situation. On the plus side, her children might be starting to live on their own, which can be good for a relationship, or not so good if her children are high maintenance.

Reader Comments
What does it feel like in your genitals
when you are sexually aroused?

"Tingling starts in my clitoris and spreads to my labia. My whole vulva starts to throb, literally. The throbbing is extremely pleasurable. Then my vulva gets swollen and almost hot. Once it is swollen, every slight touch sends lightning bolts of pleasure all around my whole body." *female age 23*

"Sometimes it's an ache not unlike having a full bladder. Other times, a sensation of heat and congestion in my labia, clitoris and vagina. If I'm highly aroused, or if my clothing is tight, I'll be able to feel my pulse between my legs. Sometimes I'll feel my tendons and muscles twitching as well." *female age 36*

"My labia feel swollen and tight; my clitoris becomes hard. Sometimes my clitoris feels like it's huge, and it sort of throbs. If I am extremely aroused, my whole vulva feels as though it's pounding, with my clitoris as the center." *female age 26*

"You know the feeling you get right before your leg or arm falls asleep? I mean, before it's annoying or hurts. It's a really intense tingling feeling. It makes my whole body feel warm and excited. There are moments, however, right before my partner enters me, when my vagina actually aches."

female age 27

When did you first make the connection between being sexually aroused and being wet?

"When I was around 10 or 11, while watching a sex scene in a film. My panties got wet, and I realized that was why. If I'm really turned on, I'll drip down to my ankles." *female age 25*

"I first connected being wet with sexual arousal when I was 13. I was watching a silent, vintage erotic film with a friend. When I went to the bathroom, I was soaked!" *female age 26*

"The first time I connected wetness with sex was when I was 9 or so and got all wet and throbby when I was watching a couple kissing at the beach. But I don't always get wet when I feel aroused; it isn't an indicator for me." *female age 38*

"When I first masturbated, I only touched myself on my clitoris, so I was very surprised when I eventually felt my vagina and it was dripping fluid." *female age 23*

About being wet...

"Being wet is hard to explain. I don't know if I can offer insight because it just happens. The most annoying thing is that if you don't wear panties and get wet, it tends to be very messy, but arousing!" *female age 36*

"For me, the degree of my wetness varies greatly from time to time and seems to be largely affected by how mentally 'into' having sex I am at that given time." *female age 34*

"If my boyfriend just starts kissing me and wants to have sex, I am not automatically wet. I need to be turned on. This could be my way of slowing down and paying attention to my body, or it could be by talking sexy, reading, looking at, or listening to erotica." *female age 26*

"It does not work when my partner concentrates solely on doing mechanical things to get me wet. Yet a simple, very tender kiss can do it." *female age 48*

"I enjoy sex a great deal, but seldom get wet." *female age 32*

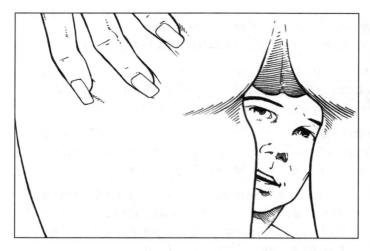

Dear Paul,

My girlfriend thinks her genitals are ugly. Is there anything I can do to help her change her mind?

Bobby in Beaver Falls

Dear Bobby,

This is part of a cultural disease. Some of the findings from this past year about the negative feelings that many young women have about their genitals has shocked me. The best I can tell you is with patient and creative encouragement on your part, perhaps her eyes will start to reflect the delight that's in yours when you look between her legs.

A Very Special Thanks to these amazing people for their help &advice:

- Claire Yang, MD, Department of Urology, University of Washington
- Christine Vacarro, DO, Madigan Army Medical Center, Tacoma, WA
- Alessandra Rellini, Ph.D., University of Vermont
- Marca Sipski, MD, Psychiatry and SCI Rehabilitation
- William W. Young, MD, Department of Obstetrics and Gynecology, Dartmouth Medical School
- Maureen Whelihan, MD, Gynecology
- Carol Tavris, Ph.D., Social Psychologist
- Ellen Barnard, MSSW, A Woman's Touch, Madison, Wisconsin
- Myrtle Wilhite, MD, A Woman's Touch, Madison Wisconsin
- Roy Levin, University of Sheffield, Sheffield England

Some of the illustrations in this chapter were strongly influenced by:
Atlas of Human Sex Anatomy, 2nd Edition, Robert Latou Dickinson 1949
A New View of a Woman's Body by the Federation of Feminist Women's Health Centers, Illustrations by Suzann Gage: progressivehealth.org

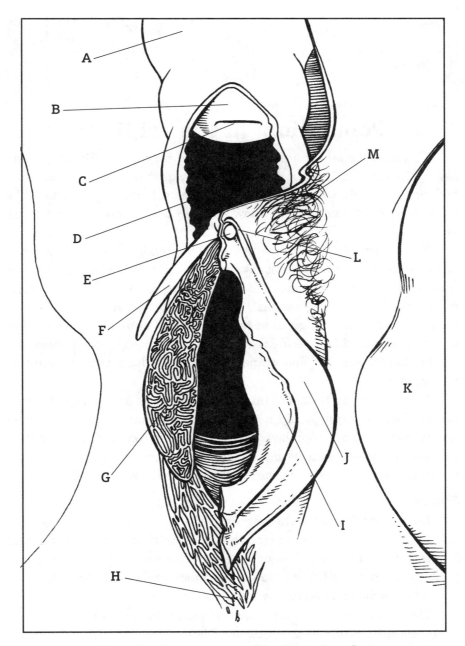

Female-Anatomy-as-Modern-Art Quiz

A–uterus; B–cervix; C–os; D–vagina; E–glans or tip of clitoris; F. crus
or leg of clitoris; G–bulb of clitoris; H–perineum; I–inner lip or labia minora;
J–outer lip or labia majora; K–inner thigh; L–hood of clitoris ; M–pubic hair

Population: In the Trillions

This book began as a series on science for surfers. But guys kept saying, "Science is fine, but how do I help my girlfriend have an orgasm?" and women would want to know about "The science of giving my BF a blowjob without having to swallow." So I've been subtle about science, until now.

The health of every woman's vagina depends on a complex world of bacteria and other organisms that's called a microbiome. But few women or men have ever heard of this. Before you say "Ewww, bacteria in vaginas," a male who weighs 155 lbs. has almost 40 trillion bacteria in his body. And it's not because he smells gross and doesn't bathe. The idea that we should be germ-free has been promoted by companies that sell antibacterial soaps and women's douche products that feature talking vaginas.

Without the bacteria and microorganisms that are so important for vaginal health, a guy would never be allowed near a woman's vagina. And if women understood how important the mircroorganisms in their vaginas are, they might be more cautious before buying sex lubes and "feminine hygiene" products that could be acting like Agent Orange.

Acidity

Except for humans, the vaginas of almost all mammals have a pH that's close to 7. This means the pH is neither acidic nor alkaline. But with humans, it's different. The pH is neutral until a girl reaches puberty. Then the pH of her vagina becomes acidic and stays that way until she reaches menopause, when it becomes almost neutral again.

The acidity in a woman's vagina is maintained by an ecosystem of microorganisms called a microbiome. Microbiomes are communities of bacteria and other tiny organisms that live inside of our bodies. They are as important as our chromosomes and blood cells. They produce substances that prevent infections and reduce inflammation. They help digest complex carbohydrates, and when the cells in our bodies are injured, they signal nearby cells to begin reproducing so we can heal more quickly. Our immune systems would be crippled without them.

Changes in Thinking

Not long ago, physicians believed that the microbiomes in all healthy vaginas were alike—as if there was one universal way every woman's vagina should be. We now know that there are five distinct communities of microorganisms that can live in a woman's vagina. While these communities are fairly stable in some women, they can transition frequently in the vaginas of other women. This means that different communities can become more prevalent at different times.

It might seem like there would be more infections in women whose vaginal communities transition frequently, but that does not appear to be the case. Researchers are just beginning to find out about the different ecosystems that are inside of women's vaginas.

Lactobacilli

One of the most important residents in the human vagina is a group of bacteria called lactobacilli. Humans are the only animals (including the great apes) who have lactobacilli as the dominant organism in their vaginas. We don't yet know the answer why.

There are many different species of lactobacilli in the world, such as those that are used to make yogurt, beer and sourdough bread. But the families of lactobacilli that live in the human vagina are unique. The only place they exist on the entire planet is between a woman's legs.

Lactobacilli in the vagina produce lactic acid and an antimicrobial compound called bacteriocin. These help kill or control undesirable bacteria, and the lactic acid helps to maintain an acidic environment that's essential for healthy functioning. The lactobacilli have tiny projections that stick out from their cell bodies. These projections clasp onto the cell walls of the vagina and prevent germs from attaching at these points.

Women who are low in vaginal lactobacillus are more likely to get sexually transmitted infections if they are exposed to them, including HIV. They are at greater risk for having miscarriages, premature babies, and suffer from pelvic inflammatory disease. This is one of the reasons why an important area of research is in how to supplement vaginal lactobacillus when it is low. The solution has proven to be nowhere near as simple as it might seem.

When There are Too Few Lactobacilli

Lactobacilli keeps the pH in the vagina low, which helps keep out unfriendly bacteria that can cause infections. When the population of lactobacilli is disturbed, the stage is set for infections and conditions that can cause itching, burning, odor and discharge.

Let's say a woman starts taking antibiotics for a lung infection. This kills off the unfriendly bacteria in her chest, but it also begins to kill the Lactobacilli in her vagina. As a result, the lactic acid in her vagina will decrease and the alkalinity will increase. The population of the friendly bacteria will begin to collapse.

As the population of the lactobacilli decreases, another of its by-products (hydrogen peroxide) will be in short supply. With less hydrogen peroxide, unfriendly bacteria will have an easier time taking up residence. Also, the Lactobacilli that was protecting the walls of the vagina will weaken. Anaerobic bacteria can more easily invade the cell walls and a woman may get a condition called bacterial vaginosis or BV.

Why Yogurt Usually Won't Help

Lactobacilli is found in yogurt, so you would think that eating a lot of yogurt or plastering it between a woman's legs would help her infection go away. But the kind of yogurt that's made from milk is specific to cow intestines. While yogurt might be good for a woman's calcium intake and maybe for her digestion, the yogurt we eat is unlikely to help with problems in the vagina.

Researchers are hoping to find specific microorganisms called probiotics to treat conditions like bacterial vaginosis. This would provide a much more elegant solution than we currently have. But it is possible that each woman will need a unique combination of probiotics to compliment the mix of bacteria in her vagina.

Too Many Lactobacilli

Another problem can occur when the population of lactobacilli begins to explode and produces too much lactic acid. Natural sugars start being fermented into carbon dioxide, alcohol, formic acid and acetic acid. This fermentation process is not dissimilar to how beer is made. But it causes itching and irritation when it happens inside the vagina.

This can cause the same symptoms as a yeast infection, including itching, burning, painful intercourse and a slight discharge. As a result, it is often misdiagnosed as a yeast infection. This is why a woman who is having problems needs both a sharp gynecologist and a good knowledge of how her vagina works. Over-the-counter drugs for yeast infections won't touch these kinds of situations.

When a woman really does have a yeast infection, it is commonly referred to as Candida. Another type of infection is caused by a protozoa known as Trich or Trichomonas vaginalis. There's also Noninfectious Vaginitis. Instead of being caused by organisms, the source of irritation for Noninfectious Vaginitis can be anything from feminine hygiene spray and body soap to premium toilet paper, laundry detergent, bike-seat irritation, and period gear.

Why a Vagina with an Infection Will Sometimes Smell Fishy

When the levels of lactic acid go down, anerobic bacteria can start to flourish. This kind of bacteria is responsible for the smell of bad breath, smelly feet, and Limburger cheese. A fishy smell is also caused by the cellular death and destruction that's going on in the vagina as part of the body's efforts to make things right again.

Fluctuations in pH

There are times when the pH in a woman's vagina will briefly rise. This can happen when she's having her period, with the pH rising to around 6 which is close to neutral. It will also go up for a few hours after a woman has had intercourse. That's because semen is alkaline and contains buffers that help keep it alkaline, which will cause the pH of the vagina to climb. A woman's own sexual lubrication can make the pH climb.

On the Distant Horizon

Researchers are looking at how a mother passes her vaginal microbiome to her infant daughter during the birth process, and the lifetime significance of this.

Some women have vaginal microbiomes that predispose them to infections, which could also predispose their daughters to vaginal infections. So there might someday be supplemental microbiomes that physicians can give to moms or to baby girls that could result in fewer vaginal infections throughout the girl's entire lifetime.

Products will also be created based on a woman's own unique microbiome that will help prevent her from getting infections and possibly even cancer.

Beware the Health Food and Vitamin Industry Probiotic Hype

The top researchers in the world are just beginning to create probiotics that will be helpful for human vaginas. The going has been slow and success has been illusive. But you wouldn't know that from the health food and vitamin industry hype on their latest and greatest probiotic pills and crotch goop. It sounds pretty good when they say one dose delivers several billion lactobacilli—never mind that these are the wrong lactobacilli.

The health food and vitamin industries can claim anything they want as long as they include a tiny asterisk with the words "This product has not been evaluated by the Food and Drug Administration. It is not intended to diagnose, treat, cure or prevent disease." Nuff said?

Are Sex Lubes 'Biome Busters?

The billion dollar sex lube industry wants women to put products inside of their vaginas that have never been tested for their impact on the vaginal microbiome or for their longterm safety. Research on this is in its infancy. For more on this, see Chapter 25: *Concerns about Sex Lube.*

Low pH Soap for Women's Genitals?

Most soaps and body washes have a high pH. Some women swear by a low-pH wash that's made for women's genitals that could be more microbiome friendly than high pH soaps. A version that is available in North America is called Sebamed Feminine Intimate Wash pH 3.8, and Sebamed Feminine Intimate Wash Menopause, pH 6.8 for women who are past menopause. Do check with your gynecologist first.

———————

Dear Paul,

My partner loves me to finger her vagina. But after a few minutes, my fingers start to sting. Do you know what's up with that?

Bernie from Vermont

Dear Bernie,

This is because your partner's vagina is acidic, which is perfectly normal and healthy for a woman who hasn't reached menopause. You might try wearing a latex or nitrile glove. Some women prefer being fingered this way because a gloved finger feels smoother than one without a glove.

A Very Special Thanks To Jacques Revel, University of Maryland School of Medicine for help that's been above and beyond the call of duty.

The Hymen

The hymen is source of myth and legend, and it remains a mystery to much of modern medicine. Not many primary care physicians can accurately locate the hymen. Few gynecologists can say what happens to the hymen of a sexually-active woman over time. And most of the research on hymens concerns sexual abuse, with some of the studies contradicting each other. So there's little credible information that's helpful regarding hymens and sexual pleasure.

This chapter presents what is currently known about sexually-happy hymens. If there are holes in our knowledge, it goes with the territory.

How The Hymen Came to Be

The hymen is a collar of tissue that's located just inside a woman's vagina. To understand how the hymen came to be, you need to know the difference between a woman's vulva and her vagina. That's because each had a hand in the development of the hymen.

VULVA: This is the part of a woman's genitals that you can see from the outside. It includes the mons pubis, the tip of the clitoris, and the lips or labia. You would need to separate the lips or labia before you can see the opening of the vagina. And you would need insert a medical device called a speculum before you could see inside the vagina.

VAGINA: The vagina is a tube-like structure that goes from the outside of a woman's body to her cervix. The average vagina is about 2.4 inches long. It becomes longer when a woman is sexually aroused.

The vulva and vagina are made from different types of embryonic tissue. The hymen is a ridge that is formed at the point where the tissue from the vulva meets the tissue from the vagina. Think of when two different land masses collide and a mountain range is created at that spot. That would be a metaphor for how the hymen was created. It's a ridge of tissue that marks the point where the vulva stops and the vagina starts.

The tissue on the outer side of the hymen (the vulva side) is sensitive to testosterone, as is the rest of the vulva. The tissue on the inner side of the hymen is sensitive to estrogen. That's because it's tissue that comes from the vagina, which is estrogen-sensitive.

It's Puberty and Not the Penis That Causes the Hymen to Change

Before puberty, a girl's hymen is often crescent-shaped, although there can be significant variations. The pre-pubescent hymen stretches across the opening of the vagina and covers much of it. It is almost translucent.

The estrogen that comes with the start of puberty causes the hymen to become shorter and thicker, more like an O-ring or collar than the former drape or wall that it was during childhood. It also becomes more elastic. This is because hymen tissue has estrogen receptors in it just like the walls of the vagina.

Since estrogen makes the hymen more elastic, our modern notion that the hymen "pops" during the first intercourse is silly. It is usually puberty that changes the hymen, not the first intercourse. It's as if nature is changing the girl's hymen to make it ready for intercourse.

From Saran Wrap into Spandex

Researchers often have trouble distinguishing between the hymens of teenage girls who are sexually active and the hymens of teenage girls who are still virgins. That wouldn't be the case if hymens were like "Cherries that pop." Still, it's hard to dispel the myth that the hymen is a seal of virginity. People continue to think of it as being like a plastic sheet that's fused onto the top of a frozen dinner.

Your First Intercourse

Most people assume there will be blood after the first intercourse. Yet far more than half of the women who take our sex survey say there wasn't any blood during their first intercourse.

Unfortunately, a number of the women who answered our survey believe the reason they didn't bleed during their first intercourse was because they had already torn their hymen while riding a horse or by doing the splits, or while their boyfriend was feeling them up. So the myth that hymens pop is alive and well.

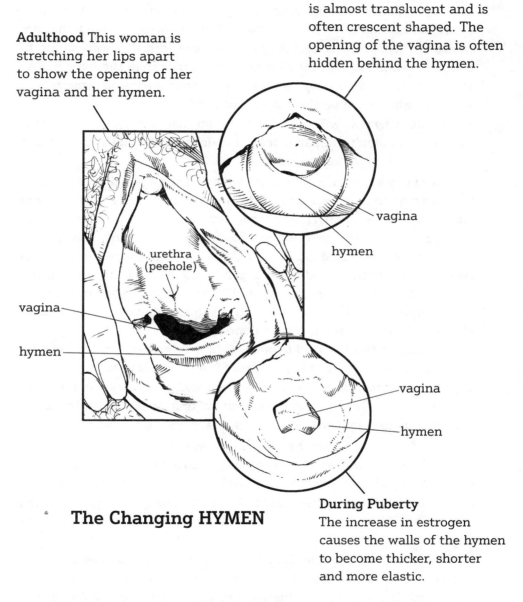

Adulthood This woman is stretching her lips apart to show the opening of her vagina and her hymen.

Before Puberty The hymen is almost translucent and is often crescent shaped. The opening of the vagina is often hidden behind the hymen.

vagina

hymen

urethra (peehole)

vagina

hymen

vagina

hymen

The Changing HYMEN

During Puberty The increase in estrogen causes the walls of the hymen to become thicker, shorter and more elastic.

Far from making hymens that break or tear, nature made the hymen ready for intercourse by changing its shape and making it more elastic during puberty.

Researchers have investigated athletic injuries in girls' crotches where bleeding occurred, including splits-gone-wrong and inline-skating related trauma. They found it wasn't the hymen that bled. In cases where the hymen most certainly should have torn if it were going to tear, it was the vagina that split and bled rather than the hymen. And why horseback riding would wear away a hymen makes no sense unless a woman was sitting on the horn of the saddle.

While a hymen will most likely be stretched during a first intercourse, it shouldn't ordinarily tear. If it does, or if there is pain, there are at least two possible causes:

Not Fully Estrogenized: In some women, the hymen doesn't become fully estrogenized or elasticized during puberty. One healthcare provider who does premarital exams says she sometimes prescribes estrogen cream for soon-to-be married women whose hymens haven't become very elasticized. So if you haven't had intercourse and are concerned, it would be a good to ask a gynecologist if your hymen appears to have been adequately estrogenized for intercourse. (No one knows if the estrogen in hormonal birth control helps the hymen become more elasticized. No research has been done.)

Clumsy or Not Aroused Enough: A first intercourse can be painful when the male partner is inexperienced, rough, has poor aim, is really big, or the woman is not sufficiently aroused and there's not enough lubrication. As a result, the hymen might tear or bruise, in the same way your gums might when you accidentally chomp on them.

Another thing researchers have discovered is how fast the hymen heals. Medical examiners have been surprised at how normal the hymen can look in girls who they know have been sexually molested. The latest research has found that tears in a hymen usually heal quickly, often within 24 to 48 hours.

Tags

A hymen can start bleeding for the first time years after a woman has been having intercourse. This might be due to a tear in a hymenal tag, which is a remnant of the hymen. These tags are like any of the other folds of skin inside the vagina, except they might look like pointy bits where there would otherwise be smoothness. Hymen tags are fairly common, but most women never detect them because they don't feel any different from other parts of the vagina.

What Happens to the Hymen Over Time

One gynecologist we consulted believes the hymen wears away with intercourse. The larger the penis, the more it wears. She believes she can accurately guess the size of a partner's penis based on how worn the hymen appears to be. Another gynecologist disagrees, saying you can't predict anything about the number of sexual partners or their girth by the appearance of the hymen.

Needless to say, research would be helpful, but one would need to examine the hymens of women who are virgins and then reexamine them a few years after they've been sexually active. You'd also need to know the dimensions of their partners' penises, how many thrusts they do per average intercourse, and how often they've had intercourse. Imagine a world where Congress would approving funding for studies like that!

The experts did agree it's not unusual to see fronds of the hymen protruding from the vagina. These might have been tags from the hymen that became stretched. Also, childbirth might be a hymen's worst nightmare.

Warranty Repair or Revirginization

Revirginization surgery, is when a surgeon takes the tattered edges of a hymen and purse-strings them together. None of our consultants were excited about it. The explicatives they used in describing the wisdom of *revirginization surgery* are not appropriate for a family book like this. However, if the alternative is being stoned in the village square...

Hymen Issues

If you have trouble removing tampons, intercourse is uncomfortable and your gynecologist says you have a *septate hymen,* a bit of local anesthetic and a small snip can often do wonders. A septate hymen is one that hangs vertically through the center of the vagina and looks a bit like the uvula at the back of your throat except it is usually attached at the top and bottom. The ridge around the head of the penis can catch on this kind of hymen during the out strokes of intercourse.

An *imperforate hymen* is more rare than a septate hymen. It is where the hymen completely covers the opening of the vagina. If a woman really does have an imperforate hymen, having it taken care of surgically is essential.

If you are having discomfort during sexplay, don't assume the problem is your hymen. One thing to discuss with a gynecologist is whether the pain is at the opening or the back of your vagina. Before blaming your hymen, you might want to rule out things like vaginismus, vulvar vestibulitis syndrome, chronic constipation, certain infections, adhesions under the clitoral hood, or when the woman is not adequately aroused or there's not enough lubrication.

Vaginsimus is when the ring of muscles around the opening of the vagina automatically clamps shut. Vulvar vestibulitis is where the vestibule and the hymen are very tender when touched lightly with even a cotton swab, not to mention an incoming penis. (For more on pain during sex, see Chapter 48: *Damn That Hurts! When Sex Is Painful.*)

No matter what your symptoms are, if a hymenectomy is suggested, get a second opinion. This is not only wise but important.

To watch our free and mostly wonderful videos about sex,
and for links to the eBook and audiobook versions of this book

please visit

www.Guide2Getting.com

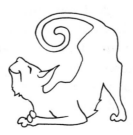

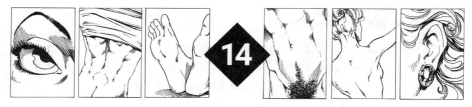

Nipples, Nipples, Nipples

While the title of this chapter is eye catching, it should have been "breasts, breasts, breasts," or "nipples/breasts, nipples/breasts, nipples/breasts." That's because for many women, the part of their breast they prefer having kissed and caressed is between the neck and nipples as opposed to just their nipples. Plastic surgeons discovered this when they were doing studies on sensation in women's breasts.

One woman might find it heavenly when a lover barely breathes on her nipples, but convulses in pain if he is the slightest bit rough. So her partner learns to traverse her tender nipples like a butterfly and becomes a master at the art of subtle stimulation. Another woman doesn't find it erotic until a lover's lips latch on like an industrial vacuum cleaner. Some women's breasts become more sensitive during certain parts of their menstrual cycle. Know your lover's body and be sensitive to the ebb and flow of what feels good and when. And don't assume it's the nipple that does the trick when it might be the area a couple of inches above, below, or to the side of it.

Another thing to consider has to do with deeper meanings. To some women, whenever lips go near their nipples they automatically feel maternal. Every sparkle of sexuality drains out them. So be sure to talk to your partner about whether she gets turned on or off by nipple and breast play, or if she'd rather you be focusing your efforts elsewhere.

Stimulation for Men's Nipples

We often assume it's only women who like breast and nipple stimulation. However, a study on nipple/breast stimulation found that 52% of males enjoy tender kisses and caresses of their nipples. Another 25% of the males were probably too manly to admit they enjoyed it. Men seem to have similar variations in nipple and chest sensitivity as women. Some men get an erection when their nipples are caressed, and some find it enhances their orgasm if a partner sucks on a nipple or caresses it at the same time their penis is being stimulated.

Six Facts about Breasts

❦ Women's breasts weigh approximately half a pound for each cup size. So if a woman has a B cup, each breast will weigh a pound, for a C cup, it's a pound and a half, and for a D cup, the breast will weigh close to two pounds.

❦ A woman's hormones influence almost every aspect of her breasts, especially the glands inside. This is why it's perfectly normal for a woman's breasts to change in consistency and sensitivity from week to week.

❦ The breasts of younger women are primarily made up of glandular tissue and not much fat. That's why they tend to be so firm. As women get older, their breast lobes are replaced by more fat, and so their breasts become softer.

❦ More than 90% of women have breasts that are asymmetrical, which means one is different from the other in size, shape or position on a woman's chest. It's usually the left breast that's larger, and in almost 25% of women, the larger breast is at least one cup size bigger than the other.

❦ Over the course of a woman's lifetime, her breast size will change up to six or seven times.

❦ As with a clitoris or penis, the sensitivity of a breast has nothing to do with its size. Small ones can be like lightning rods, while big ones might not be sensitive at all.

A Very Helpful Take on Breasts For Men

Here are some women's perspectives on their breasts as reported to Meema Spadola in her wonderful book, *Breasts—Our Most Public Private Parts,* Wildcat Canyon Press:

From Elaine, "My preferences vary constantly. What feels pleasurable one moment can feel annoying the next. Sometimes I hit sensory overload and can barely stand to have my breasts touched."

Cecilia says, "My nipples are very sensitive and I could be aroused almost to the point of orgasm just by touching them, but only very gently, almost not at all." At the other end of the spectrum is Heather, who prefers a firm touch that includes clothespins and biting.

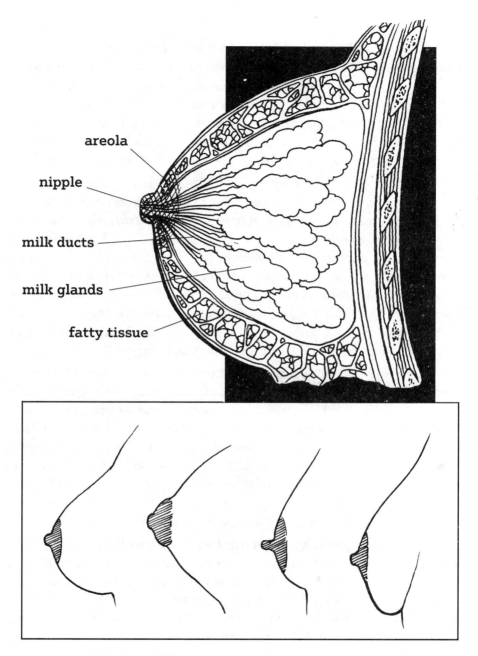

areola

nipple

milk ducts

milk glands

fatty tissue

Breasts are made up of glands, ducts, and surrounding fat. In younger women, the proportion of fat in their breasts is usually lower. It increases with age. It is the fat that gives breasts their unique size and shape. It is completely normal for breasts to feel lumpy.

There is Carrie, who was known as the girl with the big boobs. "Guys were sometimes more attracted to my boobs than to me." One day when Carrie was wearing a large rain slicker which hid her breasts behind a wall of thick yellow plastic, she met a man from out of town, and they seemed to hit it off. They talked on the phone and emailed for the first year of their relationship, with him never knowing that her bras were the size of saddlebags. Assured that he liked all of her and not just her mammaries, Carrie eventually married the man.

One woman in Ms. Spadola's book reports, "When a man touches my breasts, I feel a little removed from the whole experience—as if he's on a date with my breasts." Another woman says, "My boyfriend loves to suck on my nipples, but sometimes I get this sense that he is focusing on them and tuning me out, and I can feel a wave of resentment, almost jealousy, when he latches onto my breasts." A third woman says, "I would feel like I had this 180-pound baby in my arms, and occasionally he'd fall asleep there sucking my breasts. I'm sure he thought he was giving me great pleasure, but it just didn't do it for me."

There are women who describe their breasts as being "a place of warmth and love," and "without breast stimulation, sex is purely physical with no emotional component." Another perspective comes from Scarlet, with 38DD breasts, who says, "I can't wait to take my clothes off in bed because I know that men will get excited; they always want to suck on my breasts. They think that I get incredibly turned on by it, but my breasts aren't as sensitive as men expect. Honestly, I could be balancing my checkbook while they're doing it. It's really not a big deal. But I do get turned on seeing them getting very turned on."

Ms. Spadola quotes a woman who has had sex with men and women: "The men didn't seem to grasp that twisting them like radio dials does not work. They treated my breasts as something separate from my body. Women seem to know instinctively what to do with breasts. Women sense that there are times when you want your breasts to be touched, and times you don't. It didn't seem to occur to the men I was with that there might be mental and cultural baggage wrapped up there."

How Women Can Let Men Know What They Want

Even if a woman's partner has a big hairy chest, she should tell him she is going to touch and kiss his "breasts" the same way she likes to have hers kissed, and then do it. If there are times when she'd like it to be gentle, tell him, "This is what I like when I say *gentle*." If there are times when she likes it extra-rough, she should show him what she means when she says *rough*. If she like her nipples tugged, she should show him exactly how and for how long. And she shouldn't get bent out of shape if he requires refresher lessons. The learning process is not nearly as straightforward as you might think.

Techniques for Happy Breasts

There is no "one-size-fits-all" bra, and there are no sets of breast-stimulation tips and techniques that will work for everyone. Here are a few things to consider. Talk it over with your partner. Experiment and have fun learning together.

Making a Nipple Taut: When your partner is aroused, place your fingers on each side of a nipple, around the perimeter of it. Push down lightly and slide your fingers apart. This will make the nipple taut. Try kissing and caressing it. Some people find that their nipples are more sensitive when the skin is pulled taut.

In and Out: Pucker up your lips and use them to make a gasket around a nipple. Then suck in and out without breaking the seal—so the nipple feels alternating currents of vacuum and pressure. This method also works well on earlobes and the clitoris. However, if you are sucking earlobes in this way, be sure that earrings are removed first. As for jewelry in the nipples or clitoris, discuss suction limits with your partner lest one of her favorite gold loops or bars ends up at the bottom of your stomach.

Five-Finger Breast Grab: This works best if the breast and your hand are lubricated with massage oil. Rest your hand over the breast with your fingertips spread open. As you lift your hand, let your fingertips caress their way up the sides of the breasts until they are clasping the tip of the nipple. Pull on the nipple just a little or a lot, depending on what your partner likes and her level of arousal.

Nipple Between Your Index & Middle Fingers: Cup your hand over the breast in such a way that the tip of the nipple rests in the space between your middle finger and index finger. Squeeze the fingers together so that when you lift your hand the nipple follows, pulling the rest of the breast up with it. The ability to do this will depend upon the

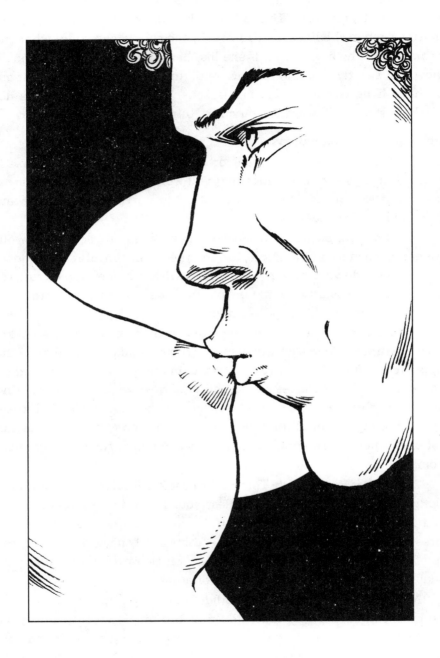

size and shape of the nipple.

Nipple and Penis: Some women find it arousing when a man caresses their nipples with the head of his penis or by pulling his foreskin up around the nipple.

All or Some? Find out if your partner wants you to lick or suck on the entire breast and not just the nipple. Remember to alternate breasts.

Hand and Mouth: Your partner probably has two breasts and you only have one mouth. Ask if she likes it if your fingers are caressing one breast while your lips are tending to the other, or perhaps she would prefer your hand to be caressing some other part of her body.

Variations in Sensitivity: Sometimes one breast or nipple is more sensitive than the other. Find out if your lover would like you to spend more time on the sensitive side, or more time on the less sensitive side

Menstrual Effects: Breast sensitivity can change with a woman's monthly cycle or if she's taking the pill. Be sure to discuss this.

Different Temperatures: An ice cube in the mouth can be a rousing way to greet a partner's breasts. Or for breasts that are already cold, drinking something warm just before licking or sucking them can feel exquisite.

Serving Tray: Fruits, desserts, whipping cream, chocolate sauce and certain liquors can be served on chests, backs, and other body parts with pleasing results. But do what you can to keep sugars out of the vagina.

Getting to Watch: Some partners find it erotic to watch a woman play with her breasts. So if you are a woman who enjoys playing with her breasts, there's no point in keeping it a secret.

Hard Nipples—Pleasure or Pain?

Let's say you are playing with your partner's nipples and they get hard. Is this a good sign? Sometimes yes, sometimes no. Until you learn more about your partner's body, don't assume that hard nipples mean happy nipples. Nipples can get hard from unpleasant stimuli such as roughness, abrasion, and cold—so be sure to ask your partner if he or she likes what you are doing. Also be aware that what a person wants in terms of nipple play can vary with their state of sexual arousal.

If You Have a Tongue Piercing or Your Partner Has Nipple Jewelry

If you have a tongue piercing, a reader cautions that dragging a steel ball across her nipples "can be a bit gnarly." Assuming your partner likes to have her nipples licked or sucked, make sure that you've coated them with a heavy layer of saliva. The extra saliva will help your barbell to glide rather than drag. Also, using the tip of your tongue when playing with her breasts and nipples will help keep the tongue jewelry away if it causes her discomfort. Get lots of feedback from your partner about this.

You'll also want to avoid sucking hard if she has nipple jewelry.

Dads and Their Daughters' Growing Breasts

Growing breasts can come between dads and their teenage daughters. This isn't something they have pamphlets on for parents at the pediatrician's office. For instance, one of a daughter's fondest childhood memories can be of wrestling and rough-housing with her dad when she was younger. But suddenly, much of the physical intimacy stops and she doesn't know why. This can be what happens when her chest develops and the physical intimacy starts to make her dad feel uncomfortable.

Hopefully, dads will understand the huge loss this can pose to their daughters. They can transform the physical closeness into involvement in other ways—such as by playing catch with a baseball or going jogging, or by taking their daughter someplace special or fun each week. The important thing is to maintain the intimacy which is so important to many daughters and dads while moving the physical relationship into a realm that's more age-appropriate.

Readers' Comments

"Kissing my breasts depends upon my mood. Sometimes I like being touched gently with fingertips and then gentle circles of a tongue followed by a very light sucking on the nipples."
female age 27

"Most of the sensitivity is in the nipple, but there are good feelings from having the whole breast caressed and sucked. Swirling your tongue around the nipple is good. Sucking the nipple is great! Biting the nipple is a MAJOR no-no." *female age 34*

"Depending on how aroused I am, I like to be sucked hard and even gently bitten on my nipples." *female age 45*

"There doesn't seem to be any logical pattern or reason behind it, but sometimes even touching the breast area can hurt. Other times, pretty much anything is okay." *female age 32*

"I had to have a breast biopsy last year for a lump. I had not thought of my breasts as pretty before. They have always seemed too small compared to what all the boys were paying attention to. With a gain in self-esteem and self-respect and with the help of my current boyfriend, I've found that I really do think of my breasts in a whole new way, especially after going through the experience of surgery. My lump was benign, but it made me think about myself in a new way and what I really have to appreciate." *female age 20*

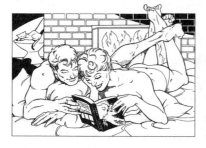

Dear Paul,

> *My boyfriend wants me to lactate for him. I am not pregnant and never been. I don't know how to lactate. I don't know if it's safe or if it is going to turn me into a hormonal wreck. If you have any advice I would be really grateful.*

Madonna in Montana

Dear Madonna,

For starters, what you are asking about is different from the breast play that some couples enjoy during lovemaking. You are talking about a situation where your breasts would be lactating and your boyfriend would be nursing on them two to four times a day, seven days a week. If he missed a nursing, you would need to pump or express the milk from your breasts. This wouldn't be a problem if you were also donating breast milk to infants, which is becoming a cottage industry in a number of countries.

Adult couples who nurse refer to it as an "Adult Nursing Relationship." It usually begins after the woman has had a baby. The father may have started nursing alongside junior, or maybe mom encouraged him to take over once the baby was weaned. There are adult couples who keep nursing for years. The child could be graduating from high school, and dad might still be sucking milk from mom's breasts.

Having to nurse so often might cause even the most eager of couples to abandon the concept. However, couples who continue this kind of nursing seem to cherish the added closeness and dependency. Not only is one partner dependent on the other for milk, but she is dependent on him to relieve her swollen mammaries. The woman's milk will often let down at the sight or sound of her partner, just as a nursing mother's breasts will let down when she sees or hears her hungry infant cry.

There are two ways that someone who hasn't been pregnant can try to jump-start her non-nursing breasts. These methods have been pioneered by adoptive moms who are trying to breast feed their adopted infants. One method involves the use of drugs to trick your body into thinking you were pregnant and have given birth. The other involves seriously intense sucking on the part of your partner, several times a day for several weeks. Even then there is no guarantee he'll be sporting a milk mustache.

If this did work, your breasts would probably get bigger, so you would need to buy new bras and blouses. As for the potential of getting stretch marks, I don't think it would be any different than with mothers who nurse infants. Also, you would need to supplement your intake of calories and calcium just as a nursing mother does. Otherwise, your body might start robbing your bones of the extra calcium that your breasts need to produce milk. And if your boyfriend didn't cut calories in other ways, he'd probably start to get fat.

As for the safety and impact of all this on your body, women have been nursing babies since the beginning of time, but would nursing an adult partner have the same impact on your body as nursing a baby? I don't know of any studies on this.

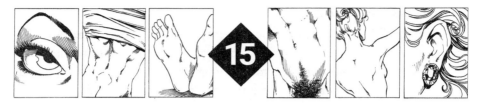

The Ultimate Tenderness

When writing this book, I tried to consider sex from many different perspectives, including mate swappers, Tantric-sex masters, born-again Christians, bondage enthusiasts, and even those whose sex lives are really boring. Having left no sexual stone unturned, one and only one universal truth about human sexuality emerged:

No matter what your sexual beliefs, fantasies, kink, or persuasion, nothing beats a good back rub.

Nobody, absolutely nobody, had a single bad thing to say about a good back rub. Ditto for foot massage.

Hard vs. Soft? Male vs. Female?

Just about every book ever written on sex loves to state that men touch women too hard, and that women touch men too soft. Nonsense. There are two types of touch that both men and women seem to like a great deal:

Feather-Light to Light: This is where the fingertips lightly dance across the surface of the skin, resulting in a delightful tingling sensation that may or may not raise goose bumps. It can also be done with the flat of the hand doing light, long, gentle strokes.

Deep & Hard: This is when muscles are kneaded with a strength and authority that chases away stress and tension. The men commented that they often fear they are doing this too hard, but their female partners almost always say it's just right or to do it harder.

For helpful resources, there are numerous books and videos on touch and massage. An hour spent reading one of these books or watching a video will do a great deal for your relationship. Pay special attention to foot rubs, hand rubs, and scalp and facial massages. These body parts are often ignored because they aren't considered blue-chip erogenous zones.

Spectators vs. Participants

To help defend ourselves from anxiety and stress, we often turn our muscles into body armor. Learning to massage and be massaged is one way to help relax your body's armor. This might be anxiety-producing at the start, so go slowly and try to enjoy the gains you are able to make.

Also, some people struggle to get fully into their bodies. They may have trouble relaxing enough to enjoy what is being shared with them. Or they need to be hypervigilant about what is going on around them. Massage can be a nonthreatening way to allow more closeness.

Combining Sex & Massage

One reader comments: "My husband often massages my shoulders while I'm giving him head. It feels wonderful and serves to relax me so I can become more easily aroused." Another reader ties her naked partner's hands together above his head. She lets him watch as she removes her satin panties and caresses his entire body with them. A third reader drags her hair across her lover's naked body and eventually wraps it around his genitals.

One man reports that the best way to drive his partner into total ecstasy is by brushing her hair or massaging her scalp with his fingertips. Another couple takes long, candlelit showers together, shampooing each other's hair and soaping each other's body.

Perhaps you have your own favorite ways of combining massage with sex play. Whatever your inclination, if there is only one thing you take from this book, it will hopefully be to make massage an integral part of your sexual relationships. Touch and massage might be the most important aspects of human sexuality, outside of the occasional need to replenish the species.

Massage your senses with regular visits to
www.Guide2Getting.com

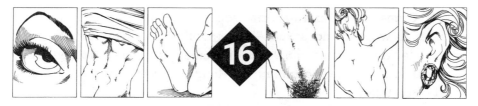

Orgasms, Sunsets & Hand Grenades

"Define orgasm? It's somewhere between a hand grenade and a sunset." —*Billy Rumpanos, friend and surfer*

One of the many nice things about sharing sex is having orgasms, also known as coming. But orgasms are not without their mystery. Perhaps it might be helpful to consider a few comments about orgasm from Dr. Frieda Tingle, the world's leading expert on sex:

Q. Dr. Tingle, what do you think of sex in America?

A. I think it would be a good idea.

Q. Do you think Americans are too concerned about orgasms?

A. Orgasm is very important for many Americans because it tells them when the sexual encounter is over. Most of these people enjoy competitive sports, where some official is forever blowing a whistle or waving a little flag to let them know the event has ended. Without orgasm, they would be fumbling around, never knowing when it was time to suggest a game of Scrabble or a corned-beef sandwich.

Q. What kind of things affect a person's ability to have an orgasm?

A. One important factor is diet. I have been told that it is impossible to have an orgasm after eating an entire pizza. Another factor is the weather. Many patients have told me that if the window is open and they are being rained on, it is particularly difficult to have the orgasmic experience.... (Dr. Frieda Tingle is the alter ego of Carol Tavris and Leonore Tiefer.)

Orgasm Defined

The best way to define orgasm is to put your hand in your pants and give yourself one. But this assumes you are able to give yourself an orgasm and you don't have six different kinds when you do. Perhaps you will find the following definition to be helpful:

👓 Orgasms are extra-special sensations that people sometimes experience while being sexual, either alone or with a partner. They occur after a certain threshold of excitement has been crossed. They can last from seconds to minutes or longer. A sense of well-being or relief often follows.

👓 Orgasms often feel as if they are being broadcast from the genitals or pelvic floor, although there is no reason why they can't come from other parts of the body.

👓 Some people experience orgasm as a single, tidal-wavelike surge with a couple of brief aftershocks; others experience it as of waves, genital sneezes, or bursts of light, color, warmth, and energy. Some describe orgasm as creeping up on them and slowly flooding their senses. Some experience it as an explosion, for others it's a whisper.

👓 Some orgasms make you feel great; others can be wimpy and disappointing. Some are strictly physical; others are physical and emotional. Some reach into the body; others reach into the soul. Some are intense and obvious; others are diffuse and subtle.

👓 The way an orgasm feels can vary with different types of sexual activity; orgasms from oral sex might feel different from intercourse orgasms. Masturbation orgasms are often the most intense, but not necessarily the most satisfying.

👓 Orgasms with the same partner are likely to run the gamut from totally spectacular to downright disappointing. It depends on the particular day, and whether your worlds are colliding or are in sync.

👓 Some people have orgasms when a lover kisses them on the back of the neck; others need a stick or two of dynamite between their legs. The amount of stimulation needed to generate an orgasm has nothing to do with how much you enjoy sex.

👓 When shared with someone you love, the feelings that follow orgasm can make it possible to experience a special kind of intimacy.

👓 Some people feel pleasantly amped or energized following orgasm, while others feel mellow and might want to sleep. For some people, one orgasm begs for another. For others, it calls for hugging and tenderness.

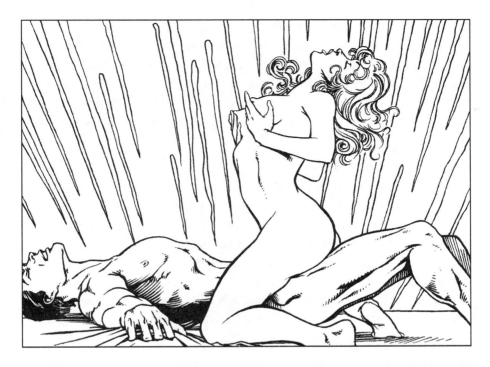

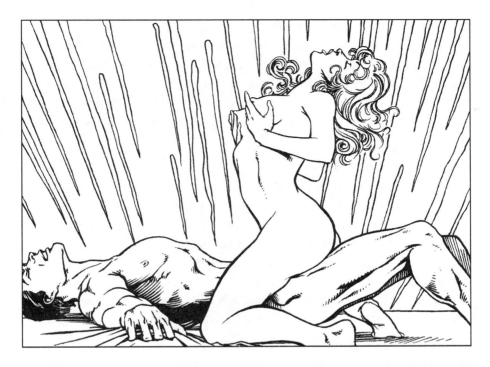Some people are easily derailed on the road to orgasm. For others, the phone can ring and the earth can shake; they come no matter what.

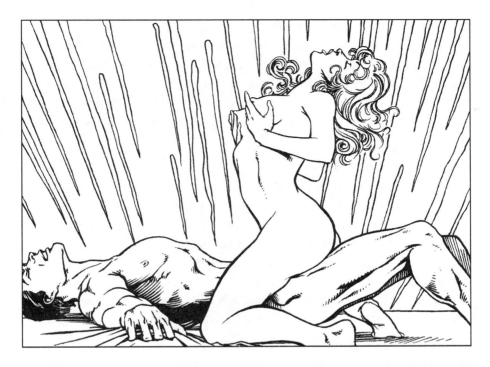Orgasms can catapult you deep into your own world. You can lose awareness of your partner, which means they're doing something right.

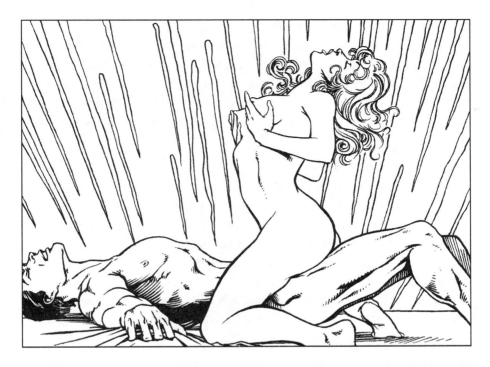It can be nice to occasionally blast off together, but it is not necessary or even desirable for partners to come at the same time. It can be wonderful to feel or watch your partner have an orgasm, which is difficult to do if you are coming simultaneously.

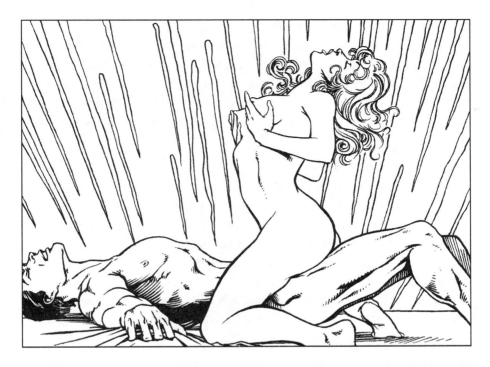Some people have orgasms with their legs squeezed together, while others come with their legs apart (innies vs. outies). People who prefer coming one way sometimes find it difficult to come the other way.

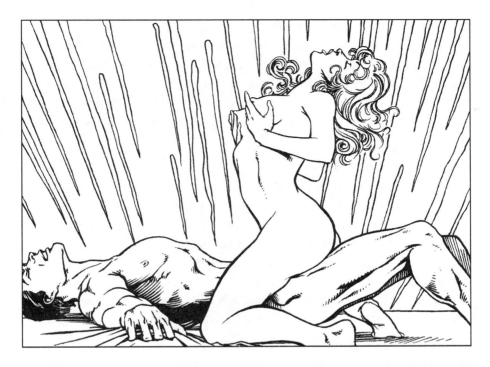Genitals can become extremely sensitive after having an orgasm. Stimulation that may have felt wonderful moments before orgasm will often feel painful or abrasive immediately after. It never hurts to ask your partner about this, since it's true for some but not for all.

Does Orgasm Alter Your Consciousness?

When people are coming, they often experience a change in consciousness. One brain researcher who has studied women's orgasms suggests that they are similar to a trance or a near seizure like experience. Getting to that point, where a woman can allow this kind of brain change to occur, might require a more nuanced process than how men arrive at the threshold of male orgasms.

Your Partner's Orgasms

We often assume that a partner who has an orgasm is fully satisfied, while one who doesn't is disappointed. Were it that simple. If wanting orgasms were the sole reason for doing a particular sex act, not many women would bother with intercourse.

Most of us can give ourselves intense orgasms when we masturbate. But not many of us can get feelings of closeness and intimacy when we do ourselves solo. For some people, it's the feelings of closeness and intimacy that are the most important part of lovemaking.

Increasing the Odds

Things that increase your chances of having an orgasm: being seriously into your partner, exercise and a healthy diet, seeing erotic images, and anything else that turns you on. (Going to college increases the chance of a woman orgasming from masturbation; guys have never needed a degree to figure that one out.)

Things that decrease the chance of orgasm: being annoyed or angry with your partner, smoking cigarettes, stress (notice how you tend to have more sex while on vacation), not sleeping enough and taking certain drugs. There's a huge list of drugs that will dent your libido or delay your orgasm, especially SSRI anti-depressants such as Prozac, Zoloft and Paxil. Hormonal methods of birth control can significantly decrease the sex drive in many women, and the combination of SSRIs and hormonal birth control has been described as the ultimate anti-sex cocktail.

Almost twice as many Protestant women as Catholic women report that they orgasm during sex. Perhaps one problem for Catholic women is the Catholic church's strident prohibition against touching yourself or masturbating, which is how a lot of women learn to have orgasms.

Information on how Catholic boys learn to have orgasms is still under litigation in many dioceses throughout the land.

Expressions, Decibels & The Way People Come in the Movies

Some people worry about how they behave when they are having orgasms. Some are self-conscious because they lose control, others because they don't. There is no correct way to come. Sexuality is an altered state of mind; what you do with it is up to you. Some people worry how they will look if they allow themselves to be overwhelmed by an orgasm. They fear their partner will laugh. Quite to the contrary. It is far more likely a partner will think:

> "Her face got all twisted and contorted. She looked like she was tripping big time. She must have had a major orgasm. Maybe I'm not so bad in bed after all...."

There are also people who have sensational orgasms but hardly show it. Their orgasms are an internal phenomenon that remains hidden from the outside world.

Many of us assume that women are supposed to make noise when they are coming, even though there is no correlation between decibels and delight. Some women sound like freight trains when they orgasm; others become completely quiet except for an occasional twitch and sigh. The same is true for men. If your partner comes in a quiet way and you would like to know more about it, why not ask?

Many of us learned to come quietly at a young age. That's because there might not have been much privacy where we masturbated. Letting out a loud bellow would have informed the entire household. This was particularly true if you shared a room with siblings, and even worse if you had the top mattress in a bunk bed. The same difficulties are faced by students living in dorms, sororities, fraternities, and in military barracks, where roommates often sleep a few feet away. So we pretend to be asleep when masturbating —a funny notion when you consider that our roommates are probably pretending they are asleep as well.

The sex-noise dilemma is also faced by parents who are making love (or trying to make love) when there's a household full of kids. Their children's response to hearing mom and dad making love can range from "Mommy sounds upset" to "That's SO gross, where's my earbuds?"

Spontaneous Orgasms

This quote is from a woman who had a spontaneous orgasm while riding public transit — a rather scary thought if you have ever taken the bus in places like Los Angeles or Detroit:

> "I've perfected this wonderful ability to orgasm without touching myself. It started one day on the commuter train when I was ovulating, and I felt myself throbbing. I started running a fantasy in my mind and discovered I could bring myself to orgasm. The only trouble with a public place is you have to control your breathing...." —*Words of a former high school homecoming queen from the Midwest, in Julia Hutton's Good Sex, Cleis Press.*

One sex therapist describes a time in college when he and his friends were talking about different ways of masturbating. One guy said he could ejaculate without touching his penis. Bets were quickly made and the room became quiet. Mr. Spontaneous whipped out his penis. After his eyes were closed for a while, his penis became erect. He began breathing faster, and eventually had an ejaculation without ever touching his penis.

Not only is it possible for some people to have an orgasm without genital stimulation, but it can even happen without sexual thoughts. Some women have spontaneous orgasms during highly charged debates or intellectual discussions that have nothing to do with sex. One female reader had her first orgasm as a teenager while her hair was being brushed, and as a 40-year-old she still has orgasms when her hair is brushed. Some women have spontaneous orgasms when working out, especially when doing crunches or exercises that involve the abs.

While not many of us are able to have orgasms without genital stimulation, the existence of hands-free orgasms does suggest that there is more to orgasm than genital contact. People who have suffered nerve injuries and can no longer feel sensation in their genitals can learn to have orgasm feelings in other parts of their bodies, such as their faces, arms, necks, lips, chests, and backs. That's because the power to experience orgasm resides in our brains and not simply in our groins.

One woman whose clitoris and vagina were removed due to cancer was able to experience the same kind of intense multiple orgasms after the surgery as before.

People who have lost one of their senses do not suddenly grow new ones to compensate. They are forced to better use the senses that remain. This suggests that many of us could achieve greater sexual pleasure from other parts of our bodies if we learned to allow it. One way of doing this is mentioned later in this Guide, where the woman stimulates her partner's penis with one hand while using her other hand or lips to caress another part of his body not normally associated with sexual feelings.

Pain, Pleasure and Orgasms

Receptors for pain and pleasure are located next to each other throughout our bodies. These receptors often fire at the same time. It is our brain's job to decide whether the overall experience feels good or bad. To make such a decision, our brain will sort through its database of everything from whether we are ticklish to how we feel about people with brown hair and green eyes like those of our partner. So our brains make their own decisions about what is pleasurable and what is painful.

For instance, one person experiences being spanked by their partner as painful and a turn-off, while another person finds the pain to be erotic. The stimulus is the same, but how we feel about it depends on how our brain interprets it.

The way we interpret pain is also impacted by our level of sexual arousal. People who enjoy being spanked during sex usually don't like the pain unless it's done when they are sexually aroused. Being aroused can cause the brain to throw routine caution to the wind, converting sensations that are otherwise painful into sensations of pleasure.

Possible Assist for Women's & Men's Orgasms

When women are about to come they often pull in or tighten their pelvic muscles. Yet trying to relax might make their orgasms more intense. Some women will hesitate to do this from fear it could allow them to pass gas or pee, but you'll both live if she does. If you consider the gas-passing habits of most couples, chances are she owes him a few.

Whether you are male or female, you might occasionally experiment with relaxing the muscle tone in your pelvis when you come. Some men find they can prolong the feelings of orgasm if they relax their crotch and anus as orgasm is about to come. Others not so.

What Was It Like?

Lovers sometimes ask each other if they came, but not what coming feels like. Sexual experiences can be hard to put into words, since they often exist on the cusp between physical and emotional sensation. But asking a partner to describe what an orgasm feels like might lead to some interesting insights and discussions.

Guys Faking Orgasm?

When the first edition of *The Guide* was published, it was assumed that women were the ones who did the faking. Yet up to 30% of young adult males have faked orgasms at one time or another. Researcher Karen Yescavage found that guys fake orgasm for reasons such as: "I was tired," "I faked it so she wouldn't see me go limp," "So she would think she was doing a good job," or "I wanted to get it over with." The reasons women gave for faking tended to fall into the "I-was-tired-bored-or-it-was-hurting" category.

A number of people who faked orgasms felt it helped increase the intimacy in sex. For them, the intimacy was more important than whether they came or not. Others feel that deceiving a partner is wrong no matter what the justification. They can't see how you can lie and feel more intimate at the same time.

The people who admitted to faking orgasms didn't fake them very often. Straight white women and lesbians fake orgasms at the same rate, which is twice as often as Hispanic women. One explanation for the disparity is that lesbians and white males may expect their partners to have more orgasms than Hispanic males do, and so the white females and lesbians felt more compelled to fake orgasms.

If Your Partner Fakes Orgasms

One of the worst things you can do when a partner fakes an orgasm is to go on a mission to help him or her have real orgasms. This usually makes matters worse. When it comes to orgasms, there is sometimes a fine line between helpful concern and obnoxious fretting, especially if the reason you need your partner to have an orgasm is for your own reassurance that you are a good lover.

Rather than trying to help your partner have an orgasm, why not try to discover the things that give him or her pleasure and comfort?

Contrary to what you might think, this could simply be holding each other for an extended time or not grabbing for your lover's crotch the minute you feel horny. If your partner has suggestions about technique, all the better, but this might not be where the issue lies.

Far more relationships crumble from a lack of emotional pleasure than from a lack of orgasms. As long as you are able to give each other emotional pleasure, there are plenty of ways to achieve orgasm. This book lists several hundred of them.

Orgasm Dementia

👓 Sometimes it's fun to count orgasms and go for it like pigs to mud. But for some people, orgasm production or procurement has a suspicious edge. Here are some reasons why:

👓 Some people get a sense of smug superiority by claiming how many orgasms they either had or "gave" a partner. They confuse sex with video games.

👓 Pleasure-giving can be a way of controlling a partner. This might not sound like such a bad problem, unless it's your job to come in order to make your partner feel like he or she did good.

👓 Some lovers expect their partners to supply them with constant sex and orgasms. A partner can start to feel used.

👓 There are people who need to have sex or masturbate many times a day to help numb anxiety or ease feelings of deadness. Flooding their nervous system with a constant stream of orgasms can be a way of keeping an emotional funk at arm's length. This should not be confused with sex that done is for fun and pleasure.

Reinventing the Sexual Wheel – Marketing & Orgasm

TV infomercials have been hawking pills and herbal concoctions for better sex and bigger orgasms, which you would be well advised to stay far, far away from—especially products that use the word "enhancement." We've also been told we should buy books and DVDs on G-spot orgasms, female ejaculation, extended orgasms, one-hour orgasms, and Tantric-sex orgasms. Some of these might help, but probably no more than talking to your partner about what feels good and what doesn't.

Reader Comments

For men: What does an orgasm feel like?

"My knees get weak and I tingle everywhere. It feels like I am numb all over." *male age 21*

"Like an energy emanating in the soles of my feet, up the back of my legs, in and through my rear end, to my belly button, and out through my balls and penis. Awesome, warm, exhausting." *male age 26*

"When I'm getting close, it feels like every ounce of fluid in my body has been forced into my penis. My whole body is in anticipation of the moment when my penis can no longer take the incredible pressure and bursts. Flames envelope the entire thing and the shock reverberates throughout my entire body." *male age 25*

"Orgasm makes me feel very connected to my lover, like I'm becoming a part of her." *male age 39*

"It feels like all your vital matter collects in your penis and then shoots out of you!" *male age 22*

For women: What does an orgasm feel like?

"Every orgasm I have is different! Sometimes I feel like I'm just melting, floating away. Sometimes I feel like I'm running or pushing into the orgasm. Sometimes an orgasm will sneak up on me; other times I will be able to control its arrival and duration." *female age 45*

"All my orgasms seem to be the same beast, but with varying levels of intensity from 'Gosh, was that it?' to an ache so sharp it's almost hard to bear. My most intense orgasms tend to come from using a vibrator but, oddly enough, they're not always the most satisfying." *female age 36*

"Orgasms range for me from a simple response in my genitals, without much sensation and even some numbness, to a mind-blowing, explosive force of nature that permeates my whole body, mind, and emotions, encircles my partner and fills the room around us. Sometimes it's the physical sensations that are the most intense part of orgasm; other times it's the emotional quality and being with my partner that take top billing. Even when the physical sensation isn't very intense, I generally feel much more whole and integrated after an orgasm." *female 47*

For women: Your first orgasm?

"With a vibrator at age 38. Finally!!!" *female age 49*

"It didn't happen until seven months after my first sexual experience. I had no idea what was happening. We were through having sex. When I began to put my clothes back on, I started to tingle and fluids started flowing out. It felt great, but I was actually kind of scared and embarrassed." *female age 21*

"I had my first orgasm during one of my first menstrual periods. The feeling of a clean pad against my genitals made me feel a warmth I had never experienced before. I rubbed against it to see if I could prolong the sensation, although I had no idea what the sensation was. I just knew it felt good!" *female age 45*

"My first orgasm took place at age 18, when my fiancé introduced me, despite my initial revulsion and disbelief, to the delights of cunnilingus. I thought he was depraved. I was sure I was going straight to hell. I couldn't wait for it to happen again!" *female age 55*

"I had an electric shaver that had an attachment which was a massager. After about an hour of moving it around on my clit (and praying that the pillow between my legs was muffling the sounds so my parents didn't hear) I had an orgasm. I'd already had sex many times with my boyfriend, but I felt like I was really sinning now!" *female age 25*

"I didn't know what was going on. My body felt like it was convulsing. I tried not to let the guy know this was happening. I didn't know at the time I was supposed to let myself go and enjoy it." *female age 26*

"The first one I had was clitoral—it tickled (I was probably 10). The second type of orgasm I had was when I was 20. I felt it more in my vagina. It was overwhelmingly emotional and I came in a flood, and I do mean flood. I thought I had peed all over my partner. Now I have both kinds of orgasms. I get to pick, let's see, lobster or steak?" *female age 26*

"My first orgasm was when I was making out in the back seat of a car. I was on top of my boyfriend and there was a lot of bumping and grinding going on, and I just climaxed, with my clothes on." *female age 49*

"I was surprised by how sensitive my clit was, but I wasn't sure the actual orgasm was an orgasm because it didn't seem nearly as explosive as what happened in the bodice-rippers I'd been reading. I couldn't believe I'd gone through all this work for that. Happily, many years of practice improved the results!" *female age 36*

"I was 20. One morning before arising I was idly rubbing my clit and fantasizing, and from out of nowhere excitement began building more intensely than it ever had before. I rubbed myself quite vigorously and for a very long time, until suddenly there was a mind-blowing explosion. I was certain that everyone in the house figured out what I was doing. I was very embarrassed. However, I repeated the experience every night—it took over an hour of heavy-duty stimulation at first." *female age 51*

"My first orgasm was by a male friend (not a lover). I told him that sex was not that great. He used his fingers to teach me what it could feel like. I remember thinking 'Oh God, this is an orgasm!' " *female age 48*

Hi Dr. Paul,

I'm a writer from a major women's magazine. I'd love to interview you for a story to ask if there's any evidence pointing to how many orgasms a woman is able to have, whether there's a "limit," and how women can achieve orgasm after orgasm after orgasm. Are you interested?

Echo

Hi Echo,

Thanks for thinking of me for your article. Here's the problem—I deal with real people who have real sex lives. You deal with editors who want sensational articles to sell magazines and generate click throughs.

The idea of "orgasm after orgasm after orgasm" sounds bizarre to me. It's one more burden we are placing on women to act like porn stars.

What should matter is if the sex is satisfying for a woman, not whether she has one orgasm, ten orgasms or none. Is the sex achieving what she wants for herself, and for her relationship if she's in a relationship?

So I'm thinking I'm not the person who's going to make your article shine, or put a smile on your editors' faces!

The Orgasm Talk

There are a lot of talks about a lot of things. But the one talk couples almost never have is *the orgasm talk* which is an honest discussion about orgasms rather than just "Did you come?"

Women's Orgasms Are the Lovemaking Trophy

One should not assume parity between men's and women's orgasms. There are reasons for this. Men's orgasms are usually a given during sex. But if the only reason a woman wanted to have sex was for the orgasms, she'd be ahead of the curve if she sent her partner off to play video games and took matters into her own hands.

For many women, it's the intimacy and full body contact of intercourse that makes sex special, not that they want a guy to ignore the importance of their orgasms. So women do not always equate sexual satisfaction with having orgasms, while for men, the idea of sex being satisfying without an orgasm is a foreign concept.

Men's orgasms tend to be obvious, while women's are not. Men are at the mercy of women to inform them if they did or didn't come. Otherwise, men wouldn't need to ask, "Was it good for you?" So it's the elusive nature of women's orgasms that elevates them to the realm of the lovemaking holy grail.

Also, a woman might need sex to be different depending on her mood. She might want sex to knock her socks off on Monday, but on Tuesday she may want sex to help her feel more grounded or connected. So orgasms might be a bigger part of sex for her on some days than others. There's no way a partner will be able to understand this unless she explains it to him.

Hopefully, in reading this chapter, you will understand why it can be helpful for men and women to have a talk about orgasms.

Recent Research Findings

Some women assume it's the man's job to provide the right physical stimulation for a woman to have an orgasm, but it's her job to get into the right mental space where she can let go of life's worries and allow an orgasm to occur. Is it really this simple?

It is unlikely a woman will forget everything that has or hasn't gone on between she and her partner during the past week just because they are about to have sex. Feelings of anger, frustration or disappointment will not evaporate the second her partner pulls out his penis. Helping to create the right mental space is just as much his job as hers.

It could also be that a man's ability to make a woman feel sexy and desired helps create the right mental space for her. Or maybe it's his willingness to be playful and to make sex fun. Acting out fantasy scenarios or being kinky could be what turns her on. Perhaps a woman wants her partner to be more "take charge" in bed. These all need to be part of the orgasm talk.

As for a man's physical skill set, just because porn makes it seem like a man should automatically know how to please a woman, it doesn't work like that in real life. Men need and often want guidance from a partner. So a woman's ability to show a man how to stimulate her physically is often the key to him being able to provide her with the kind of physical stimulation she needs to have an orgasm. Again, part of the orgasm talk.

Orgasms Before? Orgasms After?

There's been a popular notion that a man should make sure a woman comes before he does. This can be good for some women, but not for others. (Perhaps the point was to encourage men to think about women's orgasms in addition to their own, because sex is often over once a man comes.)

But prescribing who comes first can place all kinds of pressure on a woman that is not conductive to sexual pleasure. Also, some women are happy to have an orgasm after intercourse is over. They might enjoy it if a partner holds them while they masturbate with their fingers or a vibrator, or after he rolls over and falls fast asleep. That way they can enjoy whatever fantasy they'd like to have.

Discussing how and when a woman prefers to have an orgasm is a good thing to include in your orgasm talk.

Orgasms during Intercourse?

A common assumption is that the penis stimulates the clitoris during intercourse. Yet if you look at where the tip of a woman's clitoris ends and where her vaginal opening begins, you might wonder what nature was thinking. The tip of the clitoris is a ways above the opening of the vagina.

Perhaps that's why so many women need to stimulate their clitoris during intercourse in order to have an orgasm. They use a finger or vibrator on their clit while a partner is thrusting, or they grind their clitoris into his pelvic bone, or they push their clitoris down with their fingers so it gets more stimulation from his penis. So if either of you is assuming women should have orgasms from thrusting alone without added clitoral stimulation, this should be something you discuss.

Fingers Okay, But Not a Vibrator?

Men tell researchers it's okay if they or their partner stimulate their partner's clitoris with their fingers during intercourse. However, they aren't nearly as enthusiastic about a partner using a vibrator during intercourse. It seems they interpret the vibrator as a rival or as an indication of failure on their part.

Intercourse is about pleasure. What does it matter if a woman is using a vibrator instead of her fingers during intercourse? Any guy whose partner enjoys using a vibrator while he's thrusting should consider himself a lucky man. That's because she'll be having intense orgasms and she will associate them with him and the wonderful feeling his penis provides when it's inside of her.

Strangely enough, guys usually don't mind if a woman uses a vibrator on her clitoris when they are having anal sex. Perhaps one of the allures of anal sex is that it's more "anything goes" than vaginal intercourse. Men feel less threatened by a woman's vibrator during anal sex.

The Final Approach But No Landing

Women will often get close to having an orgasm, but something happens or changes in the last minute and they suddenly career away from it. So when you are having your orgasm talk, be sure to discuss what a woman needs as she's approaching orgasm. Men will often push a woman off a trajectory toward orgasm by suddenly going faster, harder, or by changing the rhythm, unless that's what she specifically wants. Talk about what she needs during the minute before orgasm.

You'll also want to find out what's best once a lover starts to orgasm. Should a man keep doing exactly what he was doing before she started to come, or does she want him to switch gears? How should he be in the minutes immediately after she has an orgasm? Some women might prefer steady pressure on their vulva after they orgasm. Others will want a partner to do what he was doing before she came, but at a greatly reduced intensity. And for some, hands off is the sensible approach.

Agony vs. Ecstasy

When I first started working in an emergency room, there was a young man down the hall who was moaning in excruciating pain. He would pepper his moans with an occasional "Oh God." If the context had been changed and someone had heard these same moans coming from a bedroom window, they would have smiled and assumed this guy was receiving the mother of all blowjobs.

How is it that pain and sexual pleasure can sound so identical? They don't feel the same, or not for most of us anyway. But it can be difficult to know when a partner is expressing pleasure as opposed to pain. This is yet another thing for the two of you to talk about. Learn your partner's signals for pleasure vs pain.

As for the assumption that women are highly verbal when they have orgasms, the opposite can be true. Some women zone out and go into another world. Hip-bucking and screaming aren't a part of it. But for other women, you might need to give the neighbors ear plugs. There is no correlation between decibels and delight.

The Bottom Line?

As you might have gathered, there's much to discuss with a partner about her orgasms. Hopefully you will not have just one orgasm talk.

A special thanks to Claire Salisbury at Western University in Ontario, Canada, to Tristan Taormino, and to Nina Hartley, who, suggests that couples should have an orgasm talk.

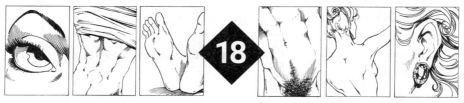

Consent

This has always been a book about consent: about asking, respecting and never pushing or pressuring a person to have sex. It doesn't matter if you are together for an hour or a lifetime, if there isn't consent, then there shouldn't be sex.

In more and more states, sex without mutual consent has become illegal. It is incumbent upon men and women to know what this means.

Then vs. Now

For too long, consent in sex has been defined as whatever you could get away with. But the excuse of "She didn't say no!" will no longer offer protection for a man who is charged with sexual assault or rape.

The new consent rules also address coercion. While it is perfectly normal for a woman to wonder if the sex was worth the effort, the last thing she should be asking herself is "was it rape?"

"I'm Not a Rapist!"

No one wants to see himself as a rapist. But if you have pressured a woman to have sex when she didn't want to have sex, it could be rape. Even if a woman didn't say no to sex, you can still be charged with sexual assault. The same is true if a woman said yes, but suffers buyer's remorse and it becomes her word against yours.

If you had casual sex with a woman who was under the influence of alcohol, drugs, or was asleep, you may have committed rape. If "all you did" was fondle or grope a woman who put your hand under her shirt but was under the influence, you could be guilty of sexual assault. Your penis never has to come out of your pants for you to be charged with a very serious felony. And you don't want to be in the position of telling the court "But she only had one beer."

If it's a "he-said she-said" situation, the chances are high the male will lose. So men need to start asking themselves if casual sex is worth the risk of being arrested for rape. I don't believe it is. If you have a penis, Title IX on most college campuses has you in its sights.

There's nothing in the new laws that say you have to buy a woman a wedding ring before asking for a handjob. But it's important that the decision be hers every bit as much as yours—without coercion, pressure, alcohol or drugs.

What Should You Do

Let's say you meet someone who you'd like to have casual sex with. Talk, flirt, ask for her contact info, then go home and masturbate. Get in touch with her the next day.

Text. Meet for coffee. Do something together besides grope and make out. If she wants to have casual sex with you, make sure she's known you for at least a couple of days and has had time to think about it. This will hopefully reduce the chances she might have second thoughts afterward. And if she does, it will be more likely because you weren't satisfying in bed as opposed to her feeling she was pressured or coerced.

If you assume "She was letting me feel her breasts, so I figured it was okay to fuck her," imagine the fun you'll have explaining that one to a police officer or to a judge and jury. You can't justify bad behavior by saying, "Women aren't always clear" or "'No' just means you need to try harder!" It is now incumbent upon the man to make sure the woman wants to have sex without being pressured.

Why the Changes?

For too long, a woman who was assaulted and had the courage to file charges against the man who assaulted her was raped a second time by the legal system. She's the one who was put on trial. This is changing. The onus for consent is being placed more and more on the male. This is fair. Males usually don't have to worry about being sexually assaulted. That's a much better deal than women have had.

No Longer Hiding in The Shadows

Until recently, people thought of sexual assault as being committed a stranger who lurked in the shadows or pried a woman's bedroom window open. No one thought of it as something your date did after the two of you started making out, or at a party among friends. But as researchers interviewed more women, they started hearing accounts of men who would not stop in spite of a woman's protests.

Rules for When To Keep Your Zipper Up
And When It's Okay to Pull It Down

An agreement to kiss is not an agreement to have intercourse. It never has been. Feeling each other up and discovering the woman's vagina is wet is not consent to put a penis in it. If a woman chooses to wear a short, sexy dress, it is not an invitation to reach underneath it or to take it off.

If you need to convince someone to have sex with you, then it's wrong. If they need to convince you to have sex with them, then it's wrong.

If a potential partner doesn't want sex as much as you do and isn't willing to say so, go home and masturbate. If the relationship is worth it, call or text the next day and talk things over.

Because someone gave you permission before doesn't mean you have permission now. Always ask. Having had sex with a person in the past is not a rain check for sex in the future.

Not being sure how far you want to go is normal. If a woman wants to get physical with you but isn't sure how far she wants to go, you must talk it over to find what she is comfortable with. In the eyes of the law, hesitation is the same as the person saying "NO!" If you proceed, you can be charged with rape.

If a potential partner who you've not had sex with before has been drinking or doing drugs, wait until the next day when she is sober and can legally consent before pursuing sex. Otherwise, you can be charged, even if she was the one who asked you to have sex.

There are men who are adept at engaging women in kissing or petting, and then assaulting them the same as "traditional" rapists who lurk in corners. Men like these can come from wealthy families who are on the social A-lists. They can be sports heroes, Boy Scouts, altar boys, and divinity students at a Bible college.

To help prevent this kind of sexual assault, the courts have pushed the limits of what consent is into a somewhat artificial and at times awkward place. The onus of stopping sexplay now rests on the male the moment a woman says, "Stop!" or "Maybe I should go" or "This doesn't feel right." A woman may have agreed to have intercourse, but if she changes her mind after 200 thrusts, a man needs to pull out immediately and not after thrust number 210.

In a decision for the State of California Supreme Court called *People v. John Z,* a woman agreed to have intercourse, but at some point while having intercourse she indicated she might want to leave. She didn't say "Stop" or "I don't want to keep doing this." The court found that she was raped because the man did not stop the moment she indicated a change of heart.

Making sure a woman can legally consent to sex is now the job of the male. Even if a woman bought the first two rounds of drinks or brought the pot and rolled the joints, she is not legally able to consent to sex if she has been drinking or doing drugs. This can be true even if she voluntarily went down on a man to help him get hard and put in the penis herself. It doesn't matter if both of you were equally drunk or stoned. The mere fact that she was drinking can turn intercourse into sexual assault in some states, depending on the situation. Also, there are times when it is not legal to have sex with a woman if you are her boss, her teacher, her minister, her physician or her coach.

Don't assume a woman is playing a game when she hesitates or says "No." Anything less than an exuberant "Yes!" should be understood as no. Never, ever, try to win a woman over by pressuring her to have sex. The courts have made it clear this will not be tolerated. If a woman does not make it clear she wants sex, a man needs to assume that sex is neither desired nor legal. Prison is no place you want to be, and it's become easier to find yourself there if you push sex on another person.

What About Dick Pics?

Never send unsolicited pictures of your dick or post pictures of you and another person having sex. These can result in your being arrested for sexual assault, stalking and multiple other crimes.

If You Know You Have a Communicable Disease

If you know you have a communicable disease and do not inform a new partner, you can be sued. Not only is it morally right to inform someone you are about to have sex with that you have a contagious condition such as herpes or HIV, but warning them will help you cover your legal bases.

Yes Means Yes

There are a number of new programs on college campuses that are designed to teach mutual consent in sex. "Yes Means Yes!" is one such program. It's where a woman is supposed to suddenly feel comfortable proclaiming to a male "I want to have sex with you, and here's exactly what I want us to do!"

This program is well intended. But for a reality check, it is being promoted by the same government that has spent more than $2 billion to fund programs that teach young women to feel shame about their bodies and shame for wanting sex. The Department of Education now expects these same women to jump for joy and shout "YES!" to sex?

These are the same young women who were encouraged to take "purity pledges" in middle school and high school, and who men in Congress are still trying to tell what they can and can't do with their bodies. These are the same young women who were called "sluts" and "hoes" if they admitted to wanting sex as much as males in middle school and high school, and they can still face dire consequences in some cultures for having premarital sex.

For a much more realistic take on "Yes Means Yes," consider this by social psychologist Carol Tavris: "How do you know what you want until you start doing something you think you want and then don't? Or do? People married for 40 years are often unable to say clearly what they want, or don't want, and we expect 18-year-olds to know what they want?"

Until society no longer tolerates men pushing themselves on women for sex, programs like "Yes Means Yes" could result in even more young women getting drunk before having sex, so they can feel less conflicted about rattling off the new mantra of "Yes, I want to have sex with you, and here's exactly what I want us to do!"

While "Yes means yes!" is something that needs to become a reality, we still have a long way to go with "No means no!" A woman should not have to repeatedly say "No!" to a person's advances.

Answers to Questions from Inquiring Minds

To Mark at the University of Georgia who feels he was misled: We've all been misled (or led on) at one time or another. Some of us have misled others. Even if it seemed like she wanted sex as much as you, the second she looked at her watch and said "Gotta go" you should have had your pants on faster than a tachyon through a crack in the cosmic egg.

To LouAnne at Texas Women's University who can't understand why consent laws apply to women as well as men: The two of you had been slamming down shots of tequila in his bedroom and his jeans were three sizes too small in all the right places. LouAnne, it wouldn't matter if he were buck naked and had a tassel on the end of his penis, when he said "No more" you needed to respect his wishes. Even if a partner has their tongue halfway down your throat, if they suddenly pull it out and wag it in a way that says "This is all you're gonna get," then you'd better stop. The same is true if the two of you have been married for ten years. A ring or wedding vow is not consent to rape.

To Randy, formerly at Fairleigh Dickinson University and currently residing in the New Jersey State Prison system: The two of you had been flirting for weeks. She invited you to a party. Both of you had been drinking when she threw her arms around you and said, "Let's go upstairs and have the sex we've always dreamed about." The following Monday, you found yourself arrested for rape. How could this be? "Informed consent" implies your partner was sober enough to make a rational decision when you had sex. If she was not sober when she put the moves on you, it is you who can be charged with a crime in some states. And even if the jury finds a man innocent, it would still cost him thousands of dollars to defend himself and the personal toll would be immense.

Why was this chapter addressed to straight males? While consent can certainly be an issue for gays and lesbians, the vast majority of consent violations involve sex that's between men and women. While plenty of women have pressured men into having sex, when the subject is rape or coercion, we are usually talking about the behavior of straight males.

The Zen of Finger Fucking

"Rubbing lightly is what I do when I masturbate, so I like it even more when my boyfriend does it. I love it when he runs his fingers along my inner lips, up and down. I also love my genitals to be rubbed and tickled when I wear jeans or corduroy. I can come from that kind of stimulation." female age 23

Some men take the term "finger fucking" literally. They think a woman's idea of a good time is having a man cram his fingers up her vagina. Or they attack a woman's clitoris as if it were a doorbell button, believing that the harder they push the closer she will come to having the big "O." The only "O" she is likely to experience is "OUCH!"

Finger fucking is not something a man does to a woman, but something he does with a woman. It's all of him — his smile, kiss, laughter, strength, and tenderness focused in the ends of his fingers.

Hopefully you will find this chapter to be helpful, especially if you are able to leave your jackhammer behind and are willing to try things with your fingers you might not have tried before. But none of it will make a difference if your partner isn't already turned-on before you reach between her legs, or to quote a reader *"There's no point in approaching my vulva and clit unless I'm already aroused. Touching me there is not the way to arouse me."*

As you will discover in reading this chapter, most of the work your fingers do will be on the outside of a woman's genitals. Only a small part of it involves putting your finger or fingers inside of her vagina.

Please forgive the term "finger fucking." It's just an expression. The last thing you'll want is for your fingers to be doing a bony imitation of a penis thrusting inside a woman's vagina unless that's what she wants you to do. If your fingers were supposed to do the job of a penis, white gooey stuff would squirt out of the tips when you rubbed your knuckles.

What This Is and Isn't

There are different kinds of finger fucking. One involves the hot-and-heavy groping that's an extension of making out. It's when a guy gets his hand between a woman's legs because she wants it there and because there's all kinds of passion and kissing and drooling going on. It's all about the moment. You don't need a chapter on that.

This is about how to please a woman with your fingertips. It's nothing you do in the dark or while you are stoned or drunk. It requires lights, looking and lots of feedback. If the stars are lined up just right and your phones are turned off and you and she are truly into each other, you might end up giving her incredible amounts of pleasure.

Altering Your Goals

Begin by banishing the usual guy-goal of giving a girl an orgasm. She'll have one if she has one; maybe you'll be the medium, maybe not. It could be she'll need to finish herself off with her own fingers or perhaps with her favorite vibrator. It doesn't really matter as long as you are able to set the stage and she takes over when the moment's right.

You'll be trying to help her walk along the edge of something intense and sweet. She might already do this when she's alone and masturbating, but it's not easy to achieve when the fingers are not her own. While an orgasm at the end of the rainbow is a worthy goal, sometimes goals can get in the way. You'll be way ahead if you stop trying to orchestrate an earth-shaking orgasm. That kind of attempt doesn't always achieve full bandwidth for a woman.

Clitoris vs. Vagina

Most of this chapter is about stimulating a woman's external genitals and specifically, her clitoris. It's the equivalent of teaching a woman how to stroke a man's penis, although you can show a partner what to do with a penis far more easily than you can with a clitoris.

Also, please watch our video on *The Clitoris:* www.Guide2Getting.com/videos. This 7-minute video has received praise from sex therapists and educators. It shows how different any two clitorises can look, and is loaded with lovemaking techniques.

The final part of this chapter is about stimulating the inside of a woman's vagina. There can be more to it than you might think.

Coaching, Patience & Practice

"I had to learn how to touch her clit... I can remember being clumsy about it early on. She'd have to stop me — I was going too fast, going too hard. I can remember her saying, 'You're in the wrong place.' 'Well, show me where. I mean physically, show me. Rub so I can see it. OK, now I understand.' Over time, I've learned where the places are. I can find them in the dark now. But early on I couldn't.... She would take my hand, or my finger, and she would put it right exactly where it was supposed to be, and she'd move it the way she wanted me to move it, and she would apply pressure to the back of my fingers, the amount of pressure she wanted, until I got the hang of it, and then she would take her hand away. If I got out of sync or something, she'd put her hand back and show me until I got it right. A few weeks later I might need some re-education, so she'd show me again." —From *Sex: An Oral History*, by Harry Maurer, Viking.

You'll want to learn how to do your partner in the same way she does herself, assuming she does herself. Start by making an agreement with her that she will provide you with lots of coaching and patience, and you will provide an eager willingness to learn.

Take heart in knowing that hands that are used to throwing a baseball, torquing down engine bolts, or abusing a game controller can get frustrated when trying to finesse women's genitals. There's knowing when to speed up, slow down, stay your course or change direction, or push softer or harder. It requires patience and practice.

Penis vs. Clitoris — Course Correction

"I've seen a couple of guys masturbate. I can't believe how rough they are with themselves!" *female age 26*

The reason this woman can't believe how "rough" guys are with themselves is because she would never dream of touching her genitals in that way. Think of how you squeeze or wag your penis when you are finished peeing. Approach a clitoris with that kind of careless abandon, and you are likely to be a dead man. Also, you can start stroking a penis when it's not aroused. But until a woman is aroused, touching her clitoris can hurt.

Ways That Women Stimulate Their Clitoris

Rub their entire hand up and down, stimulating the clitoris, inner labia, and outer labia.

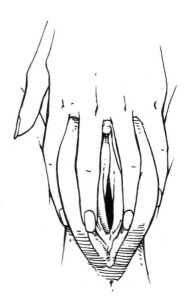

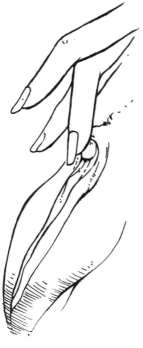

Softly stimulate the glans or tip of the clitoris.

Adapted with thanks from Sadie Allison's
**Tickle Your Fancy — A Woman's Guide
To Sexual Self-Pleasure**

Place three or four fingers
between the outer labia
and massage.

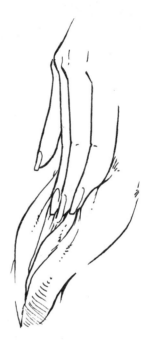

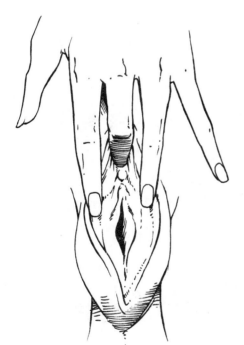

Separate the outer labia with
their index and ring fingers
while stimulating the clitoris
with their middle finger.

More Ways That Women Stimulate Their Clitoris

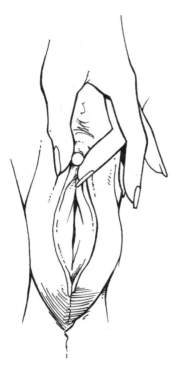

Roll, squeeze, tug, or lift.

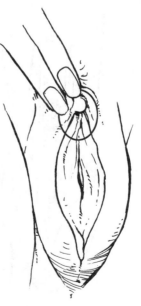

Rub along the side (up and down) or in circles.

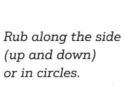

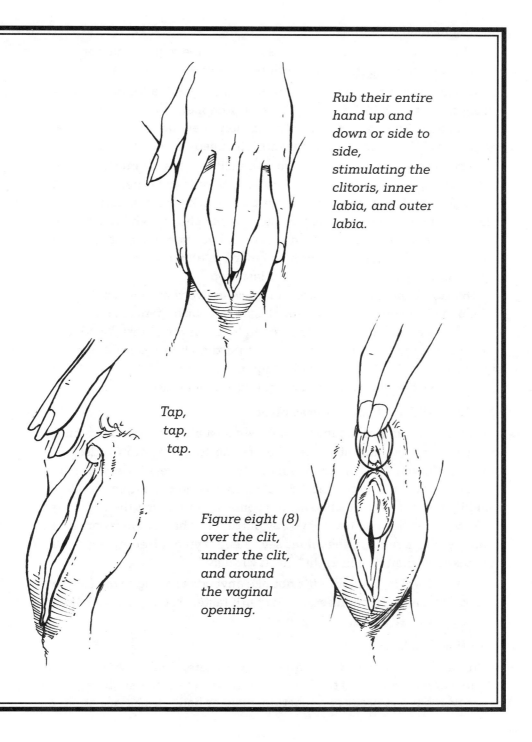

Rub their entire hand up and down or side to side, stimulating the clitoris, inner labia, and outer labia.

Tap, tap, tap.

Figure eight (8) over the clit, under the clit, and around the vaginal opening.

Showing Instead of Telling

"When women moan or gasp, it encourages me to press harder or faster on the clit. Always with poor results." *male age 41*

Never assume that if a little pressure feels good, a lot of pressure will send her through the ceiling. This may happen, but not in the way you intended. Guys also reason that if slow feels good, fast will feel even better. If faster is what she wants, she needs to let you know.

When it comes to touching a woman's clit, always err on the side of tenderness. Softer is usually better unless she tells you otherwise. Push just hard enough to move the skin back and forth over the shaft of the clitoris, assuming you can find the shaft of the clitoris. And don't even get near the naked glans of the clitoris until you've paid your respects to a woman's inner thighs, outer lips, inner lips and mons pubis. The tip or glans of the clitoris should be your last stop.

The tip of the clitoris is often more sensitive than any single part of the penis. You don't want the rough skin of your fingers to rub across it. This is why you should gently push and pull on the clitoral hood and inner lips as a way of indirectly simulating the clitoris until a woman lets you know she wants further engagement. It ultimately depends on how sensitive her clitoris is, and on how sexually aroused she is.

Why "Just Tell Me!" Doesn't Always Work

A woman's understanding of her own sexuality is sometimes on a body level and she may struggle when trying to put it into words. She might say "harder" when she means faster, or vice versa. Getting frustrated and saying "Just tell me!" does absolutely no good. She probably would if she could, but it's like asking someone to tell you the meaning of life. She may be able to show you by putting her hands over yours and guiding your fingers. Or she might say, "Keep trying different ways—I'll let you know when it feels right" or "Try it here."

Mix-ups will happen. But it's not like anybody is going to die or lose their job because you confused harder with faster. You have your hands between a woman's legs. Be happy.

Learn How She Masturbates

"It's not a dish of salted peanuts down there, don't just grab and hope for the best. It's very sensitive. Even the slightest movement can produce a reaction, good or bad." *female age 45*

When a woman masturbates, she will often rest her wrist on her lower abdomen just above the pubic bone. Try to do the same, since it will influence the way your fingers feel on her genitals. Lie next to her and reach your arm over her body until your fingers are between her legs. Or try sitting like the couple in the illustration below.

To learn how some women masturbate, grab a romance novel and have a bowl of popcorn or chips close by. Read a few pages, rub a little clit, read a few pages, eat some chips...

Here are some tips women readers have suggested:

😎 Dry fingers on a dry clitoris do not make for the best of times.

😎 Does your partner puts something inside of her vagina when she masturbates? This can provide a feeling of fullness, which can help amplify the sensations. Other women prefer external stimulation only.

😎 Try to bring lubrication up from the bottom her vaginal opening, where the lips make a "U." This is where a woman's natural lube tends to initially pool. Drag the fluid up with your fingertips, or use saliva or lube. This assumes you have made an effort to help her become aroused.

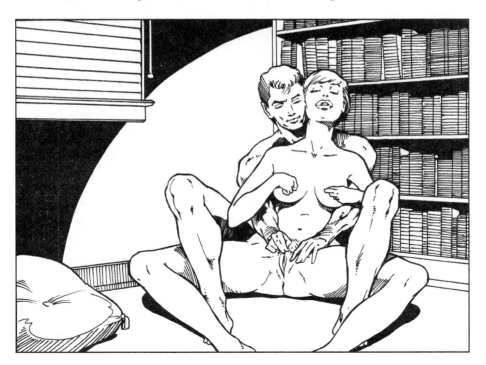

☻ Ask if your partner uses extra lubrication when she masturbates, such as saliva, baby oil, *Vaseline, coconut oil,* or store bought lube. If she uses lube, have her show you how much to use.

☻ Some women direct the stimulation to just one spot. Others might stimulate themselves in a more global way when they are masturbating, tugging and pulling on the entire surface of their genitals.

☻ Find out if your partner has a favorite side of her clitoris or labia that she likes to stimulate. Be sure to follow her lead

☻ Some women move their finger side-to-side across the clitoris, or up and down like when plucking a guitar. They will assume it's all very simple and have no idea why you don't get it.

☻ Since the shaft of the clitoris runs though the mons pubis, some women push and pull on the mons or push into it and make a circular motion with it. This stimulates the neck and shaft of the clitoris.

☻ A partner may want you to pull back the hood of her clitoris to more directly stimulate the glans or tip. This will allow for much higher levels of stimulation. Ask first and be sure she's sufficiently aroused.

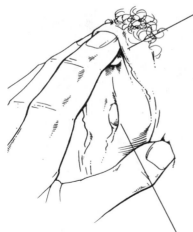

Reaching under the hood for the glans of her clitoris.

1. She needs to feel very aroused first.

2. Be sure there is a thick layer of lube between your finger and her clitoris.

3. Make very light, gentle movements.

4. Give each other lots of feedback, to find what spot feels best and how to move the finger tip over it.

5. Relube or add water to keep surface slick.

The opening of her vagina may become round if her vulva is engorged enough.

**This is a form of stimulation that might work for some women.
For others, it will be too much or too little.**

😎 A woman's pubic bone can be an excellent perch for a tired hand whose fingers are playing with the lips and folds below.

😎 When men try to masturbate women, they will often use all fingers and no wrist. When a woman does herself she will sometime incorporate her wrist into the motion, with only one finger touching her genitals. This can be a subtle but significant detail, and it requires practice. (If you think your tongue wants to fall off during oral sex, wait until you try doing the wrist-clitoris thing for twenty minutes. There are reasons why women use vibrators.)

😎 An excellent way to learn more about pleasing a partner is to rest your fingers over hers while she is masturbating. Then have her place her fingers on top of yours. She shouldn't hesitate to take a man's fingers and put them exactly on those parts of her body where she likes to be touched. Most men will appreciate the assist, and after about the 500th time, most will be able to do it just right.

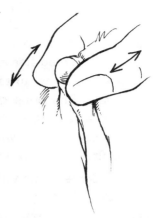

Whether you should roll the shaft of the clitoris depends on how long it is and if she wants you to.

😎 Another advantage of having your arm resting across your partner's body is it allows you to feel how her body is responding. This is important, because as a woman becomes more aroused she may need you to stimulate her in a different way. Being able to read her body's signals will provide your cue.

😎 While lying next to your partner, rest your arm across her body with your fingers on her genitals. Separate her labia with your first and third fingers and stroke between her inner lips with your middle finger, bringing lubrication up from the bottom of her vaginal opening. Also, some women like to have their vulvas tapped with fingers, and some even like to be lightly slapped on the genitals. Ask first!

😎 Try to achieve a steady tempo and rhythm with your fingers. That way, if she says "faster" or "slower," you'll have a point of reference to work from.

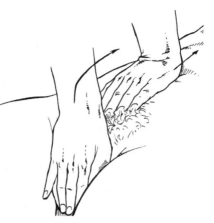

👓 Place a well-lubricated hand between your partner's legs with your fingertips resting below her genitals but not touching her anus. Pull your hand all the way up to her stomach, with your fingertips gently separating her labia with each stroke. Then do the same thing with your other hand, alternating strokes.

👓 Some women like something in or on their anus. It's not going to work if she forgets to tell you about the vibrating butt plug that she can't get off without. But be careful about going from a woman's rectum to her vagina without first washing your hands.

👓 The perineum is the groin's version of a demilitarized zone. It's between the anus and vagina. Push against it with your fingertips and see what she says. (A woman's perineum is much shorter than a man's.)

Fist or Thumb on the Lower Part of Her Vaginal Opening

To help create a sensation of groundedness in your lover's genitals, you might try pushing the thumb or palm of your other hand against the lower part of her vaginal opening or on her perineum. This helps some women to feel a sense of solidity or comfort.

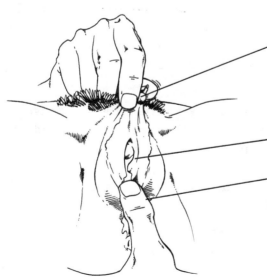

Clitoris stimulation by the hand above while the hand below puts pressure on the lower part of the vaginal opening and the perineum.

The opening of her vagina.

Thumb pressure from below might help amplify the sensations, or you might try using your entire hand against her perineum area at the same time that you are massaging her clitoris.

Genital Massage

Giving a woman the kind of genital massage that is described in the next few pages differs from trying to "get her off by hand." You will be sitting across from her instead of beside her. Rather than trying to imitate the way she masturbates, you will be helping her stay near peak levels of pleasure for several minutes or more before having an orgasm.

You can help your partner reach different levels of sensation as you change the length of your finger's stroke by just a hair, or by changing the speed, or pressure. You may eventually be able to tell from the sensory feedback you are receiving in your finger exactly where to place it and the motions to use. And you will be able to see her genitals open up, puff up, brighten, contract and perhaps even pulse.

Getting Started with Genital Massage

Your partner should be lying on her back. Sit between her legs, facing her, or to one side with one of her open legs across your lap. You'll need good access to her genitals with both hands, along with a good view so you can see the changes that are occurring as she becomes more aroused.

You might start by caressing her inner thighs to help her relax and to build excitement. The more relaxed a woman feels, the more sexually excited her body can become. This is a good time to start talking to each other, because you will need lots of feedback to learn where and how to touch. It won't work without a woman's input.

Clit Clocks—Finding Her Mark

Imagine the old-fashioned type of clock that has a big hand, a little hand, and perhaps even a cuckoo bird at the top. Mentally superimpose the clock over the tip of her clitoris. This will give you a map for how to find any special spots that you will want to focus on in the future.

Also, look at how the inner lips are sitting, their color, and observe the opening of her vagina. The landscape of her genitals will be changing as you find the right spots to massage. Visual cues will be helpful and kind of amazing. People think nothing of a penis swelling when it is aroused, but we seldom think of a woman's genitals as changing. If she's okay with it, you might snap before and after pictures with your phone so she can see the changes.

Next, put a glob of lube on the tip of your index finger. Depending on her anatomy, you might pull the hood of her clit back with the fingers of your other hand or push into the space between the hood and the tip of her clitoris. The clit-massaging aficionados from "The Welcomed Consensus" who are referenced at the end of the chapter still recommend using old-fashioned KY in the tube, and/or Vaseline on the clit itself. They haven't found anything better for direct clit massage.

Gently circle the glans of your partner's clitoris with the lube. Ask her to tell you what it feels like, and if she wants you to push harder or more lightly. Make sure you notice what her clitoris feels like on your fingertip and how it responds when you touch it. Does it make her anus contract? Observe as much as you can.

You might start by using a linear motion, as if you are flicking a tiny light switch on and off. If you find any spots that she says feel good, experiment with the pressure and the length of the "on-off" motion.

Anticipation vs. Dread

If it stops being fun for the two of you or if she starts to feel uncomfortable or overwhelmed, stop! If you go beyond what feels good, her body will tense up the next time you do this, and that's what you don't want to have happen. Anticipation can work for you, or it can work against you.

Massaging the Mons

The mons pubis is the fleshy mound above where the lips begin to open. It has hair on it if a woman doesn't shave. It's easy to ignore the mons and head straight for the clitoris, yet some women masturbate by putting fingertip pressure on the mons and making a circular or back-and-forth motion with it. She enjoy it if you knead the mons or tap on it with your fingertips. Or you can try pushing the palm of your hand against the mons and make a circular motion with it. If you are trying to amplify sensation, you might pull up on the 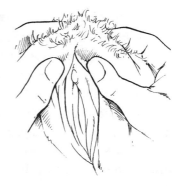 mons with one hand while gently tugging on the inner lips with the fingers of the other.

The Lip Part of Erotic Massage

To massage the outer lips, clasp each lip with a lubricated thumb and forefinger. Then run your fingers from the lower to upper, as though you were tracing one side of a parenthesis.

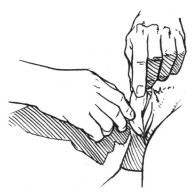

For the inner lips, try gently tugging them. They connected to the bottom of the clitoris. Or hold a lubricated inner lip between your thumb and forefinger. While squeezing just a little, pull your fingers straight away from the woman's body. Your fingers will end up in the air, as though you had pulled them off the edge of a sheet of paper.

Dry Humping Variations

There's no reason why a woman shouldn't lube up a favorite part of her lover's body and rub against it with her vulva. Some women like to do this on a man's back, thigh or hip.

Some women enjoy using the head of a sweetheart's penis for masturbating. This can be invigorating for both partners. There's also a form of dry humping where the woman presses the lips of her vulva over the penis like a bun over a hot dog. She then moves her hips up and down, rubbing her clitoris along the shaft of the penis. The penis never goes inside of her vagina as it would if this were intercourse. This was invented by Eve after she discovered that having intercourse with Adam resulted in unwanted pregnancies.

Even though a penis is not going inside of a vagina, sexually transmitted infections can be passed on this way and pregnancy is a possibility if the guy ejaculates. So he should wear a condom if these are concerns. If getting pregnant or sex germs aren't a problem, some women like to use a man's precum and sometimes his ejaculate as a lubricant to masturbate with. Some add saliva or their body's own lube.

The Extra-Sensitive Clit

Some women have a clitoris that is super-sensitive to touch. This kind of clitoris is not particularly forgiving. Even the most sensitive of lovers would feel challenged by it. Make sure the woman is highly aroused before your fingers go near her clit, and be mindful of how quickly it can go from being sensitive to totally numbing out. Try to become a master of indirect stimulation. It might be better if you caress her over her jeans or underwear than when she's naked. Some women masturbate with their fingers over their underwear rather than inside. Also, see how a glob of thick lube is used in the illustration below.

Fingers inside Her Vagina

Now we get to placing your fingers inside of your partner's vagina. In matters of love and sex, it never hurts for a man's fingers to have a sense of humor. Fingertips that tease and dance will find an especially warm welcome. Gently running your fingertips up and down a woman's inner thigh is a million times more enticing than shoving a finger up her vagina. If and when she's ready to have your fingers inside of her, she will let you know. Even then it's sometimes wise to tease and play some more.

Fingernails: Weapons of Mass Destruction

Before fingering your partner's vagina, cut your fingernails and finish up with a nail file to catch rough edges. Pry out any grease or dark gunk that's under your fingernails. If your hands are rough, put hand lotion on them every day.

You might consider wearing latex gloves. The smooth latex surface sometimes can feel nice for the woman and helps keep your fingers from stinging when they marinate in vaginal fluids, which are fairly acidic. Try putting a dab of water-based lube inside each fingertip of the glove. See if it makes any difference for you or her.

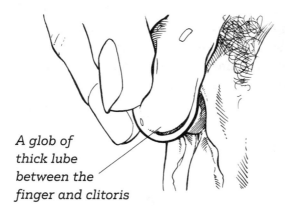

A glob of thick lube between the finger and clitoris

Never fear trying a glob of thick lube on the tip of the clitoris. This can be a good way to approach a clitoris that is hypersensitive. [Inspired by the "Illustrated Guide To Extended Massive Orgasm" by the Bodanskys.]

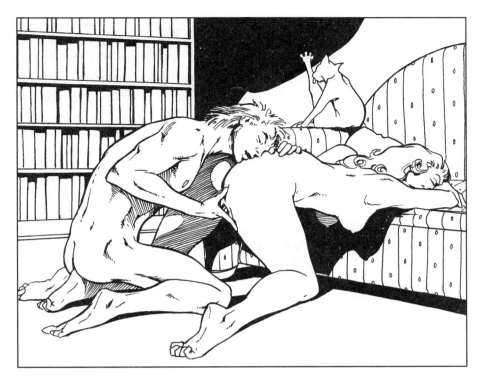

Some women enjoy being touched from behind.

Exploring a Lover's Vagina

Don't assume a woman will want you to thrust your finger in and out like a penis. When it comes to sexual stimulation, fingers and penises are two very different tools and should be used differently. And don't surprise a partner's vagina by suddenly shoving a finger into it. Ease it in slowly and in stages, one joint at a time, and only after your partner has reached a level of arousal where she's spreading her legs and arching her hips.

If you are trying to find the most effective ways of stimulating her vagina, start at the rim or opening of the vagina. Put pressure on each part of the tissue around the opening with your fingertip, moving just a little each time and eventually making a complete circle. Ask your partner to give you feedback about any spots that she might want you to revisit. Then move your finger a bit deeper inside and do the same thing over again. Keep repeating this until you have done her entire vagina.

Be thorough about exploring the first third of a vagina, because that's a part that can be most sensitive to touch. Pay special attention to the roof of her vagina between 9:00 and 3:00. A number of women report pleasurable responses in this area. If your partner has not reached menopause, there will be tiny folds or ridges on the roof her her vagina that make it seem corrugated. These are called the vaginal rug-gae. They help the vagina to expand during intercourse and childbirth.

If your partner wants you to stimulate the roof of her vagina, you might try jiggling your hand or pulling it upward. When pulling your hand upward, your finger will act like a hook. The part from your fin-gertip to your first knuckle will be inside her vagina, with your inner knuckle and hand pulling up against her clitoris on the outside. Or your partner might want you to make a come here motion with your finger-tip against the roof of her vagina, like in the illustration below.

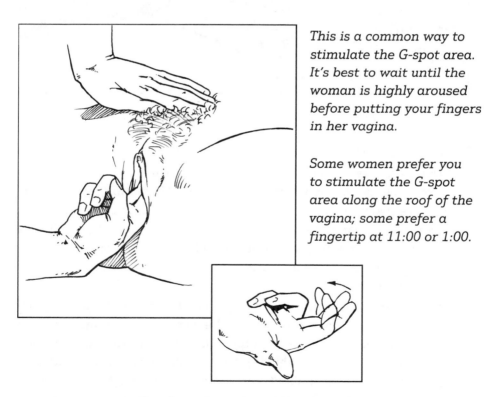

This is a common way to stimulate the G-spot area. It's best to wait until the woman is highly aroused before putting your fingers in her vagina.

Some women prefer you to stimulate the G-spot area along the roof of the vagina; some prefer a fingertip at 11:00 or 1:00.

Some women enjoy G-spot area massage, others find it to be unproductive or uncomfortable.

These structures are inside a woman's pelvis where they can't be seen.

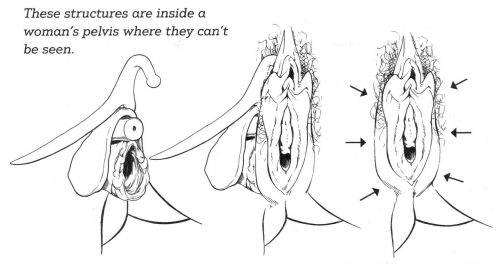

X-ray view of what's inside　　　　　**View from the outside**

Pressing your fingers into the groin where the arrows are can feel very pleasing to some women. You are not only massaging the outer lips or labia, but you could be stimulating parts of your partner's sexual anatomy that are buried far beneath her labia. Push in with your fingertips; let her feedback be your guide.

———————————

If you give each other lots of feedback, you will discover what does and doesn't work. But don't assume that what worked for a former partner will be well-received by your current lover.

If you have been stimulating her clitoris with good results and her genitals are puffed up, you might want to keep caressing her clitoris with one finger while placing a finger from your other hand in her vagina. Stimulating her clitoris and vagina may feel good for some women, but will be too much or distracting for others.

Deeper Inside: The Cervix and Vaginal Tenting

A woman's cervix can usually be found in the upper rear part of her vagina. It's easily felt if she is on all fours or brings her legs to her chest. The cervix feels like a small dome of tissue that you can run your finger around. It may also have a small cleft in the middle, like your chin. Some women enjoy it if you carefully stimulate the area surrounding the cervix. Cervical sensitivity can vary with a woman's menstrual cycle; massaging it may release some blood if she is close to her period.

When a woman is highly aroused, the back part of her vagina that surrounds her cervix can begin to balloon or tent. When the back of a woman's vagina is tenting, you can feel open space with your fingers. When your finger or fingers are in the deepest part of a partner's vagina, she might be able to feel a dull but enjoyable sensitivity. This part of the vagina is more sensitive to pressure than touch.

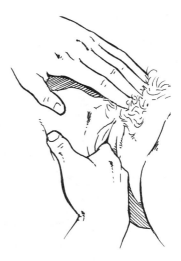

A partner might also enjoy it if you place your free hand over the lower part of her abdomen while you are exploring inside her vagina with the fingers from your other hand. Experiment by applying different kinds of pressure on her abdomen with your top hand.

Using Two Fingers Instead of One or Three

In reviewing lesbian porn movies, author Jay Wiseman noticed that when lesbian performers put their fingers in a partner's vagina, they almost always use two fingers—not one or three. Wiseman asked a number of women about this, and most replied that two fingers simply feel better. This will also depend upon a woman's level of arousal, the size of her partner's hand, and sometimes upon her body's menstrual status.

Winding Down

"The first time I felt a woman's vagina was with my first love. We were taking things very slowly, and when I would ask if I could go down her pants, the answer was no. I respected her wishes and we always did something else, usually making out. One day she finally told me I could proceed below the waistline. It was warm and wet and very soft. The wetness of her vagina was the most exciting feeling I'd ever had." *male age 25*

For some men, putting their fingers between a woman's legs is a moment of magic. There's the woman's warmth, the feel of her wetness, and the way her body sometimes tenses and squirms.

While you are considering new ways to pleasure your partner's genitals, keep in mind there are other parts of a woman's body where touch produces intense sensation. One reader reports his lover has an area

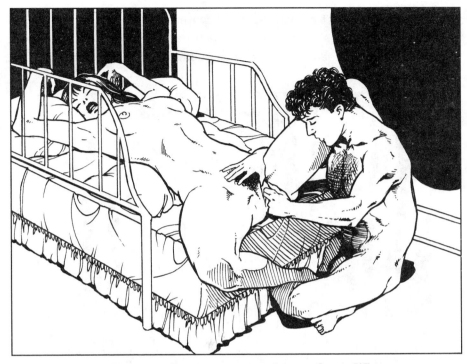

*The Prince is fingering a very happy Snow White
while the Dwarfs are away in the forest.*

on the small of her back that is so erotically charged her knees nearly buckle when he caresses it. He once nearly caused her to orgasm in the middle of a busy hardware store by caressing this part of her back.

The fingers of another reader are so sensitive to touch that getting a manicure feels like a sexual experience. And sometimes, sensation happens purely by accident, like when you have been stroking the more sensitive parts of her body, playfully caressing her thighs or tugging on her inner lips, and suddenly, an orgasm just sneaks up on her.

It never hurts to experiment with new ways to touch your partner, both with your fingers and with your heart.

Hand Held Shower Head: While not exactly finger fucking, you can't beat the hand held shower head for fun. If you don't have one of these, consider getting one. It shouldn't take more than fifteen minutes to install, unless your plumbing is really rusty. Hop in the shower and try out the various settings. When you hold the shower head point-blank against the skin, it causes the water to bubble somewhat like the jet on a hot tub. Don't point a focused jet of water directly into a vagina, as it might force air inside the body, which can be dangerous. Different brands of shower heads create different kinds of spray. Some perfect,

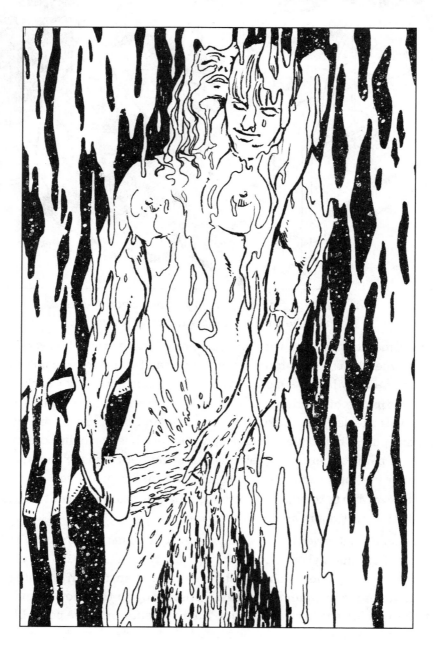

others not. Some men enjoy the feeling of the spray against the side of the scrotum, but with the pressure on low or medium.

Jets in the Hot Tub: If you haven't tried the jets of a hot tub for genital stimulation, what are you waiting for? Also, you might check with your hot-tub repair person about fitting an extension hose on one of the massage jets so you can direct the flow precisely where you want without having to sit in an uncomfortable position. Tell him it is for your grandfather's hydrotherapy.

Waterproof Vibrators: There are waterproof vibrators. These have only one conceivable purpose. Enjoy using them!

Reader's Advice on Playing with Their Genitals

"I would first tell him to approach slowly. Having someone just dive straight towards where they think my clitoris is becomes overwhelming. I like to be teased, I like a slow and sensual working up to where they think my clitoris is. If they are totally in the wrong area (just because it's hard doesn't mean it's my clit!) I have no qualms about giving directions." *female age 22*

"Wait until I'm really turned on and I'm practically shoving your hand down my pants. Then, gently play around and see what I respond to. Once you've found my spot, start out slowly with only a little pressure. Don't focus exclusively on the spot, because that gets annoying, and it makes me less sensitive. As I get more turned on (which you can tell through body language like hip thrusting and my vocalizations), increase the speed but not the pressure." *female age 22*

"Always get your fingers wet before touching where there isn't thick hair. Never, ever touch my clit dry. It hurts! Go ahead and play with my pubic hair. I keep it trimmed, but it means that every time you brush it, it sends a ripple of sensation through me. When I start arching up towards you, slip your finger just inside my outer lips and press gently, with a little circling motion. If I spread my legs more, please touch me! You should probably re-wet your fingers, either at my vagina (if I'm wet enough), or with some lube, or with your own saliva. I love being teased. Run your fingers along the edge of the inner lips, with just a little pressure. When I start moving against your fingers, caress my clit. Just barely touch me, that feels best. That finger has to be very, very wet. In a very short while I'll be calling your name and God's!" *female age 20*

"The key word is GENTLE. At least in the beginning. Caress the pubic hair, then you could slightly penetrate with a finger near the vaginal opening. Gently move your hand forward till you find the clitoris. Never directly stimulate the clitoris, it's way too sensitive. Instead, position your finger(s) on top of the hood and gently manipulate it side to side. Be sure no matter what you are doing that there is plenty of lubrication, either from my natural supply or from a bottle." *female age 35*

"Before you even think about coming near me with your fingers, please make sure that they are smooth. Long nails aren't fun, neither are sandpaper hands. I know that many men are very rough with their own members, but I do not need that. You'd be surprised what the lightest touch can accomplish. There is no need to "grind" your fingers into me. And please, when you find a pace that has me moaning, don't decide to switch to a different pace. That gets annoying." *female age 20*

Reader's Advice on Fingers in Their Vaginas

"I like a finger in there, but please, don't dig for China." *female age 48*

"I like it if he inserts one finger until the opening relaxes, then adds a second finger. When I begin to breathe faster, he should start flexing his fingers." *female age 32*

"When I am sufficiently wet, I enjoy two fingers. I like it when he puts them in gradually and 'fucks' me with them gently. But no fingernails and no rushing!" *female age 35*

"Start with one finger, then go up from there. To find the G-spot, put your thumb over my clitoris, then insert your first finger into my vagina and feel for the rough spot on the upper wall. Rub this spot!!!" *female 26*

"I don't necessarily care for fingers in my vagina. I'd rather have a penis in there." *female age 43*

"I like him to rub the entrance of my vagina in a circular fashion, but I don't like a finger all of the way inside." *female age 30*

"I like to wait until I can't stand it and beg him to put his fingers inside of me." *female age 25*

A College Sex Educator's Advice about the Clitoris

"When talking to guys about sensitivity in the clitoris, I compare it to the head of the penis right after ejaculation. The head can become so

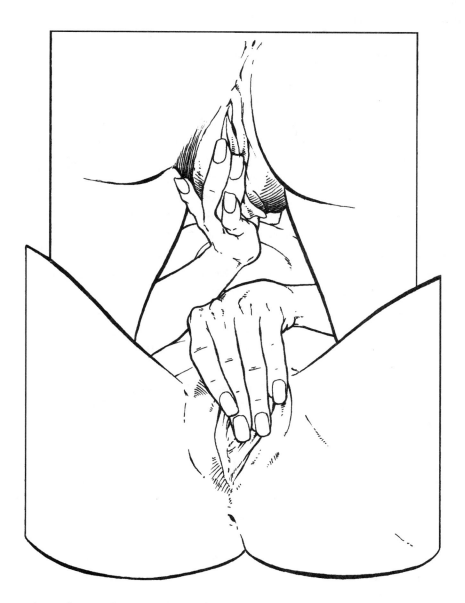

A reader said it wasn't until she'd had sex with women that she began to appreciate how different any two women's bodies can be, and what a steep learning curve this must be for men.

super sensitive that you don't want any direct contact. You can keep stroking the shaft but stay away from the head. That's how it can be for a woman's clitoris when you first touch it."

Resources for Finger Fucking Skills Enhancement:

Be sure to see our video on *The Clitoris* at Guide2Getting.com/videos

Learn everything you can from: www.OMGYes.com, PleasureMechanics.com, EroticMassage.com and www.Welcomed.com. Women will be so impressed that you won't have had time to play video games or watch porn. Here's why: 😎 www.OMGYes.com is a website that's done research on specific ways that women like to receive sexual pleasure. They have created great looking videos that show you how different women get off. An annual membership costs less than a month on most porn sites, with far greater dividends. 😎 Check out the Pleasure Mechanics very helpful video: *Guide To Fingering: How to Touch a Woman for Fabulous Foreplay & Powerful Orgasms*. At The Pleasure Mechanics: PleasureMechanics.com. 😎 There's an array of erotic massage videos at the New School of Erotic Touch: www.EroticMassage.com. This site is dedicated to different ways of stimulating and massaging people's genitals and rear ends. 😎 www.Welcomed.com a finger-fucking resource that I found both fascinating and strange. A female reviewer I asked to look it over hated it. This has been created by a pod of mostly humorless persons, consisting of five or six women and one man. Even their name is a bit unusual: "The Welcomed Consensus." They have devoted years to learning how to stimulate the clitoris, seemingly with the one man's finger, which is getting very old by now. (Nothing like ET's finger, but still...) In the first of their *Deliberate Orgasm Collection*, the members appear to be wearing uniforms from the original Star Trek series. The fourth video has the stiffest, slowest, and perhaps most awkward introduction of any how-to video in history. And if a bikini shaver ever got close to these women's abundant mountains of au natural crotch hair, its bearings would seize in horror. When one of the women said, "Can you move your finger up just a hair?" the possibilities boggled the mind. What I found fascinating at the Welcomed.com was purely anatomical—how these women's genitals changed with arousal, and how they pulsed for twenty minutes at a time. This was highly instructive.

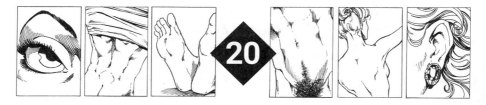

Handjobs — Different Strokes For Different Blokes

Women often ask, "Why should I give him a handjob? I can't possibly compete with the hand that knows him SO well. Besides, he can give himself a handjob any time he wants."

After reading hundreds of men's sex survey responses about masturbating vs. receiving a handjob from a lover, the vast majority of men—more than 90%, would rather receive a handjob from a lover.

Think about it: Who is he fantasizing about when he's jerking off? It's you! And that's just giving him a garden-variety handjob. There are extreme handjobs that can turn his entire body into a giant sex receptor.

What You Bring To It

It might help to explain two of the main reasons why guys masturbate. There can be lots of other reasons, these are just two.

One reason is for fun time when he's alone. It's like playing a video game, with the controller being in his pants and the display in his mind, or on his phone when he's watching porn. Some women get upset when they discover their partner does this; they view it as rejection. That's unfortunate, because people usually masturbate throughout life, whether they are in a relationship or not.

Another reason why a guy might masturbate has to do with longing for the presence and touch of a partner. He imagines a woman he loves is there and it helps him feel less alone. This is the kind of jerking off that helps a lot of guys keep their sanity until they find a partner. It's a form of sexual life support. It can also provide a sense of intimacy when he does have a partner but intercourse isn't on the agenda for the day.

Depending on the mood and the situation, your handjob might be casual and fun, like the way he does himself when it's a form of sport, or it might be to supply comfort and intimacy. Either way, it's all good.

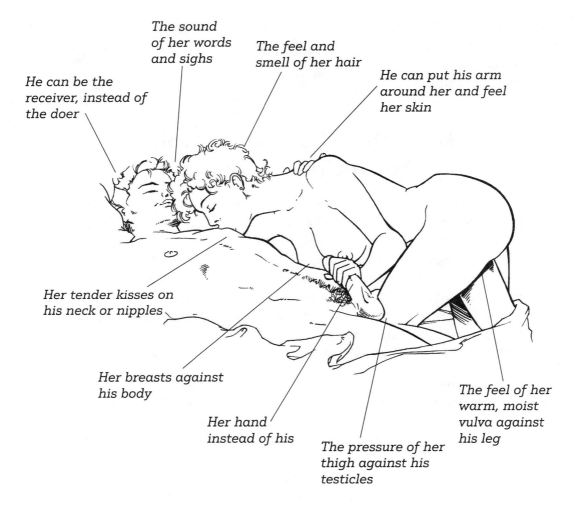

The sound of her words and sighs

The feel and smell of her hair

He can put his arm around her and feel her skin

He can be the receiver, instead of the doer

Her tender kisses on his neck or nipples

Her breasts against his body

Her hand instead of his

The pressure of her thigh against his testicles

The feel of her warm, moist vulva against his leg

Things a woman brings to a handjob.

Although your hand may be doing the same thing that his hand has done thousands of times before, it's your presence that makes your handjob superior. So try putting more into it than just moving the muscles in your arm. Make it a fun and intimate act. Take control. Cuddle close to him. Give him tender kisses on the neck or nipples. Your handjobs can be more emotionally comforting than you might know. They are an opportunity for intimacy and closeness that a lot of women underestimate. And you don't have to worry about STIs, getting pregnant or needing to swallow. What's not to like?

Hand Placement

With handjobs, hand position is everything. The way to learn the position that works best for your partner is to lie parallel to him and reach across his body. This will provide you with the same approach to his penis that he uses himself. Ask him to form your fingers around his penis in the same way he does when he's alone and thinking about you.

He probably positions his fingers to stimulate the most sensitive area of the penis called the frenulum. It's just below the head on the side of the penis that's away from the man's body when he has an erection.

Do not wrap your hand around the base of the penis. You might as well be stroking his ankle. Wrap your hand around the penis so your thumb goes over the top part, and your fingers wrap around the front that faces away from his body when he has an erection. Your fingers should be in the same position as if they were holding a cup of tea. That's how we guys learn to masturbate, by drinking tea.

Guys usually position their hand so the crook of their fingers rubs over the frenulum, as opposed to their fingertips. So rub your fingers over this pleasure spot with each stroke, especially if you plan on getting the handjob done before next year.

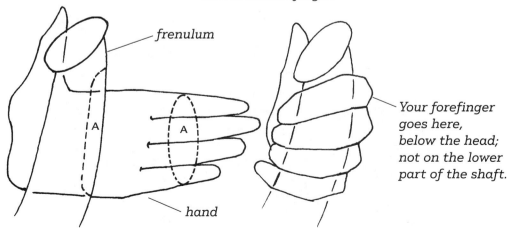

Some men grab with their entire fist, others only use their thumb and forefinger and/or middle finger.

frenulum

A

A

Your forefinger goes here, below the head; not on the lower part of the shaft.

hand

This is a rough approximation of where your hand should go. Each man will need to show you how he does it.

Getting a Grip—Learning Man Basics

"I could never move my fist that fast for so long. He really man-handles that sucker, and it doesn't seem to hurt!" *female age 55*

A frequent complaint from men about the way women give handjobs is that they use too light of a touch. There is a reason why a common slang term for masturbation is "beat your meat" and not "tickle your meat." Nor do terms like "jerking off," "slap the monkey," "bash the bishop," and "whacking off" imply gentleness.

On the other hand, the *grip of death* is not always welcome, either. So one of the first things you'll want ask a partner is how firmly to grip his penis. Does he want your hand tighter? Looser? Ask again after you've given him a couple of handjobs.

The Stroke

After your partner shows you where to place your hand on the shaft of his penis, have him show you how far up and down to stroke. This may depend on how much foreskin he has. When there is more yardage to work with, the stroking length will often be greater. That's why each guy needs to show you what works best for his particular penis.

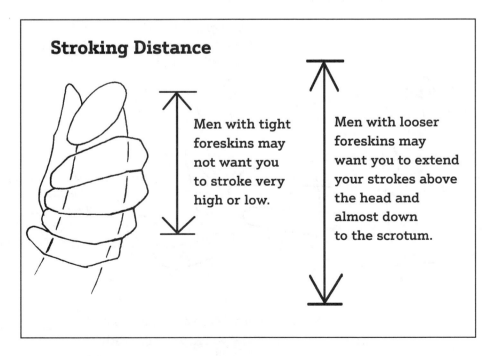

Stroking Distance

Men with tight foreskins may not want you to stroke very high or low.

Men with looser foreskins may want you to extend your strokes above the head and almost down to the scrotum.

Practice, Patience and Taking Control

Don't be surprised if he'll need to show you a couple of times before you get it just right, especially if your hand is considerably smaller than the hand he is used to (hopefully his own). If your own lover is too uptight to teach you, some of his friends might be willing to let you learn the basics on them, or maybe one of your BFFs can demonstrate on her boyfriend.

Dry or Lubed?

When a man is circumcised, it can sometimes feel better to masturbate with lube. Masturbation or a handjob with lube can help a man whose penis has been circumcised to get more sensation from the head of his penis. However, doing it dry is far less of a production to clean up and almost essential if you're giving him a quickie.

An advantage of doing a guy who is not circumcised is that an intact foreskin usually provides optimal sensations without needing to add lube.

What Does a Penis Feel Like?

When a penis is soft it can feel like human lips—more like a squid than a hotdog. Some people describe it as being squishy. The skin has a silky smooth, almost translucent texture that slides over the tissue beneath it. A soft penis is extremely flexible. It can be warm or cold to the touch.

To know what a hard penis feels like, find a fairly buff guy who lifts weights and ask him to flex his arms. A hard penis feels similar to a hard bicep, although a hard penis won't be nearly as big around. Poking a finger into a man's unflexed pecs will give you an approximate idea of what a semi-erect penis feels like. Here are some women's recollections about the first time they touched a penis:

> "It was sort of like 'Oh my God, what do you do with it?' I knew if
> you did something to it in the right way, that was good. I felt it
> very, very carefully, not sure what I was dealing with. It was like
> an alien creature that you were supposed to automatically know
> how to please. As I listen to myself describing it, I must have
> considered it as separate from the individual who it belonged to!
> *female age 34*

"It wasn't a pleasant experience then, but it sure is now." *fem. 42*

"I had intercourse a number of times but never touched it. I didn't get into that until much later." *female age 26*

"I didn't like the way it felt when flaccid. A couple of years later I finally got around to making friends with it, and it became exciting." *female age 21*

"It took me a while to figure out that you could really handle it, that it wasn't fragile." *female age 27*

Your Touch vs. His

Men sometimes view their body and their penis as two unrelated entities. They stroke their penis without caressing other body parts that could help make it more of a full-body experience. This is one of the ways that a partner's handjob can be so special. She will be adding her own special magic, perhaps by straddling him and pushing her crotch into him, or by caressing him with her other hand, or by kissing him with her soft lips, or by whispering into his ear.

Few women realize they have the potential to control nearly every cell in a man's body with each stroke. Instead, they just jerk away.

Technical Points

Some women give handjobs that are jerky. After all, it is called "jerking off," but that term is a misnomer. It may appear that when guys masturbate they use a single upstroke followed by a single downstroke, in rapid succession. But that's not how men do it. We have a more fluid motion. The hand doesn't stop or even slow down as it changes direction from up to down. The motion is smooth rather than jerky. You also might want to caress his testicles with one hand as you are jerking him off with the other.

You don't want to slow down or stop pumping as a man begins to ejaculate. Most guys will appreciate it if you keep stroking ("stroking through") although you need to ask him about making direct contact with the head of his penis after he has an orgasm. Some men might want you to milk out each drop of semen. Guys do this by pushing their fingers into the part of their penis that's between their balls. This is part of the urethra where semen collects before ejaculation. Have your partner show you how to do this if it's something he does.

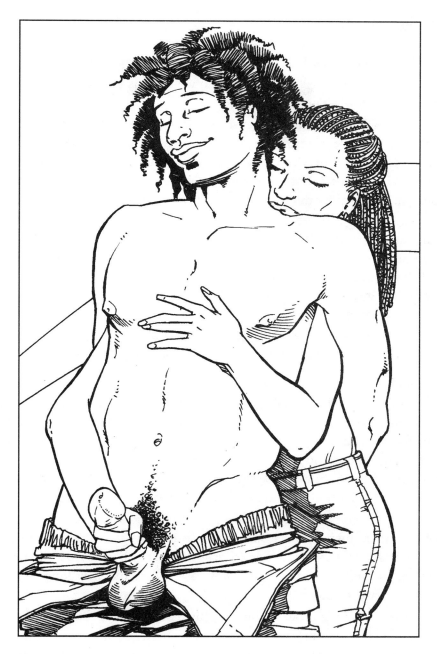

Her fingertips are wrapped around his penis rather than digging into the front. She's also kissing his neck and caressing his chest. All signs of excellent form.

Adding Some Bling

Panty Play: If he likes lingerie, take your panties off and drape them over his penis and testicles while you are giving him a handjob.

Position: Consider doing your man when he is standing or kneeling as opposed to lying on his back.

Ball Trick: Some guys will push the little finger of the stroking hand against the lower part of the penis near the scrotum. This causes the scrotum to jiggle or vibrate with each stroke, providing a secondary source of sensation. But seek a man's input if you try to do this, since your pinky might inadvertently poke him in the balls.

Alternating Caresses and Stokes: In his wonderful *Tricks to Please a Man* (Greenery Press) author Jay Wiseman suggests caressing a penis and balls for ten seconds with your fingertips, followed by one quick up-and-down hand stroke. Then caress for ten more seconds, followed by two quick up-and-down hand strokes. After every ten-second period of caressing, increase the stroke total by one.

Thigh Sensation: Have your male partner straddle your thigh so it is pushing up against his testicles as you are stroking his penis.

How a Man Can Help Himself

A man can help himself and his partner if he will turn on the lights, get naked, and let her learn about his genitals. He should have her tickle, squeeze, tug, and prod each part of his sexual anatomy so she can learn his comfort zones and become more confident in handling his penis and testicles. She should increase the pressure on each part until he says to stop, then back off a bit. Here are some specifics:

Penis: A woman should tug on it, yank it, and squeeze it until she's able to distinguish a man's *Ouch!* zone from his *Ahh!* zone. As for hand-jobs, he should show her how to grab his pens, how hard to squeeze, how far up and down to stroke, how fast to go, and how long to keep stroking after he comes.

Testicles: If the room is cold and his testicles have retracted almost to his armpits, turn up the heat and put something warm over his scrotum. Once his testicles have been coaxed back down, a woman should tickle, caress, and play with them, with the man letting her know what feels good and what doesn't. She should slowly squeeze each testicle, with him signaling the limits of his comfort zone.

Penis beneath Testicles: A woman should put a finger or two in the space between her partner's testicles and push in until she is massaging the part of the penis that's buried beneath them. She should explore a little further back, behind his scrotum. Find out what feels good.

Clean Up

Tissue and socks are the #1 and #2 things guys use for cleanup after jerking off, unless they are doing it in the shower. If you don't have any tissue handy for cleanup, tell him to ante up a sock if he's wearing them. And if you are goddess among women and are wearing dark colored bikini underwear instead of a thong, you can always use those and stuff the sticky soldier into your purse afterward, but be sure to let him know that he owes you big time.

Using light colored fabrics or bedsheets for clean up is a bad idea, because if there's lots of protein or sperm in his semen, it can stain.

Extreme Hand-job Techniques For an Extremely Good Time

The next couple of pages cover techniques for doing a handjob where the goal is to enhance sensation with each stroke without letting him ejaculate. (Let him come at the end.) Lubricating your hands and his genitals is essential. Any number of skin-friendly oils will work fine.

Lubing Him Up

The first thing to do is to get your partner completely naked. This is usually not a difficult task. The most civilized way of adding lube is to cup one hand over his genitals and drip massage oil over your hand. Gravity will pull the oil through your fingers and onto his genitals. Make sure his testicles and penis are thoroughly basted with oil. Put a thick towel under him beforehand to keep the oil from staining the sheets.

Different Strokes

When giving a man a routine handjob, it's best to be by his side so you can imitate the way he strokes himself. But when you are giving him an extreme handjob, you can sit in front of him or lean over him when he's on his back.

It is not necessary for him to have an erection. Some people think it feels best when the penis isn't fully erect, so reassure your partner that you don't expect him to stay hard. Semi-erect might feel best.

Fists Going Up: Be sure all skin surfaces are well lubed. Wrap one hand around the base of his penis, squeeze lightly and pull it up along the shaft and into the air. As this hand is making its upward stroke, grab the base of the penis with your free hand, squeeze and do the same thing. Create a fluid motion with one hand constantly following the other. Slow the pace if he shows signs of impending orgasm. Try giving a slight squeeze or snap on the upward stroke as your hand reaches the head of the penis.

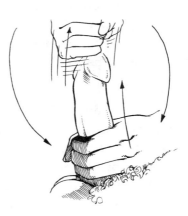

Fists Going Down: Same technique as above, only in the reverse direction with your hands going from the tip of his penis to the base. This usually requires an erection. Otherwise, his penis will just flop there in your hand. Also, don't grip as tightly as with fists going up.

All Thumbs: Face your partner and clasp your fingers together as if you were deeply in prayer, but with your hands clasped around his penis. Use the pads of your thumbs to massage the front part of the penis that has the raphe or seam going up it. Spend extra time rubbing the area where the head attaches to the shaft. Just below this juncture is the sensitive frenulum. Some people compare the sensitivity of the frenulum to that of the clitoris, although they are overstating the case.

Open Palm Buffing the Head of His Penis: Hold the shaft of the penis in one hand. Open your other hand flat and rub it in a circular pattern over the head of the penis as though you were buffing it. Make sure the palm of your hand is well-lubed.

Twisting the Cap Off a Bottle of Beer: Make sure his penis is well lubricated. Hold the shaft near the base. With your other hand, grasp the head of the penis as though it were the cap on a bottle of beer. Twist it as if you were opening the bottle, with your thumb and forefinger running along the groove under the ridge where the head attaches to the shaft. A

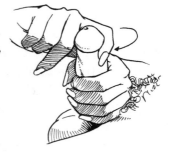

variation is to position your hands like you are wringing a towel dry.

Strokes for When The Foreskin Is Pulled Taut

The penis can usually be made more sensitive by pulling the foreskin down against the scrotum. Guys who masturbate with lubrication often use one hand to pull the foreskin taut while stroking the shaft with the other. This also helps keep the skin on the scrotum from rising up onto the shaft of the penis.

To make the foreskin taut, clamp your thumb and forefinger around the shaft of the penis about an inch above where it joins the scrotum. Pull the skin down so your remaining fingers and palm wrap around the testicles. If the man is not circumcised, reach higher up on the shaft to pull the extra skin down. If he is circumcised, you won't have as much foreskin to pull taut. Make sure the penis is well lubricated

From His Penis To His Chest: His penis should be lubricated and resting flat against his belly. Pull the skin taut with one hand, and lay your other hand flat on top of his penis. Then drag your open hand toward his chest, pulling your hand over the surface of his penis and onto the skin of his abdomen. Keep repeating the motion.

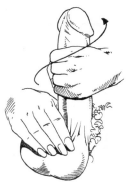

The Corkscrew: Pull the skin taut at the base of his penis. Wrap your other well-lubricated hand around the shaft, squeeze lightly and twist it upward as though you were following a corkscrew. If his penis is hard enough, you can do a reverse downstroke. This should return your hand to the same position where it started, or you can just do a series of upward strokes. *Don't hesitate to do this to the shaft of his penis when you are giving a blowjob.*

Thumbs Up Then Down: There are two ways to grasp a lubricated penis from the base pulling upward. One is with your thumb up, then rotate your fist so your little finger is up. Alternate your hand orientation after each stroke. You'll need to put some arm motion into it.

Octopus or Parachute Fingers: Pull the foreskin taut with one hand. Lay the palm of your other hand over the head of the penis and drop your fingers down along the sides of the shaft. (Your hand will look like an open parachute or an octopus.) Stimulate the shaft of the penis with your fingers as you lift your hand up and down. You can also twist your hand sideways, or do a corkscrew stroke that combines both motions.

Massaging Under the Testicles

Heat the room or put a warm washcloth over your partner's crotch until the testicles hang freely. Press into the middle of the scrotum with the pads of your fingers. You will be touching the part of the penis that is covered by the testicles. *(See the illustration below.)*

There is a single small area or juncture in this part of the penis where ligaments, muscle fibers, and nerve endings seem to converge. Putting fingertip pressure on this spot while massaging the rest of his penis with your other hand can create a subtle, warm feeling that some men enjoy. This area might be on one side of the shaft rather than in the middle. The only way to find it is with exploration and feedback. You can also massage this area when giving a blowjob.

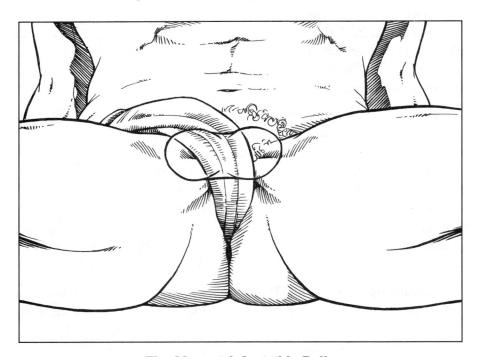

The Man with Invisible Balls

Women often assume the penis is somehow glued or stapled to the front of a man's pelvic bone. In reality, it runs beneath his testicles and anchors inside his pelvis. Some men enjoy having this part of the penis massaged. Push into the space between the testicles with your fingertips and gently rub. Also massage the space behind it (aka "taint").

Testicle Massage Techniques

Here are a few techniques to try on testicles. None of this should cause any pain or discomfort. If it does, stop. There is more information about testicles and testicle massage in Chapter 9: *Balls, Balls, Balls.*

Simple Testicle Massage: Explore with your fingertips the space between and around the testicles. Be gentle at first, and seek plenty of feedback. For some men, the right kind of testicle massage almost feels like a back rub with hints of orgasm.

Scrotum: With your thumb and forefinger, make a ring around the part of your partner's scrotum where it attaches to his groin. Squeeze gently until his testicles pop out a bit, but not enough to cause pain. This will cause the skin on the scrotum to be tight. At the same time, run the fingertips of your other hand up and down the sides of the scrotum with a light tickling touch.

Penis Up, Balls Down: Grab the lower part of his penis with one hand, and clamp the fingers of your other hand around the scrotum. This should cause the testicles to pop out a bit, and the skin will become taut. Squeeze both hands lightly. Then do an upward stroke with the penis hand while your hand on the testicles pulls gently in the opposite direction. Find a tempo that works and keep repeating.

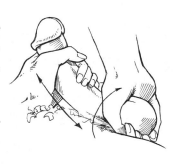

Digging Like a Dog Does: Straddle a partner's chest while facing his feet. Lay his penis flat against his belly with the head pointing toward you. Place a well-lubricated hand between his legs with your fingertips resting below his testicles. Pull the hand all the way up to his belly, dragging your fingers over his testicles and penis. Repeat with your other hand, alternating strokes as a dog might when digging up dirt.

Walking Him Along The Edge

This is where you use any of the handjob techniques for long periods of time without letting him ejaculate. Let's say his starts to ejaculate when he reaches a 9 on a 10 point scale. At that point, there's no turning back. So try to keep him between a level 7 and 8 for as long as possible. When he ejaculates, it can be intense.

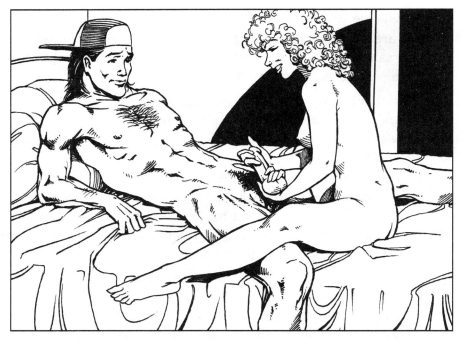

This position can be great for hand jobs with lube, but not so good for doing it dry. Worse yet, her form is poor (fingertips digging into the frenulum) and it looks like she's pulling his penis off of his body. But he doesn't care, what with his washboard abs and cool cap.

One way to keep a guy at such a high level of excitement is to learn his body language for when he is about to ejaculate: the veins in his penis may start to bulge, or his penis might give a sudden throb, the color of the head might darken, his testicles may suck up into his groin, his muscles may suddenly tighten, his hips may thrust, and he might start to groan or invoke the names of the deities and saints. As he gets close to coming, back off with the stroking. If a man can report his levels of excitement, his partner can learn when to up the pace and when to back off. Soon enough, she'll become so familiar with his body language that he won't need to tell her.

Shoulders First

The shoulders and back often become the body's collecting points for tension. There is no point in doing good work on a man's genitals when the weight of the world is parked between his shoulder blades. This is also true for women's bodies. So you might start with a backrub.

Some men believe that the only important part of sex is when a penis is being rubbed, sucked or fucked. They might not care about the tension in their shoulders. They will sometimes direct your hands straight to their crotch with the idea that an orgasm will help relax them. Think of how much more pleasure they could receive if they were relaxed to begin with.

Making It a Whole Body Experience

Handjobs can be used to help a man link the sensations in his crotch with other parts of his body. So you might stimulate your partner's genitals with one hand while caressing other parts of his body. It may help if he inhales deeply while you are doing this, as though he is sucking the warm glow from his genitals into the upper part of his body.

Or you might try kissing or caressing his neck, shoulders, or chest while massaging his genitals. At different intervals, stop stroking his genitals but continue to kiss or caress the other parts of his body. The goal is to help him experience sensation over his entire body.

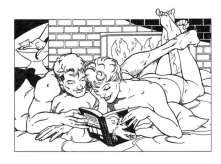

Dear Paul,

What if a guy is uncircumcised? Do you give him the same kind of handjob as a guy who is cut?

Helen from Troy

Dear Helen,

You'll find the answer and more in our video *A Woman's Guide To Men's Foreskins* at www.Guide2Getting.com/videos. It includes several lovmaking tips for partners of men who are intact.

If you want to take your handjob skills far beyond anything any guy could ever imagine, you can't go wrong with a video by The Pleasure Mechanics titled *Guide to Handjobs, How to Touch the Penis for Prolonged Arousal and Powerful Orgasms* (www.PleasureMechanics.com). And there are several erotic massage videos at the New School of Erotic Touch: www.EroticMassage.com.

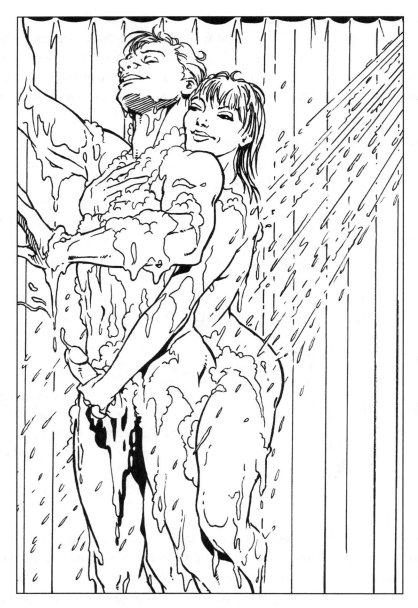

The shower is a fine place for giving a man a handjob.
(Shower drains know all about semen. They encounter it often!)
If you need lube, use hair conditioner instead of soap.
Soap burns if it gets into the urethra.

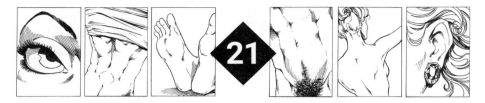

Doing Yourself In Your Partner's Presence

There is often something erotic and even forbidden about seeing your partner masturbate. This is just as true for women watching men as for men watching women. That's what this chapter is about.

Many of us have the fantasy that once we get into a relationship, we won't be playing with ourselves anymore. In some cases, that's how it is for the first couple of months or years. You're having enough sex with your partner that you can't remember why you used to masturbate so often. In other relationships, which can be just as satisfying, you don't really stop masturbating. And some women report that they masturbate more often when they are in a sexually satisfying relationship.

Playing with yourself in front of a partner can sometimes take a lot of trust. That's because masturbation tends to be more self-disclosing than other types of sex. Maybe that's why most people on our sex survey say they would rather be walked in on while they are having sex with a partner than when they are masturbating. Having sex with a partner leaves you feeling less vulnerable, even though more people probably masturbated during the past twenty-four hours than had partner sex.

Here are eight reasons why being more open about masturbation can help expand sexual enjoyment in a relationship:

👀 If your partner can see how you please yourself, it might help him or her understand more about pleasing you.

👀 Orgasms from masturbation can be more intense than other kinds of orgasm. It might increase the level of intimacy in your relationship if you can ask your partner to hold you while you get yourself off.

👀 Although the sex you have with your partner can be really satisfying, masturbating is the only way some people can have an orgasm.

👀 There are times when people feel like doing it solo. If this is an accepted part of your relationship, you won't have to hide or feel weird when you want to control your own orgasmic destiny.

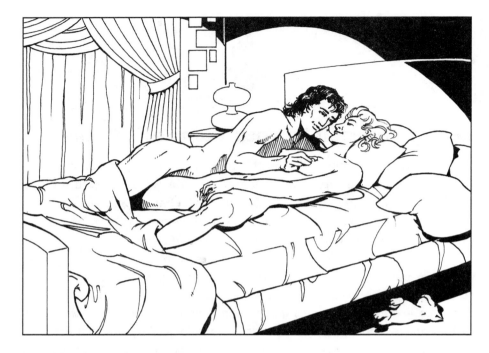

☻ People often have unreal expectations that a partner can satisfy all of their sexual urges. There will be many times when one of you
is in the mood and the other isn't, or when your partner is so pleasantly
drained by what you have just done (oral sex, genital massage, etc.)
that he or she curls up and falls asleep on the spot. It would be nice if
the awake partner doesn't have to be sneaky about masturbating.

☻ When you masturbate in each other's presence, don't forget that
a partner's pleasure might be greatly enhanced with a special assist
on your part. A man might enjoy it if his partner caresses his testicles,
chest or neck while he masturbates, and a woman might find it delightful if her partner caresses her neck, shoulders or breasts or whispers
sweet or nasty things into her ears while she masturbates.

☻ Masturbating together is an excellent way to share intense sexual feelings without the risk of unwanted pregnancy or STIs.

☻ Summers in the East, South, and Midwest are sometimes so
miserably hot and muggy that the last thing you'll want to do is hug an
equally hot and sweaty partner. Masturbating together is one way you
can share sexual pleasure without full-body contact.

Readers' Comments

"I wish he would do it in front of me more often. I've even named his penis Squeegy Loueegy." *female age 37*

"It took a while for us to get comfortable with it, but I like to watch my husband stroke his penis. He enjoys watching me, too. I often masturbate as part of our loveplay because I like stimulation in more places at once than two hands are capable of doing." *female 47*

"During intercourse one of us always has to touch me so I can have an orgasm, so in that respect, he's seen me do it. And we both chat about how we masturbate when we are alone sometimes." *female 30*

"Masturbation is the act in my life that keeps me sane. My wife even helps me sometimes." *male age 38*

"I masturbate in front of my husband, mostly with a vibrator. I still find it a bit embarrassing." *female age 35*

"I masturbate at least once a day. My lover loves it when I masturbate with him or beside him. He thinks it's one of life's great mysteries. I like to watch him masturbate, though sometimes it makes me jealous. I'd like him to take the time and attention he spends on himself and use it on me." *female age 24*

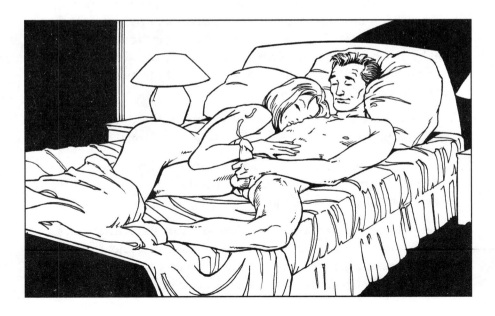

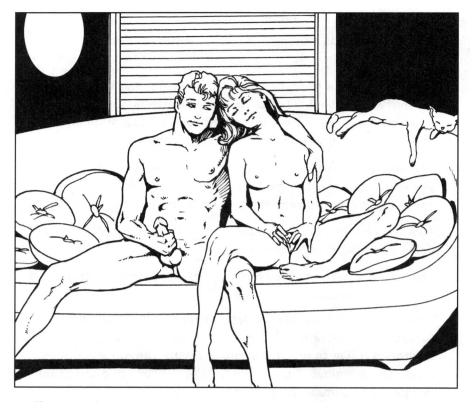

"I masturbate regularly because in the fourteen years that I have been sexually active I have never received an orgasm from intercourse. The only way I can come is from a vibrator or by my husband performing oral sex on me. Sometimes I masturbate privately, other times in front of my husband right after intercourse." *female age 35*

"I masturbate several times a week, and if she doesn't know after twenty-five years, well, I'd be surprised." *male age 48*

"I never realized it was possible for a guy to be turned on by seeing a woman touching herself. Needless to say, once I figured this out about him, I put on a good show." *female age 45*

"Sometimes, you just want to come and not have intercourse with your partner. It makes sense because you know how to make yourself get off better and faster than anybody else. You might also get to know yourself and discover new techniques."
female age 26

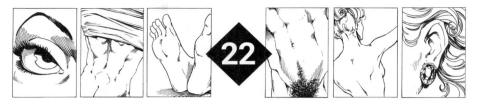

Oral Sex: Vulvas & Honeypots

There's a funny thing about oral sex, at least when you are on the giving end—the woman you are giving oral sex to sometimes disappears. All that's left is a twitching, moaning protoplasm which only partially resembles the person who was there before. You are pretty much alone. After it's over, you might want to ask, "Hey, where did you go?" but you learn not to because she will usually just give you a big smile and want to curl up in your arms or maybe she'll want to have intercourse.

You would think a chapter on giving a woman oral sex would be straightforward: place tongue on detonator (clitoris) and start licking or sucking. Then wait for the fireworks to occur. Instead, this is one of the more difficult subjects to write about. If you doubt this, consider some of the answers we've received on our sex survey from women about oral sex:

"I hate it when a guy sucks on my clit."

"I can't get off unless he sucks on my clit."

"I'm more sensitive on the right side of my clit."

"I'm right handed, but he should focus on the left side of my clit."

"My clit is omni-dimensional, left side, right side, it doesn't matter."

"I want him to lick from bottom to top with a flat tongue."

"I need him to flick the tip of his tongue from side to side, hard and fast."

"I love it when he fucks me with his tongue."

"I hate it when he fucks me with his tongue, that's what his penis is for."

"I like his mouth on my whole vulva, like he's nursing on it."

"I want him to focus on my clit, anything else is a waste."

"Women are so much better at this than men."

"I'm bisexual, and the best oral sex I've gotten is from men."

"I love it when he pushes a wet finger into my asshole just before I come."

"He better not touch my ass when he's giving me oral or it's over."

Anyone who can predict the exact type of oral sex a woman will want deserves *The Congressional Medal of Muff Diving*. One lover might have a clit that's so sensitive anything beyond butterfly kisses will push her from ecstasy to agony. She'll want you to keep your head stationary with a wet mouth and light suction might be best. Another lover may have a sleepy clit that needs the oral equivalent of an earthquake.

Given the many variations, this chapter provides you with an array of possibilities. Please give your partner a pen or highlighter. Ask her to highlight the parts that are relevant to her puss and your mouth and to make notes for you in the margins. If she isn't sure what works best, then the two of you can have great adventures learning together.

Inviting your partner's feedback will send a clear signal that you want to learn. She might not have gotten that from her former partners.

Our Survey Results: Does a Woman Want Your Penis or Your Mouth?

We have asked hundreds of women if they had to choose between receiving oral sex or intercourse, which would it be. No one anticipated that a large majority would say intercourse, even if they have orgasms more reliably when receiving oral sex. The deciding factor was usually intimacy over orgasms. For some women the best of both worlds is having intercourse after they've had an orgasm from oral sex. Some women enjoy it when a partner will mix it up with oral sex, then intercourse, then oral sex, and he finishes off with his penis inside of her.

Of the women who were not comfortable receiving oral sex, about half were concerned with the way they might taste, smell, or how their labia look. Some worried they take too long and it's asking too much of a partner to keeping doing it for what they perceived was an eternity. Other women couldn't believe a partner would enjoy having his face between their legs. And some women simply don't like how oral sex feels or can never come that way. Here's some of their concerns:

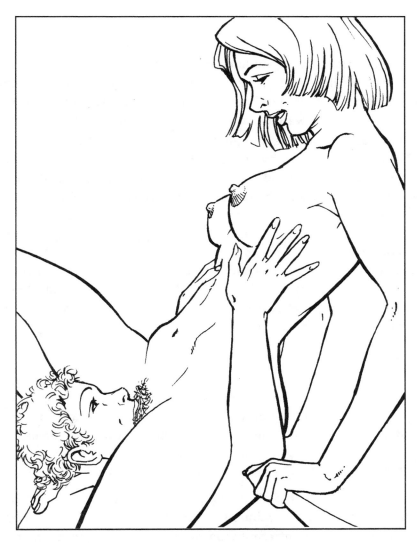

"I worry I take too long."

"I don't like his face being down there; I'm sure I smell."

"There's no way he can enjoy doing it."

"I can't relax; it makes me feel too vulnerable. I so much prefer
  intercourse!"

"I have a lot of hang-ups about it. I think the guy wants to get
  out of there as soon as possible. So I need to be reassured you
  really enjoy it. The orgasm I have with oral sex is the most
  wonderful, but it often takes a long time and would try the
  patience of anyone."

Corporations spend millions of advertising dollars trying to convince women their genitals smell so they will buy useless products for their crotches. Hopefully, if you like giving your partner oral sex, you will let her know how much you want to do it. Tell her often.

If a partner worries her genitals smell, one solution is to perform oral sex when the two of you are in the shower or right after a shower. That could help her feel she is clean enough, and sometimes it is nice to give a partner oral sex when she (or he!) has just had a shower.

Some women are uncomfortable when a man has a close-up view of their genitals. If that's the case, it could help ease your partner's mind to do oral sex with the lights out. Also, inhibition tends to decrease as sexual arousal goes up. So a partner may be more open to receiving oral sex after she's become highly aroused. And last but not least, there are women who don't have aesthetic concerns or partner worries. They just don't like receiving oral sex.

Oral Sex in Real Life vs. Oral Sex in Porn

"I give a woman oral sex for at least 30 to 45 minutes. From my experience, women don't start to relax until about 10 to 15 minutes into it. Then they go to a stage of comfort. It also depends on the amount of build-up and foreplay and the existing relationship you have. The more foreplay and better the relationship, the quicker the comfort level is reached." *male 33*

Porn gives an incredibly distorted view of oral sex. Plenty of women need thirty to forty-five minutes or longer of oral sex before they can orgasm. This is very different from what happens in porn, where oral sex seldom lasts for more than a minute. Yet there's a well known porn actress who cannot orgasm in real life unless she receives forty-five minutes of focused oral sex and she cannot orgasm from intercourse at all. But in hundreds of porn movies, she pretends to orgasm easily from intercourse and only a minute or two of oral sex. So if a woman is concerned about taking so long, please reassure her to the contrary.

When a Woman Has Been Sexually Abused

When receiving oral sex, a woman needs to give up control. While this won't be a problem for most women, others will struggle with turning the reins over to a partner. This can especially be an issue for a woman who has experienced sexual abuse. Listen carefully to her concerns. If you can't come up with a way to progress that is mutually acceptable, do not push the issue. See Chapter 50: *Good Sex after Bad– Rape & Abuse.*

Whatever the reason for a lover's concern, reassure her that you'll stop whenever she asks you to. And if she asks you to stop, stop that very moment. You'll always have time to discuss it later.

The Way Women Taste

Most carpet munchers know that some women's genitals taste great, others less so. Beyond that, men are fairly useless when it comes to discussing genital taste. Lesbian and bisexual women, however, will talk your ear off about the subject of how women taste:

> "One woman who I loved going down on suddenly began tasting different—not nearly as good. As it turned out, she had started taking vitamin pills. It was never a problem if she took herbs, but vitamin pills would ruin the way she tasted."

> "A former girlfriend was a tennis pro. Sometimes she would play tennis for a few hours and I could go down on her without her taking a shower and she would still taste sweet. There are other women whom I have gone down on right after we showered, and they still didn't taste good. In making my own inquiries, I found that the sweeter tasting women didn't eat red meat."

> "I watch my diet carefully, but the sweetest, best-tasting lover I ever had was a meat-eating, beer-drinking dietary disaster."

So much for consensus. For a thought from the cleanest lesbian in all of Hackensack, New Jersey:

> "Some women spend more time filing their toenails than they do taking care of their pussies. When I'm in the shower, I always separate the lips of my vulva and wash between them. I'm also careful about little bad-tasting pieces of gunk that collect under my clitoral hood. These are what uncircumcised males get under their foreskin if they don't pull it back and clean it."

A Q-tip dipped in mineral oil can work well to get rid of "little pieces of gunk" that stick under the clitoral hood, but it's always best to speak with a gynecologist first.

Learning to Listen: Getting Your Muff-Diving Mojo Going

During more intense states of sexual arousal, the higher functioning parts of a woman's brain begin to shut down and she moves into a trace like state of sexual bliss. This can take away her ability to verbalize and even conceptualize what's going on, and it can become difficult for her to give you helpful feedback.

While she might ordinarily know what direction your tongue is moving across her clitoris, she may reach a point where she' not be able to tell. She just knows it feels good. There's no point in getting frustrated or angry if it seems like she's not being clear or she's not able to string words together with her normal coherence. You'll need to learn what her body is telling you when it does the following:

Sudden flinching, convulsing or jolting

Hips arching

Hips bucking

Inner thighs quivering

Inner thighs squeezing your face

Crotch moving into your face

Crotch pulling away from your face

Body going limp with occasional twitching

Body going limp with no twitching

Her hand squeezing yours

You'll especially need to make sense of a woman's hand motions when she's tugging on your hair or ears during oral sex. Fingertips on the top or side of your head can speak volumes, but their movements can be difficult to understand. The same is true with gasps and cries. And it's also important to be mindful of her breathing patterns and if they change as you make changes. After you've given her oral sex a couple of times, ask her about establishing signals for if she wants you to make changes, and which changes she thinks will be helpful.

Cunnilingus Catastrophe #1 – The Porn Model

Like so much of porn, what's done on the screen should stay on the screen. The porn version of muff diving has nothing to do with pleasure. It was created for the camera to have easy access to a woman's crotch. That's why cunnilingus in porn is called "fence painting," because the person who is giving the oral sex sticks his or her tongue out as far as possible and makes licking stabs at the woman's genitals. In real life, giving oral sex is more like wrapping your lips around a juicy peach, which hides what the camera wants to show.

Orals sex in porn is over faster than a teenage boy on prom night. In real life, you should plan to be at it from ten minutes to an hour.

Cunnilingus Catastrophe #2 – Taking the Direct Route

There's only one truly wrong way to arrive at a woman's crotch, and that's by going straight to it. This is why the term "muff diving" is such a misdirect. Never dive. Begin at a woman's knees and work your way up her inner thighs, caressing and teasing as you go. Or start from her neck or shoulders and work your way down.

Approach a woman's genitals slowly with lips that kiss and a tongue that teases. Hopefully, you've already engaged your lover's favorite hot spots before beginning your descent into the valley of womanly wonder. Unless she tells you otherwise, it never hurts to make sure your partner's genitals are throbbing and moist before your lips make contact with them.

Cunnilingus Catastrophe #3 – Systems Not Aroused

A wet tongue is not an antidote for a dry puss. Fantasy, romance, teasing, kissing and caressing are your oral sex advance team. If your lover likes to walk on the wild side, add the occasional spanking, kink or rough sex. Remember to create arousal first, before approaching a lover's clitoris, unless she tells you she wants you to go right for it.

Oral Sex vs. Video Gaming

Nina Hartley, who has given oral sex to more women and men than most people alive, says she sometimes struggles to keep focus when giving a woman oral sex. So take heart, this happens to the best.

While it's doubtful Ms. Hartley is as good at gaming as she is at making porn, it might be helpful to consider how different oral sex is from playing video games, especially when many of this book's readers do both.

Video gaming is all fingers and thumbs; going down on a woman is all lips and tongue with the occasional finger assist. Video gaming is a visual feast, but when you are giving a woman oral sex, the lights are often low or you'll have your eyes closed so you can be at one with the job at hand. Gaming invites you to lean into the action and sometimes go wild, while going down on a woman requires a calm, deliberate focus. With gaming, the more successful you are the more feedback the game provides. With muff diving, the better you do, the more likely your partner will fade off into her own space. Sometimes there will be hip-bucking and cries of pleasure, but other times a woman's body goes into a state of suspended animation with occasional moans and twitches.

With oral sex, your joy is in helping your partner to drift into a world of pleasure. Once you get her there, you pretty much stop existing, which is its own special joy.

Positions for Giving a Woman Oral Sex

Each couple will find the oral sex positions that work best for them. For starters, it's hard to beat the classic missionary-style position. This is where the woman is on her back and the man is on his stomach with his face between her legs. This position allows her legs to flex comfortably, which helps her pelvis to tilt up for better access. Her thighs can be over his arms or shoulders, or under them.

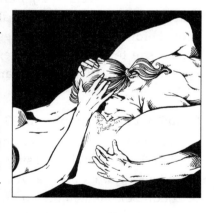

A great thing about this position is how comfortable it can be for the woman and it doesn't interfere with her ability to take long, deep breaths. It's also a position where your bodies are pointing in the same direction. Your tongue has clear access to her labia and clitoris. This works well if your partner likes you to retract her clitoral hood and lick the underside of her clitoris. It also allows you to stimulate the opening of her vagina with your tongue if that's what she likes. A disadvantage of this position is your head is looking up. This causes your neck to bend backward and it can get very uncomfortable. A variation is when you are kneeling at the edge of the bed. This allows your neck to be less bent, depending on how you position your bodies

Another comfortable position is the classic missionary but turned on your sides. This allows the man to rest his head on the inside of his partner's thigh. If she's a fan of wrestling, it lets her apply the ultimate head scissors. Some men love having a woman's thighs around their head, while others find it to be claustrophobic. One disadvantage is a man doesn't have as much access as when her legs are spread apart. Some men will start off in the missionary position, when a woman's clit might be more sensitive and mouth and tongue control are critical. Then they ask the woman to roll on her side so they can get into a more comfortable sides position and keep going for as long as she likes.

Another oral-sex position is where your partner is sitting on your face. However the term "sitting on your face" is rife with deception. While it might look as if she is sitting on your face, the human face isn't the most comfortable object to sit on. As an alternative, she might want

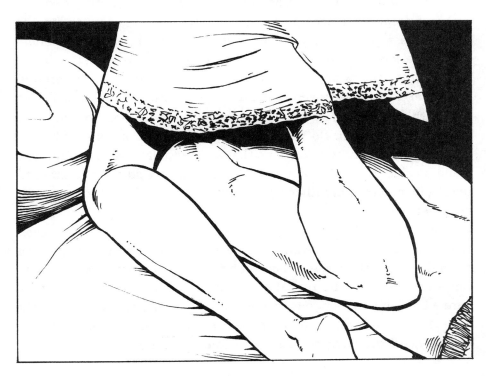

to stay on all fours, with you propping your head and upper body on pillows. This will give your face the necessary altitude to make the contact you need with her crotch.

A position that can be more comfortable for a man's neck is when a woman is sitting in a chair or on a stool with him sitting or kneeling between her legs. (See the illustration on page 249.) Some couples enjoy a 69 alignment where their heads are pointing in opposite directions.

Lock Jaw & Tongue Cramping

Tongue cramping and jaw paralysis are common side effects of giving oral sex. These usually occur moments before the woman blurts out, "There, that's perfect, don't stop!" Being able to continue when every ligament and muscle fiber in your neck and face are screaming for mercy is what separates the oral-sex men from the boys.

Protect Your Neck—You are not a Crash-Test Dummy

If your neck is in a strange position or weird angle, you won't have the stamina to do a good job. Make sure your neck is comfortable. Generally, you will be in this position for much longer than anticipated.

A strategically placed pillow under your partner's bum can provide better access to her labia and clitoris. It can raise her pelvis so the angle of your neck isn't as severe and it can help increase the sensation in her clitoris. Put a pillow under your head if it makes you more comfortable. If oral sex-related neck pain is an issue, try it with her sitting in a chair.

With experience, you will discover which positions do and don't land you in traction. Do not suffer in silence. Discuss this with your partner so you can find positions that are mutually pleasing. That way you'll be able to give her more of what she likes. And don't hesitate to give your mouth a breather by replacing the tip of your tongue with your wet fingertip.

Also, it is not unheard of for a woman in the heat of oral passion to grab a man's skull and yank it one way or another with enough force to cause whiplash. If she grinds your face into her crotch with a nose-flattening swoosh, she probably wants you to up the tempo or pressure a bit. But don't let your tongue go full throttle, because this might cause her to whip your head in the opposite direction. Learning to shift tongue-gears gradually can add years to the life of your neck.

The Thermal Envelope of a Woman's Crotch

Besides porn, the second worst source of information on how to give oral sex is the movies. When you see an actor with his face between a woman's legs in the movies, his head is almost always covered by sheets or a blanket. This has to do with ratings, not comfort.

Once a woman begins to feel sexually excited, the heat signature between her legs increases. This means you will start sweating like a pig if you put a blanket over your head while giving her oral sex. It can ruin what should be an enjoyable experience. So be sure there is plenty of air circulating around your face and head. If your bedroom is cold enough to be a home for penguins, turn the heat on while you're giving oral sex.

Slobber

Oral sex can throw salivary glands into overdrive. Instead of swallowing or letting the saliva pool in your mouth, you might want to let it flow wherever gravity takes it. But this requires preparation, as you will need to place a towel or two between your partner's bum and the bed. Otherwise, one of you will end up sleeping on a really big wet spot

Be sure to talk to your partner about saliva abatement. Does it feel okay to let your slobber flow between her legs? If not, does she want you to blotter it up every so often with a towel? Some women will appreciate it if you push the edge of a towel against the area that's just below their vagina so your saliva won't trickle down their butt crack.

Also, some women will want a generous coating of saliva between your tongue and her clitoris, while that won't allow for enough friction for others. With proper feedback, you'll be able to get it just right.

Avoiding Beard Burn on a Woman's Thighs

Grunge is not good on a woman's thighs. Five o'clock shadow is killer. If you are one of those guys who grows a shadow ten minutes after shaving, drape a towel over each of your partner's thighs, like mechanics do over the fenders of cars when they are working on the engine.

And clean shaven or not, oral sex is about your lips and tongue, not your chin in your lover's vagina. Less chin is better when it comes to oral sex.

Oral Sex Cheat Sheet

The Mons is a mound of tissue that's over the pubic bone. Try massaging the mons with your fingers before starting oral sex. Pushing the mons up with your fingers during oral sex can change the angle of the clitoris and provide better access.

The Vestibule is the area between the inner lips. Explore this sensitive area with the tip of your tongue. Try grasping her clitoris between your tongue and top lip and gently nodding or shaking your head. It will stimulate the vestibule.

The Inner Labia or Lips can thicken and darken when a woman is sexually aroused. Try sucking on them or pull and tug them with your lips. You might also try to gently tug on them with your fingers while licking or sucking on a woman's clitoris.

When a woman has large inner lips...

Taint or Perineum This is the space between the genitals and anus. It is much shorter in women than in men. While a woman might find it very enjoyable if you lick this area, be careful not to dip your tongue into her anus and then back into her vulva. If you are going to rim, it's best to rim and only rim.

The Outer Labia or Lips are made from the same type of skin as the scrotum. Kiss them. See if she like you to suck on them or tug on them with your lips.

This Can Be a Good Place to rest your upper lip when focusing on the clitoris.

The Clitoris should be an end point, not a place to start. It responds better after a woman is aroused. Some women like a gentle sucking or nursing motion on the clitoris, some a flicking with the tip of the tongue across it or in circles around it, some prefer long licks with a flat broad tongue from the fourchette to the mons. You won't know without asking.

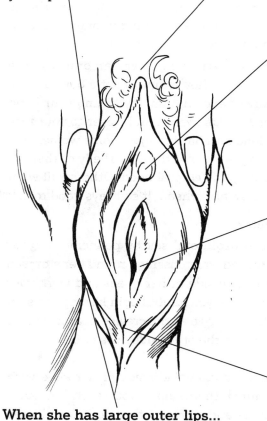

The Vagina The part of the vagina that is sensitive to touch is around the opening. Try making circles around the opening with the tip of your tongue. If she likes you to thrust deeper, you don't need to push your tongue in very far. She won't feel much past the first inch.

The Fourchette is where her lips come together at the bottom of her vagina. It's where some of the lubrication pools. Try massaging it with your fingers before using your mouth. Then massage it with the tip of your tongue or by pushing your mouth into it.

When she has large outer lips...

Furrows and Folds Try running the tip of your tongue up and down the furrows between the inner and out lips, and then between the outer lips and inner thigh.

The Tip of Your Tongue

You won't believe how much you can learn about giving oral sex by licking the palm of your hand. Notice how quickly the end of your tongue goes dry. So much for the fantasy that the human tongue is always wet.

A dry tongue creates drag or friction. Nature did not create the clitoris with a high tolerance for friction. This is why you'll need to coat your tongue with saliva first. After a few minutes, saliva from your mouth should automatically run down your tongue and keep things well-lubricated, but not at the start. (There's nothing wrong with keeping a bottle of water or good-tasting lube by your side.)

The last thing you want to do when giving a woman oral sex is to lick her genitals like they show in porn. Her vagina is not a bowl of milk and you are not a cat. But by way of explanation, try licking your hand with a soft tongue. You may need to push your hand closer to your face because a soft tongue is not as long as a hard tongue. Some women will prefer a softer, more rounded tongue against the underbelly of their clitoris, given how it isn't insulated by the clitoral hood. Others will want the tip of your tongue to feel like an arrowhead. It's always good to ask.

Northern Route or Southern Route?

It rarely shows good form to begin oral sex by pouncing on your partner's clitoris. Once she is aroused, start kissing around her stomach and work your way down, or on the inside of her knees and work your way up. With the stomach-down route, you might begin kissing the skin over her hip bones. You'll eventually arrive at the crevice near her inner thigh. Then return to the hip bone on the other side, kiss circles around it, and work your way down.

With the knees-up approach, smother the inside of her knee with kisses. Work your way up her inner thighs until you reach her outer labia. Then move to her other knee and start smothering it with kisses, working your way up to ground zero. By then, your partner will hopefully feel that life will stop if you don't begin giving her oral sex.

Ground Zero

Maybe you know more about troll rogues than going down on a woman, or perhaps you are an oral sex pro. Regardless of your skill set, here are some things to consider about giving really good oral sex—as long as you get reliable feedback from your partner.

🐛 As a woman flexes her legs, her pelvis arches forward. This can provide better access for oral sex. A lot of women will do this themselves by putting their legs over your shoulders, or by planting one or both feet on your shoulders. Some pull their legs up to their chest. You can also wrap your arms around the back of a woman's thighs and push them forward.

🐛 Some women provide all the oral access a man needs by simply spreading their legs. Or you may want to separate the outer labia with your fingers. This provides a direct route to the inner lips, and can sometimes feel like the difference between kissing a woman whose mouth is open versus one whose mouth is closed. Some women will offer a helping hand by separating the lips themselves.

🐛 Lavish her outer lips with licks and kisses. Try running the tip of your tongue up and down the furrows between the outer and inner lips.

🐛 The mons pubis is the mound of flesh that sits directly above the labia. It is where the bulk of the pubic hair grows. Pushing or pulling up the mons while doing oral sex can heighten the intensity for some women, and some might want you to nibble gently on the mons. If a woman doesn't shave, it can feel good when you lightly tug on her pubic hair.

🐛 The inner lips of women's genitals tend to be longer around the vaginal opening. You might try clasping them between your fingers and tugging on them gently while your mouth is focused on the clitoris. A woman who is highly aroused may enjoy this, but be sure to get feedback.

Her Clitoris

"Don't immediately dive into the clitoris and stay there. Warm up by licking all of the vaginal area. Suck on the labia. Then turn your attention to the clitoris. I like my clitoris to be licked, flicked and sucked. Sometimes I get off faster if my partner licks lower on the clitoris, rather than at the top of the hood. It makes for a different kind of orgasm." *female age 25*

No matter how small a penis is, nobody should have trouble finding it. Not so with the tip of the clitoris. Some are in clear view, others play hide 'n' seek. Sometimes all it takes to expose the tip is a lone finger to pull the hood up. Other times it takes both hands and a litany of prayer.

To find the tip with your tongue, separate the outer lips with your fingers. Make sure your tongue has plenty of saliva on it for lubrication. Take a long slow lick from the bottom of her vagina to the top where the big lips meet. Somewhere along the way you will most likely feel a small knob or slight protuberance. Find out from your partner if this is the tip of her clitoris. Have her explain to you exactly how she likes it licked, assuming she likes it licked.

As your partner becomes aroused, the tip of her clitoris will swell. Some swell predictably; others not so much. This can be challenging until you become familiar with the way her clitoris changes. She might want you to lick on a specific spot or location. You might need to go on faith and past experience.

"Gentle teasing brings me to an orgasm. I like him to start off gently, with light licks and kisses all over my vulva. I can't take too much pressure on my clitoris, though, and sometimes that ruins it for me." *female age 23*

You would think the surest way to arouse a woman would be to start at the tip of the clitoris, since that's where so much of the sensitivity can be. But with some women, you never touch the tip at all, while others might want you to throw a lip lock on it.

Some women enjoy it if you kiss their entire genitals in the same way you do their mouth. Others crave gentle nursing action that's focused on their clitoris. Some like it if you flick the tip of your tongue over the clitoris in a sideways direction; others prefer an up-and-down motion as though you were rapidly turning a light switch on and off. Some like a circular motion. These motions may seem awkward at first, but you'll get the hang of it. Some women will want you to speed up or change locations as their arousal grows, others prefer a constant motion from start to finish.

When it comes to the clitoris, less is sometimes more. Stay simple and steady unless she advises to the contrary. Your partner might have a favorite side of her clitoris where she wants you to lick. To help improve access to the favored side, she might try flexing one leg while the other lies flat and a bit to the side. Other women have an ambidexterous clitoris that welcomes an approach from any side.

The clitoris sometimes disappears soon before orgasm. No one knows why. With input from your partner you will learn how to respond; in the meantime, when a clitoris disappears, you might try giving a little suck to pull it back out.

After learning more about your partner's responses, experiment by puckering your lips around her clitoris and making a light vacuum. You can then push the clitoris in and out of your mouth either with your tongue or by reversing the suction every couple of seconds.

Your partner's clitoris and the area around it may begin to pulse once she is highly aroused. This is usually an indication to stay your course. Problems start when you decide to up the tempo or go harder.

When a woman begins to orgasm, her clitoris will usually start to contract. The contractions happen less than once a second. Some people say to time the movements of your tongue in synchrony with the contractions. Good luck making that one work.

Some women prefer to receive different kinds of stimulation depending on the time of the month. At one point in her menstrual cycle you might need to avoid the tip or glans, but two weeks later you can flick the tip silly. This is nothing you're going to learn during a one-night stand.

If you are focusing on other parts of your partner's genitals besides her clit, you don't need to be as careful with your movements. But when you are mostly focused on your partner's clit, precision can be the key. As Nina Hartley says, "With women, millimeters mean everything."

Landscape Mode vs. Portrait Mode

Most men can flick their tongue from side-to-side longer and better than they can do it up and down. Rapid up-and-down flicking often brings out your tongue's inner spaz. If up-and-down flicking is what your partner wants, you might experiment with changing the angle of your head from portrait mode to landscape mode. With your head turned sideways, side-to-side flicking will feel to her like you're doing it up-and-down.

One Change at a Time

When you make changes during oral sex, try only one new thing at a time. Wait for your partner's reaction before making further changes. For instance, if you want to speed up, don't speed up and change direction at the same time. Otherwise, you won't know what worked.

Passive Sucking While Your Partner Controls the Movement

There maybe be times when a woman won't want you to move your tongue, but only apply pressure to her clitoris with your mouth or pull a light vacuum with it. Your partner can then move her hips back and forth or up and down, controlling the sensation herself. It takes less than an inch in any direction to achieve a very pleasing effect.

This can work especially well if you aren't sure what to do, or if the two of you aren't able to get into a good rhythm. You provide light suction while she provides the movement.

The Urinary Meatus

When it comes to oral sex, using terms like "urinary meatus" or "the area around her peehole" can cause an aesthetic flat tire. However, the part of a woman's genitals between her clitoris and vagina is called the urinary meatus. It is worth exploring with the tip of your tongue. For some women, this might be the difference between good oral sex and great oral sex. For others, it might cause irritation or pain. So be sure to get her feedback.

Also, keep in mind that the head of your penis is one big urinary meatus. Also that kissing her genitals is usually more hygienic than kissing her on the mouth.

Tongues and Fingers Inside Her Vagina?

The opening of the vagina is in the lower half of a woman's genitals. A man might occasionally feel compelled to stick his tongue far into his lover's vagina. But this can cause his tongue to cramp, and she's not likely to notice because the nerves that register touch only go in as far as the first inch. So if she wants tongue thrusting, find out how much is "just right" so you don't end up going farther in than is necessary.

As for putting your fingers inside a woman's vagina as you are giving her oral sex, you must absolutely ask her first. Some women say there's no more surefire way to kill an orgasm than for a man to stick

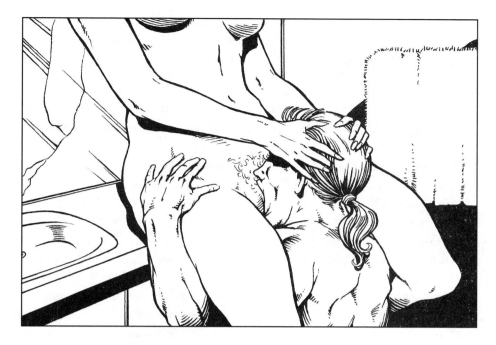

his fingers inside their vagina during oral sex. Other women treasure one or two fingers inside their vagina, but not until they have reached higher levels of arousal. Some might like a thumb pushing down on the floor of the vagina.

As for what to do with your fingers once they are in her vagina, your partner might want them to stay perfectly still or she may want you to twist, jiggle or thrust your fingers in and out. There could be special spots in her vagina that she likes having stimulated.

The back of the vagina often balloons open during sexual arousal. Some women enjoy having this area filled up. A dildo can work well to accomplish this during oral sex. Also, a woman might fantasize about having one man's penis inside her vagina at the same time that another man is licking her clitoris. Adding a dildo to the mix can help satisfy this fantasy unless a second lover is handy. There are also oral sex dildos that strap on a guy's chin. They look like a trip to the orthodontist that went terribly wrong.

All of Her in Your Mouth

If a woman enjoys this, open your mouth wide and put your top lip just above her clitoris. Put your lower lip at the bottom end of her vagina. Then push your face in and begin to suck all of her into your mouth. The emphasis is on gentle suction, unless she wants you to amp it up. Keep repeating and never blow air into her vagina.

If She Starts Bucking

It's not unusual for a woman who is receiving oral sex to start bucking her hips with pleasure when she is having an orgasm. This kind of motion can knock a guy off her mound.

A work around is for a partner to rap his or her arms around her thighs from behind, as in the illustration above. He then puts his hands firmly on her hip bones. The female hip bones provide a perfect handle and were probably put there for this very purpose. This way, she has to lift the weight of his upper body in order to buck. This will help keep her pelvis still enough so he can give her more of what's causing her to buck in the first place.

However, don't assume that bucking and hip flailing means a woman is receiving more pleasure than one who is mostly still during oral sex. A woman who orgasms quietly may be having a more intense experience than one who is expending energy to sound like a porn star.

Ass Play during Oral

When a woman is about to have an orgasm during oral sex, a finger tip gently inserted into her anus can launch a cascade of pleasure, or it can be the worst thing you could possibly do.

If you decide to try this, there is no need to stick your finger in very far. Just putting pressure on the rim around a lover's anus might light up thousands of nerve endings. A variation is to insert a well-lubricated butt plug or vibrator in your partner's rear before given her oral sex. Or your partner might want you to firmly squeeze her butt cheeks, but stay away from her anus.

You can always go for a triple play: lips on her clitoris, a finger or thumb in her vagina and one up her rear, although a lot of women will find this to be overly stimulating and not in a good way.

If She Has Genital Jewelry or You Have a Tongue Piercing

Genital piercings can be an important player in oral sex if you learn how to use them correctly. If your partner's clit or hood is pierced, experiment with sucking her clit into your mouth and flicking the jewelry with your tongue. Her response may depend on how close to a nerve bundle the piercing lies. With the proper feedback, you'll learn exactly how to use a woman's genital jewelry to provide her with exceptional oral sex. But be careful about the jewelry coming apart. It's not the kind of thing you want the doctors to be fishing out of your stomach.

It is possible to give wonderful oral sex when you have a tongue piercing, but only as long as you know where the ball is and what it's up to. Try flicking your tongue across the palm or back of your hand. This will help you learn to steer your ball better. The last thing you want to do is bang a steel object against a woman's nerve endings. You will need to flick your tongue more delicately than a guy who doesn't have a tongue piercing. According to a woman who has dated a couple of guys with pierced tongues, flicking a pierced tongue across a woman's vulva can feel really cool, but only if the man is extremely gentle and acutely aware of the impact that a pierced tongue has. She also cautions against probing inside a woman's vagina with a tongue that's pierced.

Mixing Up Oral and Intercourse

Some couples enjoy it when a guy goes down on a woman for several minutes, then they have intercourse for a few more minutes, then he goes back down on her, then they have more intercourse. There is no rule book. Figure out what works best for the two of you and enjoy it.

It Ain't Over until It's Over or She Pulls Your Face Away

Just because your lover has had an orgasm, there is no reason to come up for air. Keep doing what you were doing until she relieves you from duty; don't leave your post until instructed by her hands pulling on your head.

But remember that the slightest movement can feel abrasive after a woman has had an orgasm. She may want you to slow to a crawl or call it quits, or lay off for a minute or two, then gently rev it up. Or she may want you to put your penis where your mouth has been. When you are with a partner long enough, you will learn her post-orgasm protocol.

Oral Information

👓 Your partner's face is not an oral-sex tachometer. A woman usually wants to be able to zone out when she's receiving oral sex rather than having to watch you looking up at her for reassurance that you are doing okay. Learn to feel what's happening by the way her body responds instead of looking for visual cues, which can often be confusing.

👓 Find out if your partner likes you to play with her breasts or other body parts while you are going down on her. One reader loves her partner to squeeze her toes when she is receiving oral sex—it can be the difference between coming or not for her. Try that on another women, and she might think you'd lost your mind.

👓 Here's a game suggested in *Ultimate Kiss*: Bring your lover to the edge of orgasm with oral sex and then pull your mouth away for a count of fifty. Then bring her to the edge again and pull your mouth away for twenty-five seconds. Then bring her to the edge and pull your mouth away for ten seconds. Be sure to explain the game beforehand.

👓 Give your partner oral sex when she is still wearing her panties. Start with your lips on her inner thighs, work up to her underwear, and then sneak your tongue under the material. Some women might like it if you blow warm moist air through the front panel, but never blow air directly into a woman's vagina.

👓 Consider pulling your lover's panties off with your teeth. Be careful not to leave holes or rip the material, given how lingerie can cost an arm and a leg; it's best that she not remember you as the one who destroyed her favorite undies.

👓 Think nothing of crawling under your lover's dress while she is standing to plant tender kisses in places where other guys only dream of going. But she'll need to sit or lie down before you go further. It's difficult to do oral sex when a woman is standing.

👓 Place the tip of your tongue on the side or bottom of her clitoris. Then push the tip of a small vibrator on the bottom of your tongue.

👓 A subtle way to make your tongue vibrate is to hum while placing it on your partner's clitoris. A well-hummed aria can push some women into orbit. Others will start laughing.

👓 Separate her outer lips with your fingers and lay your tongue flat against the lowest part of her vagina. Take a slow, long, wet lick upward from the base of her vagina to her belly button that lasts for at least ten seconds.

😎 Some women enjoy having several pillows under their lower back and rear end so their entire body is on an incline with their crotch angled upward. This provides great access, a wonderful view, and your neck won't cramp as much when doing oral sex for long periods of time.

😎 On a hot muggy day, ice cubes can spice up oral sex play. During the cold of winter, sipping a warm drink before kissing a woman's genitals can also have a nice effect.

😎 There are swings that are great for doing oral sex. They can be hung from a door jamb or ceiling rafter. The swing spreads the woman's legs and places her at the perfect height for a man to give her oral sex while he is sitting upright, with his neck straight. Beware: many swings are poorly made and uncomfortable. The better ones aren't cheap.

😎 Some women have a problem with being kissed on the face after being kissed on the crotch. If that's the case, keep a wet washcloth handy. Run it across your face after giving her oral sex.

Safety Note: It can be sexy to blow warm moist air over your lover's genitals, but very dangerous to blow air into her vagina. Never lock your lips on your partner's vulva and blow air into it.

When a Woman Gushes

Some women expel fluid around the time they have an orgasm. If your partner gushes and you have a problem with it, take solace in knowing that it wouldn't be happening if you weren't doing something right.

Does Anyone Really Use Dental Dams?

Years ago, someone decided the way to safely go down on a woman was to spread a latex dental dam over her crotch. Why not just use neoprene or Naugahyde? You have no clue what you're licking. And try whipping your tongue back and forth over latex. No matter how much slobber you throw on it, your tongue drags and your RPMs tank. Some people find plastic food wrap to be a more satisfactory barrier. You can see through it, it doesn't slow your tongue, and you can always re-use it afterward to cover a casserole. If following safe sex guidelines is important in your situation, do a browser search on the CDC website and other credible sources for what's currently being recommended for oral sex.

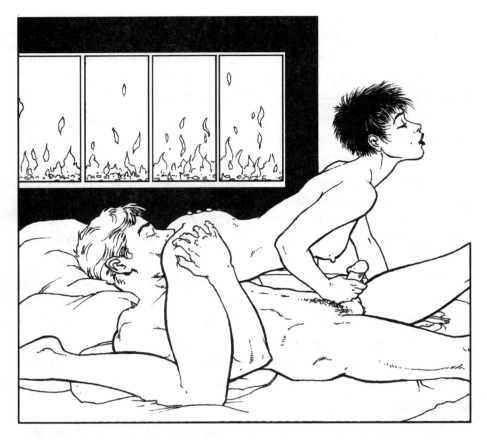

Maintaining a Hard-On While Giving Oral Sex

When a guy is giving his lover oral sex, he needs to keep doing it long enough to get her off. But this can require the kind of concentration that isn't always conducive to maintaining an erection. And giving oral sex is one time when a guy doesn't have to worry if he does or doesn't have wood. So a woman should never assume that no boner means her partner is unhappy or unexcited about giving her oral sex.

Unfortunately, some men who feel they absolute must have an erection will stop giving oral sex the moment they feel their hard-on starting to go and try to have intercourse before it's "too late."

Things a Woman Can Do to Help a Partner Who Is Going Down on Her

Tugging on Your Bush: If you have pubic hair, take a moment to tug on your bush before receiving oral sex. You'll pull out loose hairs that would end up sticking to the back of his throat.

Shaving Duties: A woman who shaves or waxes shouldn't hesitate to put a lover in charge of muff maintenance, if he's good at it.

Labia Laundering: Separating the labia and washing between them once a day will help to keep genitals clean and tasty. Some women find that just using water works best, others like a mild soap like SebaMed.

Not Helpful: If a woman fears her genitals don't taste good, she should ask her partner. If she feels there is something bad about her genitals, she should tell her partner lest he feels hurt by her rejecting behavior. Perhaps his reassurance will be helpful. But if it's something that genuinely makes her feel uncomfortable, he should not persist.

Feedback: If a man's ego is so fragile he can't handle a woman's feedback about oral sex, perhaps he would do better with a mindless partner who has no input to give. If you aren't equal partners in sex, you aren't equal partners in the rest of your relationship.

Playing with Yourself: Don't hesitate to reach down and masturbate while your partner is doing oral sex. Let him know about it.

Humor: Humor is one of the most important sex aides there is. Try not to forget this.

Oral Sex When a Woman is Having Her Period

Some couples are fine with oral sex when a woman is having her period. Here are some solutions if you want the action but not the flow:

Flex Disc, Softcup, Diva Cup and other Menstrual Cups: These are tampon alternatives that collect menstrual flow as it comes out of the cervix and before it flows through the vagina. They work well for oral sex during your period. See Chapter 27: *Surfing the Crimson Wave* for details.

Tampons: A fresh tampon will usually catch most of the flow. You must take the tampon out if intercourse is going to follow.

Diaphragm: Some women get a diaphragm for the sole purpose of having sex during their periods. The Softcup or Flex disc will do most of what a diaphragm will, and you don't need a gynecologist to fit it.

Plastic Wrap: A simple way of dodging menstrual flow is by putting plastic wrap over a woman's genitals before going down on her.

STI NOTE: Little is known about the risks of HIV transmission when doing oral sex on a woman who is having her period, but it can be a way to give and get hepatitis.

Sixty-Nine

69 is when a man does oral sex on a woman at the same time she does oral sex on him. Some couples enjoy 69, but not all. A lot of women find 69 to be an unpleasant distraction. For them, oral sex is about being able to receive. Shove your dick in their face, and it's suddenly about a woman having to preform. So ask first.

Readers' Comments

"Get a good rhythm going. Don't suck or lick too hard on the head of the clit. Also, either be smooth-shaved or have a beard, but no in-between. Beard burn really kills down there!"

female age 45

"Stubble on the face is not welcome in tender areas down below."

female age 48

"Please quit when I say so; it gets really tender and ticklish after I come." *female age 43*

"Lick around the area of the clitoris, not directly on it, until I am more aroused and then only part of the time." *female age 35*

"Start out slowly, working around the outer area with your tongue. Don't just push in. Do a lot of gentle rubbing and caressing on the insides of the leg. Gradually probe the vulva with your tongue. Develop a rhythm and keep going until I come."

female age 32

"If my partner's tongue gets tired, he uses his finger and sometimes it feels the same." *female age 25*

"I like a man to first shave me smooth, then gently kiss and finger me." *female age 34*

"It's great when he puts a finger into my rear while giving me oral sex. It makes for quite the explosion!" *female age 38*

Oral Sex: Popsicles & Penises

Some women enjoy giving a man oral sex. It can give them a feeling of power and control over their partner's body. It can also provide feelings of intimacy and closeness that can be both soothing and exciting. Other women don't find anything special about it but will go down on a guy if he enjoys it. And some women would rather suck on a rusty pipe than let their lips stray south of a man's beltline.

Whatever your preference, this chapter offers tips and techniques about giving oral sex to the male of the species. It starts with a candid discussion about male ejaculate. It offers techniques for giving splendid blowjobs and it includes suggestions for the man who is receiving oral sex to help make it a good experience for his partner and himself.

When Gay Guys Blow

Women get the feeling they need to swallow a guy's ejaculate in order to give a truly fine blowjob. If this were true, you'd think it would apply just as much in the gay community, where the giver of the blow-job knows exactly what it feels like to receive a blowjob. But that's not the case. Gay guys don't always swallow when giving blowjobs. As one gay male reader says, "No way am I going to do all that work getting a partner to come and not watch him ejaculate. Besides, I don't exactly love the taste."

Swallow only because you want to and not because there's some *Miss Manners of Blowjobs* who says it has to be.

To Swallow or Not to Swallow—That Is the Question

Considering what usually happens if you suck on a penis for long enough, a woman eventually has to decide if she wants to swallow semen. For some women the salient factors are how they feel about the guy and how they feel within the relationship. For others, it's the taste and texture.

Different guys come in different flavors. As a female reader states: "My current lover tastes great, I like swallowing his ejaculate. But when my former boyfriend came, it felt like battery acid in the back of my mouth." Another reader says she has no problem with the taste or texture of male ejaculate, but that it sometimes upsets her stomach. That's probably due to the prostaglandins in semen. A British sex expert who sounds like the queen says that male ejaculate is an acquired taste, like swallowing raw oysters. As for the smell of male ejaculate, it's like a weak solution of bleach—original scent as opposed to Lemon Fresh or Spring Rain. (For all things semen, see Chapter 6: *Semen Confidential.*)

Who knows what to advise about swallowing except that a man shouldn't push the issue unless he is willing to swallow a mouthful of his own, although the actual amount is closer to a teaspoonful. (See page 269 for how to give a really good blowjob without swallowing.)

Swallowing and Hormonal Considerations

Women sometimes wonder if they are getting a dose of male hormones when they swallow semen. While the testicles produce the lion's share of male hormone, this goes directly into a man's bloodstream and not into his semen. You don't need to worry about sprouting a beard or growing a big Adam's apple from swallowing cum. And the only way you will gain weight from male ejaculate is if it makes you pregnant.

Regarding your health, the main concern about male sex fluids is whether the man has a sexually transmitted infection. If there's any chance of that, use a flavored condom when you are blowing him.

Have an Understanding

The important thing to remember about giving a blowjob is that it is going to feel pretty wonderful to your partner. So lighten up and loosen up. Stare his one-eyed snake in the scrotum and say, "I'm the one with the teeth, so behave yourself and do as I say!" Giving a good blow job is about being in charge. Enjoy it and have fun calling the shots.

Quick & Easy

Going down on a man isn't as much a mystery as going down on a woman, given how the penis is pretty much in your face. The childhood experience of sucking on popsicles will give you an idea of how to begin. However, popsicle-sucking does not make for an excellent blowjob.

There are different kinds of blowjobs. Some women like to include lots of kissing and licking; others mainly suck on the penis. Using your hands can add an extra dimension.

Blow Jobs in Porn vs. Real Life

Have you ever noticed that porn actresses never gag when giving blow jobs, and it's not like they're sucking on small penises? Maybe it's something they learn in porn acting school. Or maybe they've had the nerves that cause the gag reflex surgically removed. Either way, blowjobs in porn often seem like they are more about humiliating or objectifying women than they are about sexual pleasure.

As for a man who wants to ram his penis down a woman's throat like they do in porn, why not find a girlfriend who is a porn actress? Although it's unlikely she'll want to do at home what she does at work.

Gag Prevention

Here are four suggestions to keep yourself from being gagged while giving a blowjob. The most important suggestion is the first:

Tell Him! If he thrusts and it gags you, let him know. Women who gag when giving oral sex seldom tell their partner about it. So if gagging is a concern, tell your partner the two of you need to work on it, because he'll be getting way more blowjobs if you don't have to worry about gagging. Be specific! If a little thrusting is OK, help him recognize the difference between that and thrusting that will cause you to gag.

Fist on Shaft: Make a fist around the shaft of your lover's penis, with your little finger resting on his pubic bone. This will give you an entire first worth of buffer. If your partner has an average-sized penis, there should be no way he can gag you. If he is luckier than most, use two hands instead of one, like when you are holding a baseball bat. Keeping your fingers around the shaft also allows you to pump it or pull the foreskin taut. More on why you might want to do that later.

On His Back: Some guys thrust involuntarily when they come. To deal with this, keep your partner on his back and position your body between his legs. When he is close to coming, keep both of your hands around the base of his penis and your forearms flat against his pelvic bone. If he thrusts, his pelvis will pull you up along with his penis.

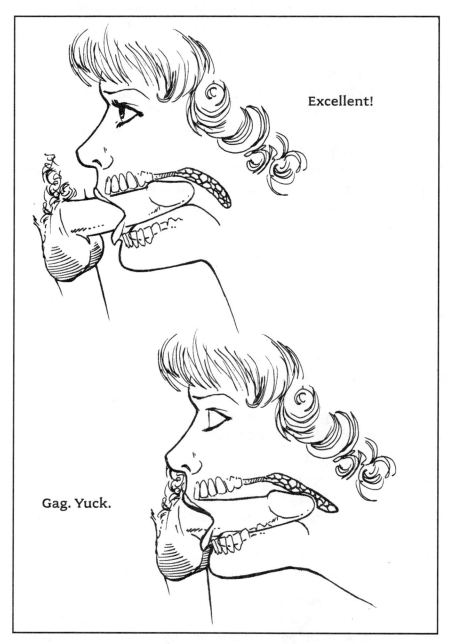

Excellent!

Gag. Yuck.

Inspired by illustrations from Violet Blue's "The Ultimate Guide To Fellatio" 2nd edition

Grab Him By the Balls: Clamp your thumb and forefinger together around the upper part of the man's scrotum where it attaches to his groin. This will place the testicles in the palm of your hand. Some men find this pleasurable, especially if the woman gently pulls downward. If he thrusts more than you want, increase the downward pull.

Positions

An excellent position for doing oral sex is to place yourself between your partner's legs, facing his body. This gives your tongue direct access to the most sensitive parts of his penis and scrotum, and the angle minimizes the tendency of the penis head to bang against your tonsils. It's a comfortable position for most women and it lets him watch you giving him head, which is a turn-on for some men. A variation is to sit, kneel or crouch in front of your partner while he is standing or sitting.

A woman might also straddle the guy's chest, facing southward as though they were doing 69. This can be nice if staring at a partner's crotch and rear end provides a man with an extra turn-on. But it places her tongue in contact with the upper side of his penis (that part that faces his stomach), which doesn't allow for maximum stimulation.

Another way of doing a blowjob is where the woman keeps her head still and the man moves his penis in and out of her mouth. The fancy term for this that nobody but priests ever use is "irrumation," which is Latin for "altar boy, hold still!"

The position a woman sometimes takes in irrumation or "face-fucking" is to lay on her back with her head propped up on a pillow. The man straddles her upper body and thrusts his penis in her mouth. He does the work of thrusting and she has good access to his testicles and rear end. She can also stimulate her clitoris at the same time. But some women feel claustrophobic with the guy on top or they fear he will thrust too deep. Putting your hand around the shaft of his penis will decrease any chance of this.

Some couples enjoy lying on their sides facing each other. That way, the woman can lay her head on a pillow while she is giving him oral sex.

Deep-Throat Myth

Truly great blowjobs have nothing to do with deep-throating a man. Deep-throating is more of a novelty than something that makes a penis feel great. If your man insists that you deep-throat him, buy a vegetable that's the same size as his erect penis. Hand it to him and say, "Let's see how you'd feel if I shoved this thing down your throat."

As was said in the porn movie *How to Perform Fellatio:* "The most sensitive part of the penis is the top part, so stop wasting your time on the bottom," and the male porn actor who uttered this profound statement had a penis with a great deal of bottom part as well as top part.

The Most Sensitive Parts of the Penis

The average penis has areas that are sensitive and other areas that are mostly for show. The part you will want to focus on is a sensitive nickel-sized area called the frenulum. It's just below the head on the side of the penis that's away from his body when he has an erection. Many men can be brought to orgasm by stimulating this area alone. (See the illustration on page 269.) The seam of the penis that runs from the scrotum to the head also responds to tender kisses, as does the entire scrotum.

For some guys, especially those who are not circumcised, the head can be really sensitive. Find out how he likes you to suck or lick the head right before and after he has an orgasm. The head can become painfully sensitive after orgasm. Ask him about this.

Blow-Job Basics Whether He Is Circumcised or Not.

Slobber: People who are neat freaks often try to swallow all of their drool when they give blowjobs. This can result in near drowning. Let gravity carry your saliva down a lover's penis. You can use your saliva as a lubricant for pumping the bottom part of his penis with one hand while doing the upper part with your mouth. Place a towel under your partner's rear or wedge one behind his testicles so there won't be a big wet spot on the mattress, chair at the library, seat of the plane, bus or where ever he's lucky enough to be receiving a blowjob.

If It's Still Soft: Some women enjoy sucking on a soft penis. They like feeling it grow inside their mouth. But even if it stays soft, each kiss, lick and suck will feel just as exquisite. One of the few times when a man can be totally passive and feel no need to perform sexually is while he is receiving a blowjob. Don't assume it's a negative sign if he takes a while to get hard or if he doesn't get hard at all.

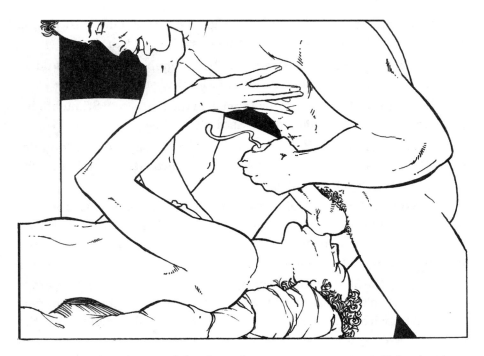

This position is also good for deep throating your partner if that's what you want to do. That's because it helps to straighten the pathway down your throat. While this position may be better for deep throating and teabagging, it's not nearly as good for regular blowjobs.

Lubrication for Licking: When you first lick a man's genitals, coat your lips and tongue with extra saliva. If you suffer from the dreaded pre-blowjob dry mouth, try sucking on a mint beforehand to help kick-start your salivary glands. The mint might also help take the edge off the taste. It never hurts to keep a glass of water nearby.

Teeth: Some women make a ring around the penis with their thumb and forefinger. They push their lips against their fingers to make a gasket that can help keep their teeth off the shaft of the penis. Others wrap their lips over their teeth when giving a blowjob, given how the mere hint of teeth on the penis scares some men. But a set of sexy choppers can sometimes be erotic, as long as the woman is not in a pit-bull mood.

Little Kisses & Flickering Tongues: Never hesitate to lavish a man's penis or any other part of his body with flicks of the tongue or sweet kisses. Kissing his penis can give your jaw a much needed rest during the middle of a blowjob, especially if he has a lot of girth.

Twisting Your Head: Twisting your head when going up and down (in a corkscrew pattern) creates a higher level of stimulation.

Twisting Your Head, and Your Tongue on the Frenulum: Stimulate his frenulum with your tongue while twisting your head.

A Shirley Temple: Soften your tongue and give his penis a long flat lick with it. This is called a "Shirley Temple" because it's similar to the way a person licks a big lollipop.

The Long Lick Nature: left a seam on the penis that runs from just below the head to halfway down the scrotum. Never hesitate to take a long, wet lick from beneath your partner's testicles all the way to the tip of his penis, along the length of the seam.

Pumping the Shaft: While your lips are focusing on the upper part of the penis, there's no reason why you can't be pumping the bottom part of the shaft with your hand or fingers. Let your saliva flow down the shaft, lubricating it and your hand. Then start pumping. Some women synchronize the shaft pumping with their head bobbing, so their hand follows just beneath their lips at all times.

The Vacuum (Hoover Fellatis): Some men like it if you draw a slight vacuum with your mouth. One way to draw a vacuum is to take as much of the penis in your mouth as feels comfortable. Then make a seal around the shaft with your lips, and suck some of the air out of your mouth. Then, as you pull your head back, a vacuum is created.

Man Nipples: Some guys' nipples are highly sensitive. Caressing them with your finger while doing oral sex might add to the man's pleasure. Experiment and seek feedback.

Inner Thighs and Other Places: The inner thighs of both men and women can be extremely sensitive. There's no reason why you can't alternate a blowjob with licking and sucking on your partner's inner thighs, or caress them with a free hand.

Fingers in His Mouth: While you are blowing him, you might try sticking your fingers in his mouth. Some men find this to be erotic.

Perineum (between the Testicles and Rear End): There is an area behind the testicles called the perineum that is often overlooked but has the potential for good feelings. Licking this area can light some men up. Gentle finger massage down there can also be good.

The Blow Hole: Explore the slit in the head of his penis with the tip of your tongue.

Rear End: Some men welcome a finger on or up their anus when receiving oral sex. (See the illustration on page 383.) Some say their most intense orgasms are during oral sex while a finger is on their prostate. Other men hate this. Also, a small vibrator up a man's butthole might catch his attention, and some men greatly enjoy being rimmed.

Visual Assist: Plenty of men enjoy watching a woman give them head. Some women might be offended by the notion, thinking it has something to do with submission. The chances are that the man is way too appreciative to be thinking about gender-power issues when you are giving him a blowjob. In her video on how to give blowjobs, porn star Nina Hartley comments, "It took me a long time to be able to do a blowjob in the light and not get embarrassed." She apparently got over it.

Oral Intermission: If your mouth gets tired, do your partner by hand for a while, or run your hair over his genitals. Or let him watch you play with yourself or put one of your nipples in his mouth. Don't be afraid to let him know about it if you are turned on. It may help speed things up.

Tap & Hum: Try to occasionally hum or tap the shaft of the penis when the head and frenulum are in your mouth.

Hot, Cold, Etc. Suck on ice cubes to make your mouth cold, or drink hot liquids to make it extra-warm before and during oral sex.

Going Down after Intercourse: Some women find it erotic to suck on a penis after it has been inside of them. Others not so much.

Help from Your Friends: If you have a friend who is more experienced at giving blowjobs, consider asking her or him for pointers, but keep in mind that you will soon be evolving your own style. What you do will also vary depending on the man you are doing it with.

Blowjob Tips for When Your Partner Is Intact (Not Circumcised)

If Your Partner Isn't Circumcised #1: Without retracting his foreskin, hold the sides of his foreskin with your fingers and stick the tip of your tongue inside of it. Run your tongue in a circle around the head of his penis. Depending on how much yardage there is, you might also be able to pull his foreskin up around your tongue.

If Your Partner Isn't Circumcised #2: By varying the level of vacuum in your mouth, see if you can make the foreskin come up and down over the head of his penis as you bob your head.

If Your Partner Isn't Circumcised #3: Ask your partner at what point he wants you to retract his foreskin (pulling the extra yardage down the shaft so the head is bare). If you don't retract his foreskin, the blowjob will last a lot longer because he's not getting as much stimulation.

Making the Foreskin Taut: This applies as much to men who are circumcised as for those who aren't: Wrap your thumb and forefinger around the shaft of his penis an inch or so above the scrotum. Then pull it down to the scrotum. This makes the skin tighter and usually increases the sensitivity in the upper part of the penis. It might also help him to come sooner if he seems to be taking forever. If he isn't circumcised, you may need to start higher up the shaft before pulling the foreskin down.

Fingers during Blowjobs

Fingers are as important to blowjobs as they are to sign language. Try caressing his testicles when you are giving him a blowjob. Also, the part of his penis that runs under his scrotum might also respond nicely to fingertip massage while you are giving him oral sex. Massaging this area with your free hand can increase the sensation for some men. (See the illustration on page 222.) If you make hand play a part of oral sex, he's not as likely to notice when your mouth needs a rest.

Teabagging or Cojones by Mouth

> "I love my boyfriend's testicles. I like taking them into my mouth one at a time and sucking on them. The skin on the sack is really soft and feels great in my mouth." *female age 23*

Some men will appreciate it if you take one or both of their testicles in your mouth. Don't fear doing this. Just go slowly until you get the hang of it. The skin around the testicles (scrotum) also loves being licked and kissed. If your partner doesn't have an erection, you might be able to fit his testicles in your mouth as well as his penis.

Right before He Comes

There might be things you can do just before a man starts to come that will increase his pleasure. Some women wrap a hand around the bottom part of the penis. Others place their fingertips along the seam on the front side of the penis and apply a bit of pressure. You might be able to feel the ejaculate surge through his penis when you do this.

Some men appreciate it if you increase the vacuum in your mouth as they are about to come, but be careful about sucking the ejaculate into your sinuses as it spurts out. Some men enjoy it if you hold or caress their testicles or massage the part of the shaft that's beneath them. Let him know that you would like to experiment and seek his feedback.

A sex worker who helped with this chapter said plenty of men like to have their nipples pinched or caressed as they are about to come.

Learn When He's Coming

If you know the right signs to look for, you can often learn when a man is about to come. This will give you options to get your mouth out of the line of fire if you don't want to swallow.

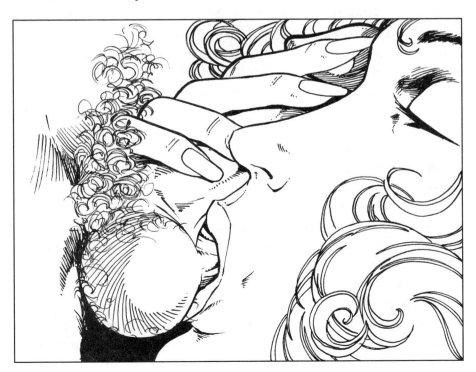

As he's about to ejaculate, his penis will start to swell. You can feel this in your mouth. A hand over the testicles may be a good source of information, as testicles usually draw closer to a man's body when he is about to come. Also, his rear end or abs might tighten up or his hips might give a thrust when coming is inevitable.

Oral Sex with Men of Size

Oral sex may be problematic if your partner's penis is enormous. Never fear. The illustration on the following page shows how you can give great oral sex without having to dislocate your jaw. Use your hands to pump the shaft while focusing your lips on the frenulum.

If You Don't Like the Way He Tastes

If you're not going to swallow, keep one of your hands around the base of your partner's penis. As he's about to ejaculate, free your mouth from the line of fire and slide your hand up the shaft. Then start pumping his penis with your hand. Use a firm grip and pump fast and furious. Don't stop pumping just because he starts to ejaculate.

Here are other suggestions if your taste buds are at war with semen:

Toothpaste, Mints, or Sweet Liquor: Sticking a dab of toothpaste in your mouth before inserting a penis can improve the taste greatly, or try sucking on a mint beforehand. Try sipping on your favorite sherry or liquor, unless you are a confirmed whiskey or tequila drinker. Or you might try glazing his yam with honey, jam or whipped cream. Champagne blowjobs can be fun, although they can result in hangovers. If you enjoy minty liquors such as creme de menthe, do a small test patch on the side of his penis first. While a little mint or menthol on the skin can feel great, too much can burn. It takes a few minutes for the full intensity to peak, so wait before declaring your test a success.

Slobber and Punt: When Old Faithful about to blow, mobilize a pool of slobber in your mouth. The saliva will help thin the ejaculate, making it run out of your mouth faster. Make sure there's a towel underneath to catch the mess.

The Back of Your Tongue: If you are going to swallow but want to decrease the taste, place his penis as far back in your mouth as you comfortably can, then start swallowing fast. This keeps the semen from coating your taste buds.

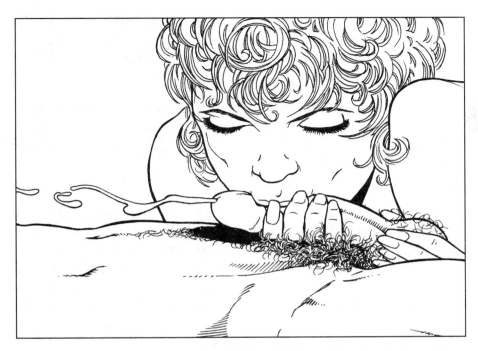

An Effective Way To Get Him Off Orally When You Don't Want To Swallow or When He's Too Big to Fit in Your Mouth

This feels so good that a lot of guys won't be able to tell you aren't swallowing unless they are looking. The trick is to focus your lips around the sensitive frenulum area (just beneath the head) while cradling the rest of his penis with your hand. Use lots of saliva and put plenty of tongue into it—almost like you are French kissing this part of his penis. Occasionally fill your hand with hot steamy breath.

Sublingual Ejaculation: This tip is in the excellent book *Tricks—125 Ways to Make Good Sex Better* by Jay Wiseman. When it feels like a man is close to coming, put your tongue over the head of his penis. He won't know the difference, but the first splash will hit the underside of your tongue where there aren't any taste buds.

Let Him Help: Some guys won't mind finishing themselves off if you have taken the time and energy to give them a really good blowjob. It might be a special treat if you kiss or suck on his testicles as he pumps himself to orgasm. (See the illustration on page 263.)

Bag It: There are flavored condoms made especially for blow jobs. But never use the same condom for intercourse, as it's easy for your teeth to make tiny rips in the condom without you knowing.

Jewelry on Your Tongue or On His Penis?

If you have jewelry on your tongue, experiment with ways of focusing it on parts of his penis for an added effect. If he has jewelry on his penis, explore ways of working it with your tongue or mouth, but don't suck on it; you don't want to risk swallowing it.

Putting a Condom on with Your Lips

An experienced partner can slip a condom over a man's penis with her mouth and he will never know it is there. In her book *The Ultimate Guide To Fellatio,* Violet Blue suggests you wet your lips and put the unrolled condom up to your mouth. Pull just enough vacuum to suck the reservoir tip of the condom into your mouth. This should hold the rest of the condom against your lips. Bend over the penis and push the condom against the top of the head. Then walk the unrolled part down the shaft either with your lips or fingers.

A key to this is getting flavored condoms. Be sure to check the consumer reviews, as some flavored condoms taste pretty bad. Also, if you don't mind the taste of the lubricant, condoms made of polyurethane might transmit the warmth of your mouth better, and feeling the warmth of your mouth is one of the best parts of receiving a blowjob.

WARNING! Do not put a condom on a man's penis with your mouth if it's for intercourse. Your teeth can easily make micro tears in the condom, which will render it ineffective for birth control.

When a Man Balks about Using a Condom

If you want a man to use a condom while giving him a blowjob, but he refuses, say loud and clearly, "Forget it, Charlie! If you think it tastes THAT great, suck on it yourself." (Although he probably would if he could, and he has probably even tried.) To help increase the sensation, hawk a small wad of spit or lube on the head of his penis before, Then put the condom on him and squish the lube around the entire head. Also, polyurethane transmits warmth way better than latex, so use a condom made of polyurethane if you don't mind the taste of the lube. He'll hardly know it's on.

While He's Coming, and Afterward

If you are keeping his penis in your mouth, find out if he wants you to do as he's coming, for instance, to suck harder, suck less, pump his shaft with your other hand, or what. Then get a sense of how sensitive his penis becomes right after he ejaculates. For some men, the head can become painfully sensitive. Ask if he wants you to keep his penis in your mouth, and if so, how much stimulation to apply.

When a man is masturbating and he has ejaculated, he might push his fingers into his scrotum to rub the hidden part of the penis that's between his testicles. This will help push out any remaining semen. It's the equivalent of wagging his penis after he pees. You might ask him about this. Perhaps he can show you how, assuming it's what he does.

Pre-Cum Jitters

Some women who are giving oral sex experience a brief paralysis or mini-dread right before their partner ejaculates. If this keeps happening, try to talk to your partner about it. Maybe he can give you early warning before he's going to come so you can stop sucking and start pumping by hand. Perhaps it will help to put a condom on his penis before giving him a blowjob, Or use the position that's illustrated on page 269 for giving a no-swallow blowjob.

If He Can't Come From Oral Sex

This is where one woman's blessing is another woman's curse. Some men don't come from oral sex no matter how wonderful a blowjob is. Even if a woman doesn't like to swallow, she's likely to assume she didn't do a good job. So he will need to reassure her how good her blowjob was, and that he's simply wired in a way that this isn't how he has an orgasm. You will also need to settle on how long blowjobs should last.

His Hands on Your Head

Men will often put their hands on a woman's head when she is giving oral sex. For most guys, this is a loving gesture which can also be used to let a partner know what feels good and what doesn't. However, some men will put their hands on a woman's head in an attempt to push it down onto the penis. This is rude, and you need to tell him to stop.

Counterpoint: One woman says, "It can be particularly exciting when a man pushes my head down on his penis. But I would never have sex with a man who I didn't love going down on. Also, you make a joke out of it when a woman grabs a man's head and pulls it into her crotch in the other chapter, but call it assault when a man does this to a woman. You present a double standard that says we women are either more fragile than men or more easily offended when it comes to sex."

Research Findings

One of the more interesting articles about the hazards of oral sex was published in a medical journal by a group of military dentists. (Bellizi, Krakow and Plack. Honest; Dr. Plack is a dentist). The article is titled "Soft Palate Trauma Associated with Fellatio."

The article tells about the daughter of an officer who was taken to the base hospital because she discovered a black-and-blue blotch in the back of her mouth. Several dentists converged on the mystery blotch, trying to discover its origin. After eliminating all other possibilities, the dentists asked the officer dad to leave the room and then popped the question: "Gotta boyfriend?"

In the back of the mouth near where the tonsils are is a highly vascularized mass of tissue (vascularized means lots of small blood vessels). The head of an erect penis hitting against this tissue can cause a bruise. It goes away like any other bruise, but it is a reminder that the woman, and not the man, should control the thrusting during a blowjob.

Ejaculate-Related Sinus Infections

Some women like to create a vacuum around their lover's penis. This can feel heavenly. However, when a man comes with the head of his penis in the back part of a woman's vacuum-pulling mouth, the vacuum can draw ejaculate into the woman's sinus cavities. This can create a cum-related sinus infection. If this is an issue, the couple should work on keeping the head of his penis in the middle part of her mouth when he is coming. Another solution is for him to wear a condom.

Lasting Shorter vs. Lasting Longer

"Why is it when you are giving men head, they take forever to come, but are so much faster when having intercourse?"

female age 29

During intercourse, most guys will make an effort to last as long as their partners want, sometimes successfully. This is not appreciated nearly as much during oral sex. When a man is receiving oral sex, he should not try to delay his climax. If your partner is one of those lucky guys who can orgasm at will, you might devise a signal for when you'd like him to come.

Things a Man Can Do to Help a Woman Who Is Giving Him Oral Sex

To help a partner give you the best blowjobs, it's important to give each other feedback. Here are some other things, as well:

Smells: Based on thousands of sex surveys, the number one complaint women have about giving guys oral sex is smelly balls. Whether you are going out on a first date or have been married for twenty years, if you want to receive oral sex, shower and don't wear the same underwear for more than a day without washing them. If everyone including your cat runs out of the room when you take your shoes off, use foot powder or foot spray. Deodorant can also be a wonderful thing, as well as brushing and flossing your teeth. (Kissing often precedes and follows a blowjob.) If you wear cologne, ask your partner how she likes the smell of it, as well as how much you should use. Some guys smell great from just bathing alone, or she might like you marinated with a citrus or spice.

Uncut? All good things have their downsides, and smegma is a downside of having a healthy, intact penis. Why not establish a pre-blowjob routine where you go to the bathroom, retract your foreskin, and tidy up a bit around it?

Pube Tug: Tug on your pubic hair ahead of time so you'll pull out the strays that might end up in your partner's mouth.

He Who Gives, Gets: To get great oral sex, give great oral sex.

Avoid Arrogance: Never take blowjobs for granted. Be thankful whenever you get one, even if your partner loves doing it. Tell her how good it feels. Ask yourself, "What have I done lately to deserve a blowjob?" Did you give your partner a full body massage? Did you help her with a challenging project? Have you done your share of the housework? Did you respond kindly in a situation where most people wouldn't have?

Attitude: Never cop an attitude such as "My last girlfriend blew me really well. Why can't you?" There are reasons why you aren't with your former girlfriend.

The Deep-Throat Fantasy: A throat is not a vagina. If a woman gags on your penis, she won't be excited about sucking on it again.

Feedback: The best oral sex requires a doer who is willing to accept helpful feedback and a receiver who is willing to give it.

When Is Asking for Oral Sex Okay?

Every once in a while you might have a horrible day and are in desperate need of a blowjob lest you totally fall apart. If you don't abuse the privilege and have a loving partner who hasn't had an equally hideous day, it could be fine to ask or beg for a blowjob. However, it's rarely a good idea to routinely ask for oral sex. Few women take well to being pestered for blowjobs. Talk to your partner about whether it's okay to ask for oral sex, and if so, under what circumstances.

Improving the Way Your Ejaculate Tastes

It is certainly possible that ejaculate, like cow's milk, can take on flavors of what the beast eats, including its favorite vices. Unfortunately, there is no science to guide us on this matter.

It has been said that dairy products make ejaculate taste bad, but not nearly as bad as asparagus. Curry is a spice of interest. Smoking and/or drinking coffee might cause ejaculate to taste strong or bitter. Perhaps Starbucks can formulate a new blend and call it "Sweet Wad."

Some people claim that vegetarians, both male and female, taste better than their carnivore brethren. However, it is likely this is just propaganda from cows and chickens. One woman said that her partner's ejaculate tasted good unless he was under a lot of stress at work. Then it would start tasting bad. Perhaps adrenalin and hormones associated with stress might cause semen to taste funky.

Drugs are another possible culprit. Whether it's over-the-counter drugs such as antihistamines, prescription drugs, or recreational drugs like speed, people claim that drugs can taint the way semen tastes.

One common suggestion for improving the taste of male ejaculate is to eat sweet fruit such as pineapple and apples. The sugar in the fruit is supposed to give semen a sweet taste. Perhaps this is just folklore. But if this is what a partner asks you to do with the carrot of giving more blowjobs, most guys would become the pineapple industry's best friend. If your partner is willing to be the taster, why not experiment with different combinations of food? Does ingesting a little cinnamon make a difference? What happens if you drink less coffee or eat less broccoli or garlic?

If your ejaculate is extremely bitter, consider seeing a urologist to screen out the possibility of an infection in your prostate gland. Although you might not be feeling pain, it's still possible to have an infection. It might be embarrassing to call a doctor's office and say, "My girlfriend says my cum tastes bitter." So just tell the receptionist or nurse that you'd like to rule out a prostate or urinary-tract infection. Then tell the physician the real reason once you see him or her in private. You shouldn't take antibiotics for this unless tests have been done and show a problem. Antibiotics are not breath mints for your penis.

Readers' Comments

"I am certain that women would give more blowjobs if they didn't feel like they had to swallow." *female age 43*

"Cum is not a gourmet treat, but not unpleasant. I'd rather be eating mocha-chip ice cream, but getting there isn't half as much fun. My partner's orgasm is often a total turn-on for me, and occasionally just a relief that the blowjob is over with." *female age 47*

"If he smells bad down there, it's a turn-off for me." *female age 34*

"It is a major power trip for me if he comes in my mouth. I like knowing I have the ability to turn this big strong man into a sack of Jello." *fem 37*

"I used to tell my partner that I was semen-intolerant." *female age 26*

"I like running my tongue around the head and sliding it in and out of my mouth. I like to take his penis in my mouth as far as possible and rub my tongue on the underside of it, pushing the head into the roof of my mouth. It seems to drive him crazy." *female age 37*

"More than anything it feels so good because I am in control." *female 43*

"When it comes to blowjobs, let the lucky son of a bitch treat you like a queen, honey, because you are." *female age 48*

"I never was very good at blowjobs until I had a lover who had a small penis. Then I felt comfortable with him in my mouth." *female age 34*

"It feels very sensual if he lets me take it at my own pace. I think the penis has the most wonderful velvety skin." *female age 38*

"I like to give head, so I don't need much persuasion. I get really wet from giving someone that kind of pleasure, and I always feel so powerful when I do it." *female age 23*

"I only like it if I can keep the hair out of my mouth. I enjoy it only because I know he enjoys it so much." *female age 35*

"I like it. I especially like the little leaks before he comes. I think cum has an interesting taste, sort of fizzy." *female age 38*

"I have discovered that we both find it erotic to have him come on my face or on my breasts when I give him head. I don't care for the taste of his semen." *female age 22*

"If I'm in the mood it's really sensual. If I'm not it's like a job." *female 43*

"I really don't like it when he comes in my mouth. I kind of gag on it."
female age 26

"It's fun to suck on a limp penis until it hardens." *female age 37*

"One thing that's really neat about sucking on a guy's cock is watching it change shape and color and get harder. You're right up there in the front row. You don't get that with intercourse." *female age 42*

"I've observed that not all guys come as much; some have very little, and others lots and lots." *female age 27*

"Never forget to caress and tickle the balls." *female age 44*

"My mouth and hand work as a team. As I pull away with my mouth, I twist my hand almost like a corkscrew." *female age 26*

"I love to give head, but I hate to feel pressured into doing it. Also, remember what goes around comes around. If I'm the only one going down, I'll be less likely to do so again." *female age 26*

"Please don't do it like they do in the porno flicks, where the girl just about bobs her head off. Not a turn-on." *male age 46*

"Don't be fooled by the name. Blowing has nothing to do with it."
male age 26

Condoms: For The Ride of Your Life

Besides the seriously hot illustration on the next page, there's not much that's sexy about condoms except for the sex you have after you put one on. Like athletic cups and bicycle helmets, condoms are something you should use but don't necessarily want to. If it weren't for saving your life from sexual infections and helping prevent unwanted pregnancies, no one would use condoms except maybe for anal sex.

So from the start, *The Guide* is being more straightforward with you about condoms than just about anyone else. Hopefully you can trust that what follows is honest and true.

Making Condom Use Sexy — It Can Be Done!

"It would really help if I could finger her while she put the condom on me." *male age 24*

Few lovers talk about ways to help each other stay aroused when putting on a condom. Here are some possibilities:

Anticipation: A woman slips a condom into her partner's pocket followed by a welcome kiss, fingertips across the front of his pants, and a few words about what she's looking forward to once the condom is on.

While Masturbating: Some women find it arousing to watch a guy put on a condom and stroke himself. Or as a special treat, he gets to watch her playing with herself while he's putting on a condom.

While Sitting On His Face: She puts the condom on him while straddling his face, like in the illustration on page 254. Or he can put the condom on while she kisses his testicles, but she should avoid getting saliva on the base of the penis where the condom needs to grip. *Putting on a condom with your mouth is a bad idea unless it's just for oral sex, as it's easy to leave tiny nicks in the condom with your teeth.*

Grinding: She can rub her genitals against his thigh or another part of his body as he is putting the condom on.

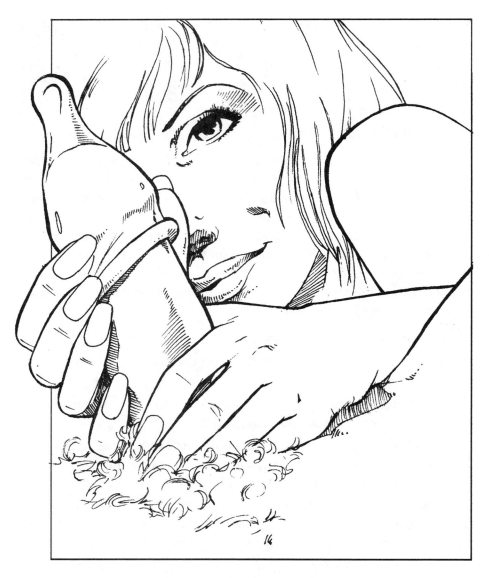

Talking Dirty: If the couple finds talking dirty to be arousing, she can be telling him about some of the things she wants them to do as he's putting the condom on or as she's putting the condom on his penis.

Hand Action: She caresses his penis and testicles, then opens the condom package but puts it down and strokes and caresses some more, and then after enough teasing, puts the condom on his penis. Keep in mind that precum can transport sexually transmitted infections.

If a Woman Feels Awkward Putting a Condom On Her Partner

A lot of women would like to try putting the condom on, but feel awkward asking. This is something a couple should discuss. Fortunately, putting on a condom can become a turn-on for both partners instead of an interruption, and when a woman puts a condom on a man, it's an important signal that the sex is consensual and mutual.

Foreskin Wedgies? Getting It Wrong from the Start

When a question about condoms for men who aren't circumcised was posted on a listserve for sex educators, the mass reply was, "Get extra-large condoms," as if guys who are uncut should be wearing condoms that are extra-large. Can you imagine if a woman posted a question about bras and instead of asking for more information, the fashion experts told her to "Buy the biggest bra you possibly can!" Unfortunately, when it comes to foreskins, sex educators in North America are sometimes in the dark ages.

Penises come in different sizes and shapes. Fortunately, condom companies make condoms that come in different sizes and shapes, from snug fitting to condoms with extra headroom. This lets the head of the penis slosh around inside the baggy part of the condom, which can feel really nice. You might like these whether you do or don't have a foreskin.

Part of your job as a couple is to explore using different kinds of condoms and find a few brands that work best for the two of you. Visit www.Guide2Getting.com for links to different condom sampler packs (enter "sampler" in the search box). Once you find a couple of favorite brands, stock up on them. Also try the female condom. Some men who are intact say the female condom feels great.

Condoms work well for the vast majority of men with foreskins. However, if you are uncut and are having condom-related problems, you might try retracting your foreskin if it retracts and put a drop or two of lube on the head of your penis before putting the condom on. After you put the condom on, work the foreskin back and forth over the head of your penis with your fingers to get the lube all smushed around.

If you are intact and would like to see an excellent video on how to put on condoms for men with foreskins, go to Guide2Getting.com and enter "condoms" in the search box. It's for gay men, but so what?

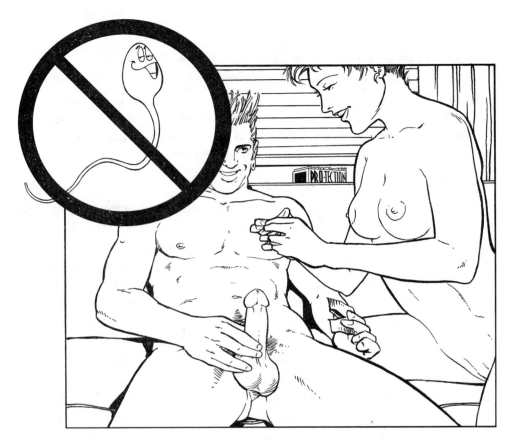

If You Are a Woman Who Doesn't Like the Feel of Condoms

You won't believe how many of the women who take our sex survey say they don't like the feel of condoms. So if you are a woman who isn't crazy about how your partner's penis feels when it's got a condom on, you are not alone. This is why it's important for women to weigh in on the matter of which condoms to buy. They notice how condoms feels, and some will feel better to them during intercourse than others.

Some women like the feel of condoms with baggier heads, others prefer condoms that fit more snugly. Some might like the feeling of condoms made of polyurethane because they transmit warmth better. Some might like condoms with nubs or ridges, other might hate them.

Condoms for Birth Control?

If the sole reason you are using condoms is for birth control, please consider more effective methods like the IUD. But if there's any possibility that you could possibly get HIV or other sexually transmitted infections, use condoms no matter what, in addition to a more effective method of birth control.

Need Extra Large Condoms? Some Do, Most Don't

The following account from a reader explains what can happen when a guy who needs a bigger condom isn't using one:

"The one traumatic thing about sex with my first partner in high school was using a condom. I'm on the larger side. The first time I tried to use a condom, it was so tight I could barely get it on and it felt like a tourniquet at the base of my penis. It was awful and I couldn't keep an erection with one on. Unfortunately, I'd read that the whole "the condom's too small" excuse is not valid because someone once squeezed 17 oranges into a condom so it's silly that a guy can't fit into one. So of course I was convinced that something was wrong with me. I kept trying, and once broke two condoms while trying to get them on! I didn't even know that they made large condoms at the time—all I knew was that if I tried to use any condom, sex would end in disaster. All they needed to say was, 'Larger condoms are available for those who need them' and my adolescence would have been a lot less stressful." *male age 26*

While it's easy to blow up a condom to the size of a watermelon, that doesn't mean you can roll a condom over a watermelon. When you first start to unroll a condom, there is a thick ring of condom material that doesn't stretch very much. Good luck getting it over the head of a penis that Nature super-sized. It's only when a condom is fully unrolled that it stretches to obscene proportions, and even then, it might not feel good on a penis that's on the wider end of the spectrum.

On the other hand, if you are buying condoms the size of a circus tent just to impress your friends or a partner, the truth is going to come out once your pants are down.

Lubing Protocol

When you are wearing a condom, you are putting a waterproof barrier between two body parts which nature designed to share fluids. To help compensate, some couples add lubrication to the outside of the condom. For increased sensation, you might also try putting a dab of saliva or a small amount of lube on the head of the penis before you put the condom on. After you've rolled the condom down the shaft, smush the condom material around the head so you are spreading out the lube. This will allow the head of the penis to slip and slide inside the condom during intercourse. (Some condoms now come with lube already on the inside.) Make sure the lower part of the penis is dry and has no lube on it. If you are putting a condom on right after receiving oral sex, be sure the shaft of the penis is dry so the condom won't slip off.

Unless you are using a condom that's made of polyurethane like the Supra or Avanti, be sure the lube is compatible with latex. If the lube doesn't say "safe for use with latex condoms," don't use it.

Tying Condoms Off

Be sure to take a condom off as soon as you pull your penis out of whereever it's been and tie off the end of it. Semen liquefies and becomes watery in a few minutes. It will run out the end of the condom if you don't tie it off.

Marathon Sex and Rough Sex

Condoms usually dry out during marathon sex, so lube up accordingly. However, after you've initially applied lube, try adding water to rehydrate the lube. If you add more lube, you could end up with a gunky, glue-like mess and the woman could get friction burns from the lube.

Intense thrusting shouldn't cause a condom to break if you are wearing the right size and are using lube if you need it. So you shouldn't need to go gentle if both of you prefer a rougher ride.

Reasons Why Condoms Break

One of the most common reasons why condoms break is from damage due to blunt puncture. That's when the condom material gathers more tightly around the head of the penis with each thrust, until the penis bursts through the condom.

If you feel a condom tightening around your penis, pull out right away and make sure the condom material hasn't stretched over the head of your penis. If it has, assume that damage has been done to the condom material, and put on a new condom.

Another reason why condoms break is when couples use lubrication that is not safe with latex condoms. *Do not use Vaseline, petroleum jelly, Nivea, Jergens, hand creams or lotions to lubricate latex condoms.*

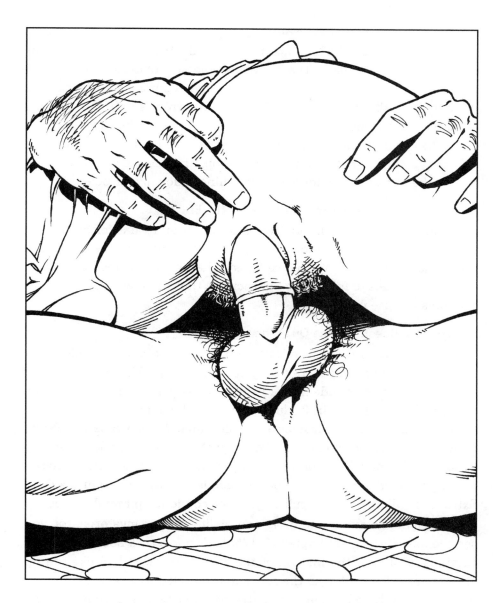

Wearing the right sized condom counts. If your penis is of the jumbo variety, use condoms that are larger. If your penis doesn't cast the biggest shadow in town, wear condoms that are snugger fitting.

Teeth, nails and jewelry can cause tiny nicks in condoms that you can't see but sperm love. Do not open condom packages with knives, scissors or your teeth, and check the date. Latex does not last forever.

Reservoir Tips May Be Irrelevant

Some condom brands make a big deal about having reservoir tips to hold a man's ejaculate. There are a couple of problems with this concept. The first is that most reservoir tips hold about 2.9 ml. of ejaculate. While half of all guys produce 2.9 ml. or less, there's still another 50% of men who produce more than 2.9 ml., which means their tips runneth over. The other problem with reservoir tips is the unproven assumption that they really do hold the fluid. Reservoir tip or not, try to squish the air out the end of the condom before rolling it down your penis.

Do You Need To Leave Extra Material at the End?

Conventional wisdom advises to leave an extra half of an inch at the end of the condom before rolling it over the head of the penis. But there has never been any science to say whether this is good or bad. So the best advice is to follow the instructions that come with the brand of condoms you are using.

If a Condom Doesn't Come Out When You Do

For a condom that doesn't come out with the penis it rode in on, take solace in knowing there's no place for it to go. The condom might play a mean game of hide'n'seek behind the woman's cervix, but that's about it. The first step in finding a jettisoned condom is to wash your hands and make sure your nails are well-trimmed. The woman might lie on her back with her knees up, like when she's at a gynecologist's. This is no time for modesty: the farther apart her legs, the better. Explore her vagina with your index finger. If lube is necessary, use just a little. Extra lube will make it difficult to grab the condom. Spit might be better.

If female sexual anatomy is one of life's great mysteries for you, see the illustrations in Chapter 11: *What's Inside a Girl.* Look at how the cervix is located at the far end of the vagina. It might feel like the tip of your nose. Try exploring the space in the back of the cervix with your finger. It's likely to be there. If so, try to dislodge it and edge it into a more accessible part of your partner's vagina.

Once you have a good handle on where the condom is, you might try inserting your index and middle fingers in the hopes of snagging the rim of the condom between your fingertips which will act like pincers or tongs. Condoms are stretchy, so pull it out by the rim slowly but

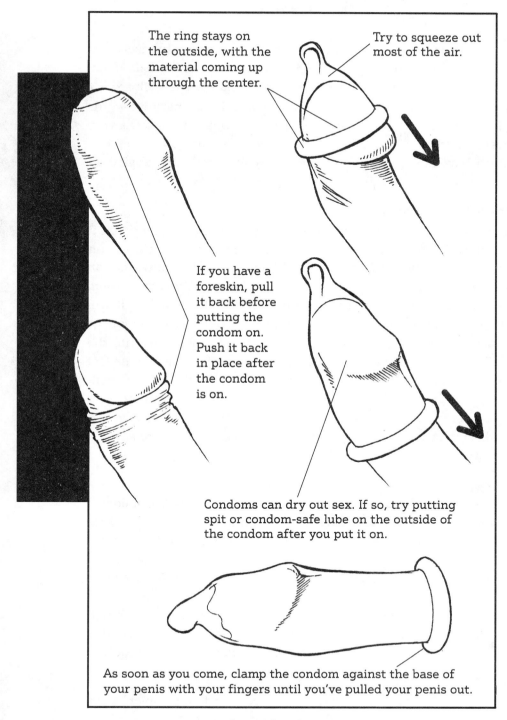

The ring stays on the outside, with the material coming up through the center.

Try to squeeze out most of the air.

If you have a foreskin, pull it back before putting the condom on. Push it back in place after the condom is on.

Condoms can dry out sex. If so, try putting spit or condom-safe lube on the outside of the condom after you put it on.

As soon as you come, clamp the condom against the base of your penis with your fingers until you've pulled your penis out.

For the Ride of Your Life!

firmly. If your partner clamps down when you are trying to insert two fingers, go slowly and gently. Her vagina is not going to implode if you take an extra ten minutes searching for the buried latex treasure.

If you were using the condom for birth control, the operative words are *Emergency Contraception, Plan B, Ella,* or a *Copper IUD.* At the very least, use emergency contraception right away. Do not wait until morning. If you have any questions or concerns, call your doctor or visit an emergency room. For condoms lost during anal sex, see page 390.

What to do if a Condom Breaks

If you were using a condom for birth control and discover that it has broken while in service, immediately take emergency contraception. *Ella* and *Plan B* are two different pills used for emergency contraception that can be very effective in preventing pregnancy if you take them right away. Better yet, consider having a Copper IUD installed. It will provide you with years of highly effective, hassle free contraception.

In the meantime, do not inject birth control foam or jelly into the vagina. The pressure might push sperm up the cervix, which is the last place where you want it to go. The same is true for douching. Wash your external genitals and pee. And if you honestly think that douching with Pepsi, Coke or Mountain Dew is going to do anything but prove you're not the brightest bulb on the planet, nothing this book has to say will count for much.

Who Brings the Condom? Reasons for Mistrust

Researchers have found that males don't always trust the condoms that females supply. One fear is that a woman may have poked a hole in it if she wants to become pregnant, as if this is every woman's secret dream. A second concern is that she may have had the condom in her purse since she was in junior high. Women sometimes mistrust male-supplied condoms as well: How old is that puppy? Did he have it in the same pocket with three jump drives and his car keys? Did it go through the wash? These problems can be greatly reduced if you talk about it first and perhaps order condoms online or buy them in a store together.

Resources

For an outrageously large list of links for condom sampler packs, visit www.Guide2Getting.com and enter "sampler" in the search box.

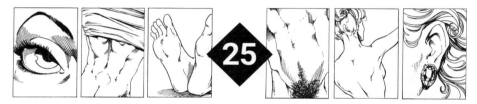

Concerns about Sex Lube

The billion dollar sex lube industry wants people to believe that using sex lube will make sex better whether a couple needs it or not. Yet we know nothing about the impact of sex lubes on the colonies of bacteria in the vagina that are so essential for vaginal health, including the prevention of infections. That's because research on this has just begun.

It could be that women will be advised to avoid sex lubes unless they truly need to use them. Or different ingredients will need to be used in lubes than those that are used today. And please don't assume that lubes which are organic, natural or "friendly to sperm" are any better for women's vaginas than lubes with chemical-sounding names.

We also know little about the impact of sex lubes on the anus and rectum. It could be that some sex lubes make it easier to get sexually transmitted infections in both the rectum and vagina. For more on why we should be concerned, see Chapter 12: *Population: In the Trillions.*

Who Uses Lube and Why?

It's surprising how many young couples are using lube. You'd think they would be dripping wet without store-bought lube. Perhaps this is due to advertising that makes it seem like sex is always better with lube. Or maybe it's because porn has made us assume that women shouldn't need more than a few minutes of kissing, caressing and sexplay before having intercourse.

As for some real reasons why people need lube: medications such as hormonal birth control and antihistamines can make sex drier than it would otherwise be. Some antidepressants can make it take forever to have an orgasm. Condoms can make intercourse dryer than normal. Marathon lovemaking sessions will often require lube, as can size discrepancies that make for a tight fit. Couples may need lube for menopause-related dryness, and lube can be a must for sex if you are receiving chemo for cancer. The lack of estrogen during a woman's period may cause her vagina to produce less natural lubrication than normal, so some couples need lube for period sex. Sex toys often require lube. And good luck having anal sex or fist fucking without using lube.

Also, no matter how sexually aroused they are, some women don't produce enough lube to have intercourse. Combine this with a partner who is wearing a condom, and lube can be essential.

Don't Spit on Spit!

I contacted a professor of gynecology at a medical school and asked, "What about the old standby of saliva for sex lube?" This professor checked in with one of the world's leading experts in vulvar pain, and both shared the same opinion that saliva can be an excellent sex lube as long as you don't need something that's very slippery.

If you wonder why these experts might recommend saliva over the pricey stuff, here are the ingredients in a well-respected lube that is water-based, hypo-allergenic and fragrance free. These are the chemicals in the lube that will end up inside your body:

> Propylene Glycol, Isopropyl Palmitate, Dimethicone, Cellulose Polymer, Polysorbate 60, Sorbitan Stearate, Stearyl Alcohol, Glyceryl Stearate NSD. B.N.P.D, Di Sodium EDTA, Phenoxy Ethanol, Methyl Paraben, Butyl Paraben, Propyl Paraben, BHT

Fortunately, only a couple of these ingredients are listed in the Hazardous Chemicals Desk Reference. And why do they call it hypoallergenic when paraben and glycol are known allergens for some women? A staff member of the FDA who I contacted couldn't find any criteria for what a hypoallergenic lube is or how the FDA defines "hypoallergenic."

Until recently, sex lubes have been classified as cosmetics. So they did not evaluate them for use in mucus membranes such as the vagina, rectum or urethra—where absorption of chemicals into the bloodstream can be quite high. Also, no agency checks to make sure that what's in the bottles of sex lube is what's listed on the label. A few years ago, a researcher found toxic chemicals in one of the lubes he tested. And a large pharmaceutical company was selling vaginal moisturizer for humans whose active ingredient was too dangerous for use in cow vaginas. Does this mean you shouldn't use store-bought lubes? No. But it does speak well for spending a few extra minutes of kissing, caressing and other forms of sexplay before automatically grabbing for lube.

Lube Basics #1

People confuse sex lubes with automobile lubes. With auto lubes, you want to eliminate as much friction as possible. But if you eliminated all of the friction when having sex, no one would ever have an orgasm. Sex needs friction in order to feel good. With too much friction, sex hurts. With too little friction, there's not enough sensation. So the best sex lube for you is not necessarily the lube that's the most slick.

Some lubes are thin, which allow you to feel more sensation, others are more cushioning. Rub the lube between your fingers. Can you still feel the ridges? If so, it's a thinner lube that will act more as an assist to a woman's natural lube. If you can't feel the ridges, it's a more cushioning lube that might be better for weekend-warrior sex or anal sex.

Silicone Lubes

People say that some of the best sex lubes currently available for general sexplay are silicone-based lubes. But this could change depending on what we learn from research on how lubes impact vaginal health.

If you have ever been on the receiving end of a penis that's wearing a pre-lubricated condom, you've had silicone inside of you. Unlike water based lubes which tend to dry out quickly, the silicone keeps the lube slicker for longer. Many people prefer it for anal sex as well as for vaginal sex and handjobs. The downside is it doesn't come off very easily, which is one of its upsides for use during sex.

Put a condom on silicone sex toys before using silicone lube. Otherwise, the outcome will not be pretty. Silicone lubes can also stain your sheets. Try treating the stains with Dawn dish detergent or a fabric-safe degreaser, but the prognosis is poor. (Lube-stained sheets on the bed are especially uncool when your parents are visiting.)

If you are into electric sex with probes and electrodes, never use silicone-based lubes. The silicone acts as an insulator. **And** silicone lubes become a slipping hazard if they drip on the floor, especially if you use them in the shower. The shower floor can become ice-rink slick. So apply it to your genitals before you get in the shower or tub.

Natural Products as Sex Lube – Coconut Oil vs. Olive Oil

If you want a natural oil for sex lube, and don't care that there's no scientific research to say if it's safe, the current choice seems to be coconut oil. However, it's not very slippery. While coconut oil sounds better for a vagina than propylene glycol, hydroxymethylcellulose, sorbitol and polysorbate 60, there's no science to guide us.

Olive oil can collect around the cervix, resulting in a rancid-smelling crotch. A recent study that evaluated the use of olive oil for skin massage found it significantly damages the skin barrier. While olive oil can be great on vegetables and salads, do not use it for sex.

Glycerin in Lubes

Lubes that are glycerin-based tend to be slicker than other lubes, which means if you rub them between your fingers you won't feel the ridges. People who prefer lubes with glycerin say they feel "really fast." One problem some women have with glycerin is that it's similar to glucose, which is one of the things that yeast feeds on inside a woman's vagina. So if you are prone to yeast infections, are immuno-suppressed, or have diabetes, consider a sex lube without glycerin.

Propylene Glycol, pH and Petroleum Jelly

The propylene glycol in some lubes can be an irritant for some women. So can lubes with a high pH. As for petroleum jelly, what limited research there is indicates that it's not a good choice.

Friction Burns from Sex Lube?

Believe it or not, women can get friction burns in the vagina when a lube is too gloppy or gets thick from drying out. So avoid gloppy lubes if you are experiencing discomfort. If you are having sex and your lube is getting gummy or is drying out, try adding a few drops of water or saliva to rehydrate it instead of adding more lube.

When a Woman Feels Too Wet

Some women lubricate so much that they can't feel the penis going in and out. If you are having this problem, have your partner pull out every now and then and dry the both of you off with a towel. Some people suggest trying an over-the-counter antihistamine to help dry up your natural lube if it's a problem, but check with your healthcare provider first.

Lubes for Anal Play

Historically, the lube of choice for all things anal was a famous brand of vegetable shortening called Crisco. Then came the '80s and the plague, and since then the sex-lube wars with sex lube manufacturers fighting for market share. (You might not think of your anus as a profit center, but companies that make sex lube certainly do.)

Nowadays, just about everyone who is into anal sex has a "slippery top ten." Good luck finding a consensus on which is best and research on which is the safest.

Vegetable shortening remains the standard that anal-sex lubes are trying to copy, but without its many downsides, eg: vegetable shortening has no antibacterial properties, so dipping fingers with fecal matter on them back into the can might contaminate it; vegetable shortening melts latex condoms, which are thought to be safer for anal intercourse than polyurethane condoms; and vegetable shortening leaves rancid-smelling sheets with wicked stains. Also, there might be problems with vegetable-shortening-fecal-ooze dripping from a woman's anus into her vagina if she is in an ass-over-tea kettle position when having anal sex.

There are no warnings on the side of vegetable shortening containers that say, "Use only in your oven and not in you ass." But there are also no scientific studies on the safety of vegetable oil for anal sex. So while there are plenty of opinions, no one really knows what's best. As for the lubes for anal sex which say they use "FDA-approved ingredients," this means absolutely nothing, as the FDA does not have a list of approved ingredients for anal intercourse.

Silicone-based lubes are the current front runner for anal sex. They should do the job for anal sex without your butt dripping grease like the grill at McDonald's. As for specific brands, ask around, do a browser search, and check the reviews on Amazon.

Be careful with lubes that contain numbing agents. They have names like Anal-Eze, and Tushy Tamer. Using lube with numbing agents is like disabling the smoke alarms in your home. Pain during anal sex is an important indicator that you are being too rough, aren't relaxed enough, aren't turned on enough, that your partner is too big, or that anal sex is not for you. Also, if something numbs your ass, it will numb your partner's penis, which means more thrusting rather than less.

Gnarly Poop Warning: Sorbitol and glycerin are used in a number of sex lubes. They are also an active ingredient in laxatives and suppositories. Don't grab just any lube for anal sex.

Lubes for Handjobs and Masturbation

Avoid hand creams for handjobs and masturbation. Most hand creams and moisturizers are designed to be absorbed by the skin so people won't feel like greased pigs after they use them. As a result, hand moisturizers are poor performers for sex or massage.

Whether it is for giving your partner a handjob or just for jerking off, you'll want a lube that stays wet and slippery. A popular and nearly legendary jerk-off lubricant is a facial cleanser called Albolene. **J-Lube Precaution:** J-Lube is a powdered veterinary lube that is water activated. It is also used for jerking off. Beware that a tiny amount of J-Lube in the peritoneal cavity (gut) of a horse or cow will quickly kill the animal, as in a few final moos and all four hooves are sticking straight in the air.

Men who are not circumcised are less likely to use lube for masturbation. Their factory-equipped foreskins usually do the job.

Women's Genitals (On the Outside)

Women have used saliva for masturbating since the beginning of time. Coconut oil might work well for masturbation or vulva massage. Scented lubes and anything containing nonoxynol-9 should be avoided If you like lube with oral sex, why not try food-grade coconut oil, unless you are following up with latex-condom intercourse.

Vaginal Moisturizers and "Arousal Creams"

Vaginal moisturizers are for situations like vaginal atrophy or post menopausal issues as opposed to when you need a lube for sex.

Estrogen creams are often prescribed for vaginal dryness. Do not use estrogen products or an Estring as lubes for intercourse! These are for vaginal atrophy, which is different from the dryness a 21-year-old might have.

As for "arousal creams," would five minutes more of kissing before intercourse have the same effect as arousal creams, which sometimes smell like old bacon grease or feel like rubbing Vicks VapoRub on your clit? Then again, if you like it and the product works for you, more power to it and you.

Most Effective Methods of Birth Control
Less than 1 pregnancy for every 100 women in 1 year.

—BEST—

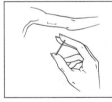
implants

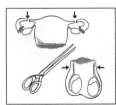
sterilization

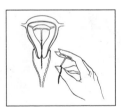
IUDs

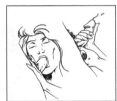
oral sex & hand jobs

—VERY GOOD—

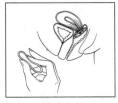
NuvaRing

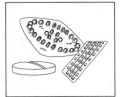
The Pill

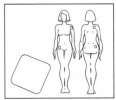
The Patch

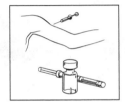
injections

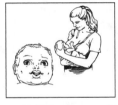
LAM (if done correctly)

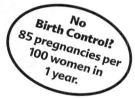
No Birth Control? 85 pregnancies per 100 women in 1 year.

—OKAY—

 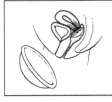
diaphragm

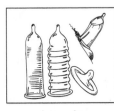
male condoms

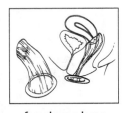
female condoms

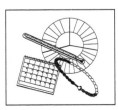
fertility awareness

Much Better Than Nothing ▶

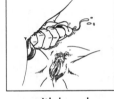
withdrawal

Highly Questionable ▶

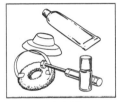
spermicides

 # Least Effective Methods
More than 30 pregnancies for every 100 women in 1 year.

Don't Forget about Birth Control & STIs!

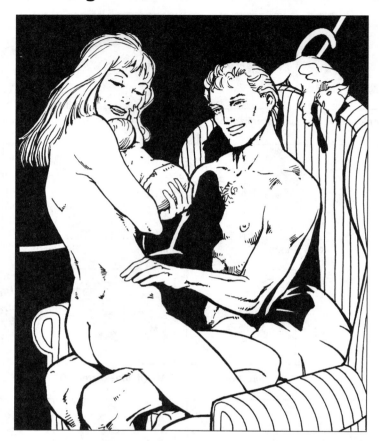

If you, your partner or your relationship aren't yet ready to be full-time parents, consider a highly effective, hassle free method like the IUD.

Birth Control Options

For a description of different methods of birth control shown on the prior page, including links to manufacturer's websites and what to do when you forget to take a birth control pill or two, please visit www.Guide2Getting.com/birthcontrol

Sexually Transmitted Infections

For the latest information about sexually transmitted infections and relevant links to the government's CDC website, please visit-www.Guide2Getting.com/gnarly

Intercourse: Horizontal Jogging

Intercourse can mean different things. It can be an intensely private and delicious act. People can use it to honor and expand their relationship at the same time they are doing fun things with their bodies. It can be a commodity for making money, and a means for achieving protection or status. It's the only way some people make physical contact with another human being. It is also what couples do when they want to create new life.

Dick, Laura & Craig

To learn more about the role of intercourse in sex, we have invaded the privacy of three young adults, Dick, Craig, and Laura. Laura used to go out with Dick, and now she's involved with Craig. Here's their stories:

DICK

Dick is a very nice-looking guy who won his fraternity's "Mr. All-America" title two years in a row. Dick has a nice job, a nice socia```l manner, drives a nice sports car, wears nice clothes, has nice biceps, triceps, and pecs, and goes out with "hot" women. Since this is a book about sex, you might as well know that Dick has a tree trunk of a penis that stays rock hard from dusk to dawn. A former girlfriend referred to it as "the sentry."

CRAIG

Craig is the same age as Dick. Craig is a sports writer. Craig is no longer eligible for the Mr. All-America contest. During a football game a few years ago, Craig went airborne to catch an overthrown pass. He got sandwiched between two spearing linebackers. Craig's spinal cord snapped, and he hasn't been able to walk or have an erection since.

LAURA

Laura is a young woman who just left a big corporation to form her own company that makes sporting gear. Laura's had sex with both Dick and Craig. Let's see what she has to say about these two different men.

"Dick's the kind of guy that many women have been raised to worship. Parading him around your friends or taking him home to your parents would win you the female equivalent of the Breeder's Cup. I've always really enjoyed sex, and until recently I could never understand why a woman would want to fake an orgasm. But it didn't take too many nights with Dick before I started faking orgasms. There was Dick, Mr. Right Stuff, making picture-perfect love. I didn't want him to think there was something wrong with me since I couldn't get into it like he was, so I started faking orgasms."

"Craig is nowhere near as perfect as Dick, but he has a great sense of humor and he is genuine. Craig is able to laugh at himself, which Dick never could. Craig has taken the time to learn exactly how to kiss, touch, and caress me, and the sex I have with him is great. When I'm with Craig I don't need to fake a thing."

"This may not seem relevant to your question about sex, but I work in a male-dominated business. I have to think like a guy from morning to night. Sometimes it leaves me feeling alien from my femininity. With Craig it's easy to find it back again. Craig never wakes me up at 3 a.m. with a hard-on poking in my back, but he feels just as masculine as Dick. With a lot of guys there's a huge difference between how they treat you in bed and how they treat you the rest of time; with Craig that's not the case. Maybe that's another reason why sex is so nice with him, even if it's not intercourse."

Okay, so here we have Dick, more functional than a Sidewinder missile. He fulfills everybody's definition of what a sexual athlete should be. Then we have Craig, who redefines the term *sexually dysfunctional*. If Craig had the same erection failure but no spinal-cord injury, therapists would collect a small fortune trying to make him "normal." He would be taking boner pills like they were M&Ms and other medications as well.

And there is Laura, a woman who enjoys sex a great deal. She is telling us that the man who can't get it up is a more satisfying lover than Mr. Erectus Perfectus.

In telling you about Laura, Dick and Craig, the intent was not to dump on intercourse. Intercourse, when it's good, can be one of the sweetest things there is. What this book is dumping on is the assumption that intercourse is good just because it's intercourse and that a man is a man because he can get hard and fuck, or that a woman is a woman because she can get wet and fuck him back.

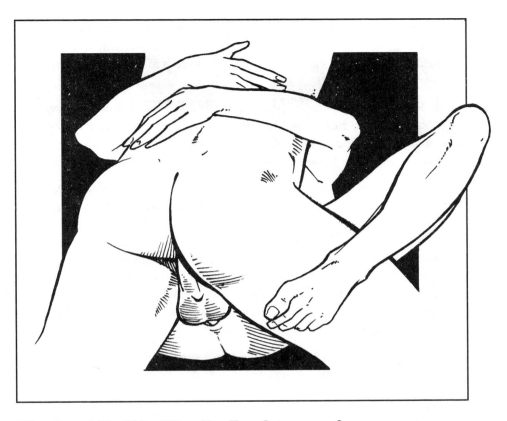

What Does It Feel Like When You Have Intercourse?

"Oh God—It's like describing the universe. It feels like I might explode and can't wait to but at same time want it to last forever. Breathless, hot, turned on in the extreme. I want to engulf and squeeze his penis, get it in me as much as possible. I love the connection of it." *female age 48*

"When his penis first enters me I want to feel every inch of it because it is exquisite. I feel like I need it inside me and I don't know if I can describe that. The actual sensations of his penis sliding in and out of me are sometimes over-powered by the pleasure I feel all over my body, so I don't necessarily concentrate on the intercourse." *female age 23*

"As he enters me I feel myself spreading open to accommodate him. Emotionally it feels right that he is inside of me. I have a feeling of fullness when he is inside me. I can feel the head of the penis as it slides in and out and can feel my vagina collapse or expand around him. If he plunges deep I can feel the head of the penis bump my cervix, a not altogether unpleasant feeling. From rear entry I can feel the penis more acutely rubbing the top of my vagina." *female age 37*

"It feels different every time. Sometimes it is very satisfying. Sometimes it hurts inside my vagina if I'm not lubricated enough. And sometimes when his penis hits my G-spot it takes my breath away!" *female age 34*

"At first I feel the light pressure of my partner's penis against my unopened vagina. It is often deeply pleasurable to feel the head penetrate, and then a slow, smooth slide all the way in, and a jolt of excitement when my lover's penis is completely inside me. The most sensation is around the outer part of the vagina, but there is also a pleasurable feeling of fullness when he is fully inside me. My hips want to move and match his strokes, or create my own rhythm for him to match. Different strokes and rhythms create different sensations." *female age 47*

"I'm strictly a clit person. I love having sex with men, but I don't like intercourse." *female age 36*

"My favorite part of intercourse is when he comes; his entire body stiffens." *female age 55*

"The first thrust is the most vivid for me. I like to slowly slide down his cock and feel it go up me. I love it when he is trying to hold back from coming; I can feel him get more swollen and hard and I get very excited when I feel that. It's when my vagina gets the most pleasure from intercourse." *female age 23*

"It depends on how sexually excited I am and whether I'm in the mood or if I'm just doing it because he wants to. If I'm into it, it's like ecstasy!" *female age 43*

"I enjoy the pumping and grinding a great deal. I love it when we are rubbing our pelvic bones together and when the penis is in deep." *female age 21*

At the Start—New Relationship or New to Intercourse
For some couples, it takes time and familiarity for intercourse to get that sloppy-intimate-erotic edge that makes it so much fun. This

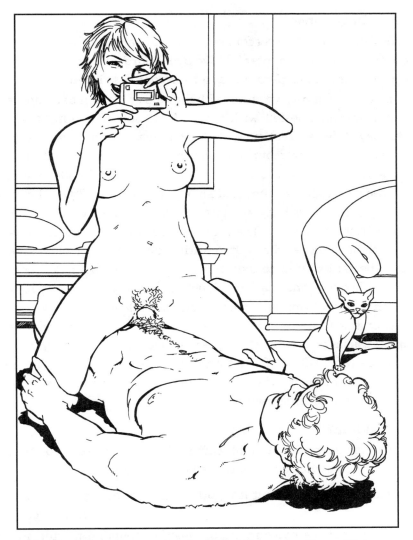

This family moment was inspired by photographer Trevor Watson.

means intercourse won't necessarily knock your socks off. It may not even feel as good as masturbation at the start. And each partner brings his or her own hopes and expectations, as well as physical anatomy and body rhythms. Patience can be a virtue.

Some couples who are having dynamite intercourse during the fifth year of their relationship had lousy sex at the start. And even when the sex is great, there will be times in any relationship when desire falls flat. Hopefully you will continue to grow as a couple during those times.

Your First Intercourse

The Guide has a chapter for people who are about to have intercourse for the first time: it's Chapter 36: *Bye Bye V-Card — Losing Your Virginity*. Here's why there's a separate chapter for your first intercourse:

On our sex survey, we've asked hundreds of women to compare how their first intercourse felt with how it feels now. While most of these women say it feels great now, it is an unusual woman who says she cherished her first intercourse, even if it was in a loving relationship.

In a study on first intercourse that included 659 college students, 79% of the men reported they had an orgasm, but only 7% of the women had an orgasm. Men had far more overall pleasure than women during their first intercourse. The mean age for first intercourse was 16½ years, although those who waited until they were 17 or older reported having a better experience than those who were younger. A year or two of added life experience can go a long way when you are only 15 or 16.

Both men and women experienced more pleasure if they had intercourse for the first time in a more serious or long-term relationship than in a casual or brief one. People who used alcohol during their first intercourse (about 30% of the total) had less pleasure and more guilt than those who did it sober. Those who used contraception reported more pleasure than those who didn't.

Who Sticks It In?

This may seem like a dumb thing, but the issue of who sticks the penis into the vagina can sometimes be significant.

"I generally prefer to put it in; otherwise we seem to miss a lot."
female age 32

"I like to put his penis in me because it seems no matter how many times we have had sex, he still misses a little bit when aiming. Also, I find it exciting to hold him while he thrusts into my vagina." *female age 23*

"She always does. No matter how many years we've been doing this, I still manage to miss!" *male age 43*

"He prefers to put it in, because if I do, he thinks I think he doesn't know where in the heck that hole is." *female age 38*

"It's really whoever grabs ahold first." *female age 36*

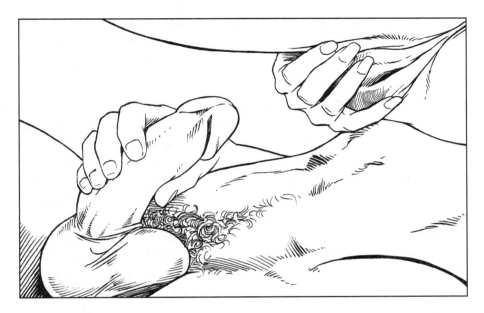

A rule of thumb is that either the woman, or the woman and man together, should stick it in the first few times. That's because only a woman knows when she is ready to have a penis inside, and all those years of inserting tampons have taught her exactly where the head of a penis needs to go.

Some women might be shy about grabbing a penis and guiding it in for a landing. This kind of reticence is silly but understandable. Once your penis-to-vagina guidance system is up and running, all bets are off regarding who puts the penis in. Whoever puts it in needs to make sure the woman truly wants it and her vagina is wet enough to take it.

If you are using lube and it starts to dry out, a drop or two of water or saliva will give it new life, while more lube will just gum things up. The women at Good Vibrations suggest keeping a water pistol handy for just this purpose, although women without humor will find this offensive, and wives of NRA members should be careful not to grab the Glock by mistake.

The First Thrust

In reading women's sex survey responses, an amazing pattern emerged. A large number of women said the part of intercourse they like best is the first stroke. For many women, it seems like the first stroke is a near religious experience, assuming they were fully aroused and eager for the thrusting to begin.

If you are a man, do not hesitate to ask your partner how she likes you to do your first stroke. Does she like you to start by teasing her with short little thrusts, going in only an inch or two? Or does she like one big straightforward glide for the gold?

Legs Bent or Straight, Open or Closed

The biggest variable in the physics of intercourse is often the position of the woman's legs—whether they are straight or bent, open or closed, over your shoulders or in your face. When a woman's legs are straight, penetration is not as deep, but the tip of her clitoris might receive more stimulation. When a woman bends her legs and brings her knees closer to her chest, the penetration is deeper. This can be nice if she likes more pressure in the back of her vagina.

If a woman's legs are together, the penis is hugged more snugly. This might create more clitoral stimulation, because the penis will push and pull on the inner labia with each thrust of intercourse (the inner labia are attached to the bottom of the clitoris.) If a woman's legs are apart, there is more skin-to-skin contact between her genitals and the man's genitals, and more bouncing-testicle action if he is on top.

Some couples enjoy intercourse with one leg straight and the other flexed. Some women keep their legs together while flexing their thighs to help achieve an orgasm. Many women stimulate their clitoris with their fingers during intercourse, and some push their clitoris against a partner's penis as it strokes in and out.

A woman's decision to keep her legs straight or bent might vary with the length and thickness of her partner's penis. A woman whose partner has a really long penis may find she gets poked in the cervix if she opens and bends her legs during intercourse, while a woman whose partner has a short penis might prefer the feeling of deeper penetration that bent knees allow.

Hopefully, you are getting the idea that there are many possibilities. You need experiment and find out what works best for you as a couple.

A Fix for When a Woman Feels Pain Due to Deep Penetration

There can be times during intercourse when a penis collides with the cervix, leaving a woman feeling like she's been punched in the stomach. Any woman who is experiencing sexual pain should consult with a gynecologist. But if it's determined the pain is from a penis hitting her cervix, there are things you might consider.

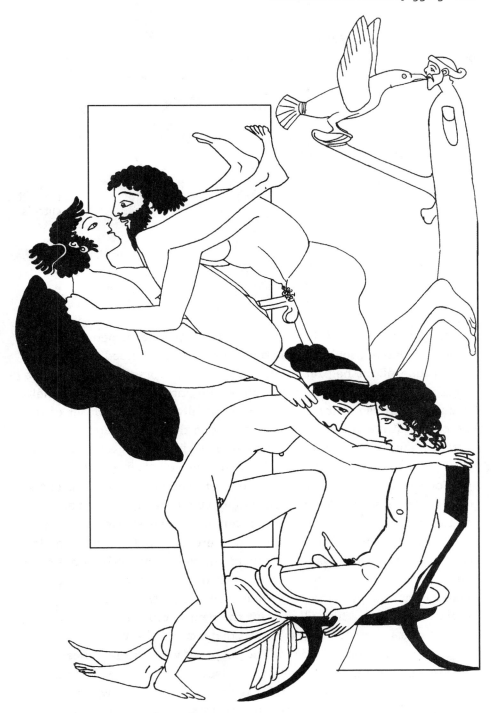

Intercourse in the old days.

Each couple's anatomy is different, so it's not possible to say which positions will be best.

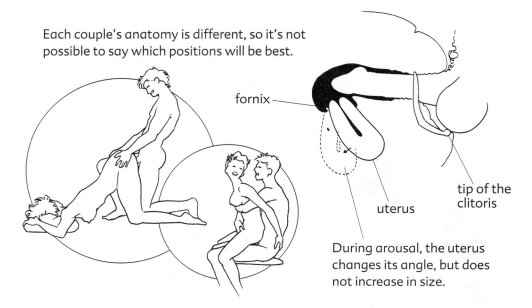

fornix

tip of the clitoris

uterus

During arousal, the uterus changes its angle, but does not increase in size.

It's not necessarily the biggest, baddest or longest penis that will cause this kind of problem. Sometimes it's an average sized penis. While adding lube might help, it might make things worse. Waiting until a woman is more highly aroused before starting intercourse may help, because an aroused cervix raises up, hopefully taking itself out of the line of fire. It may also help to try positions that discourage deep penetration, like rear entry when a woman is laying on her stomach or on her side with her body straight. Or, she might do better on top.

You can also jerry rig a donut or gasket to go around the base of the penis to decrease the depth of thrusting. One type of sleeve that some couples recommend is called a "universal silicone sleeve for a penis pump." While using this sleeve during intercourse was not its intended purpose, it can work well. Or, you might get a masturbation sleeve called "Maven" by Vibratex. Cut an inch or more off the end of it to make a donut-shaped ring that you can slide onto the base of the penis before intercourse. This will prevent the penis from thrusting too deep, and the extra pressure of the Maven material on the woman's clitoris can provide a welcome dividend. The people at **www.SexualityResources. com** recommend the Maven over other sleeves because the material can be cut without falling apart, and it is not so snug that it will act like a cock ring. Many of their female customers have this type of pain and this is the one solution they tend to rave about.

The male's pubic bone can push or grind against the clitoris in the missionary position, adding stimulation.

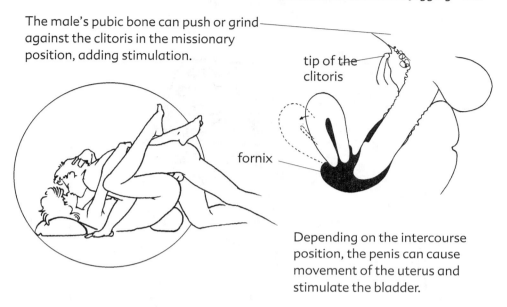

tip of the clitoris

fornix

Depending on the intercourse position, the penis can cause movement of the uterus and stimulate the bladder.

Thrusting—Shallow vs. Deep

The walls of the vagina change shape with each thrust of intercourse. This means that with each stroke, thousands of nerve endings are being pulled and tugged, which, neurologically speaking, can feel quite nice. (It doesn't feel half-bad for a woman's partner, either.)

There is a difference between the kind of nerve receptors in the first part of the vagina versus those in the back. The first inch of a woman's vagina is sensitive to touch. After that, it's more about pressure.

Because of its sensitivity to touch, stimulating the rim of an aroused vagina with a finger or the head of a penis can be a nice way to begin intercourse. Shallow thrusting allows the ridge around the head of the penis to stimulate this first part of the vagina. The art is in not pulling out too far and having your penis fall out. Another benefit of doing shallow thrusting is that the snuggest part of the vagina will wrap around the most sensitive part of the penis, which is just below the head.

Beyond the first inch, the vagina can feel stretching and pressure more than it feels touch. As a couple experiments with different positions, they will discover which parts of a vagina respond to pressure from the head of his penis. While the classic missionary position works well for many couples, others might benefit from some of the more exotic positions like the ones they show in Cosmo. (A problem with Cosmo is how they describe the more bizarre or gymnastically difficult

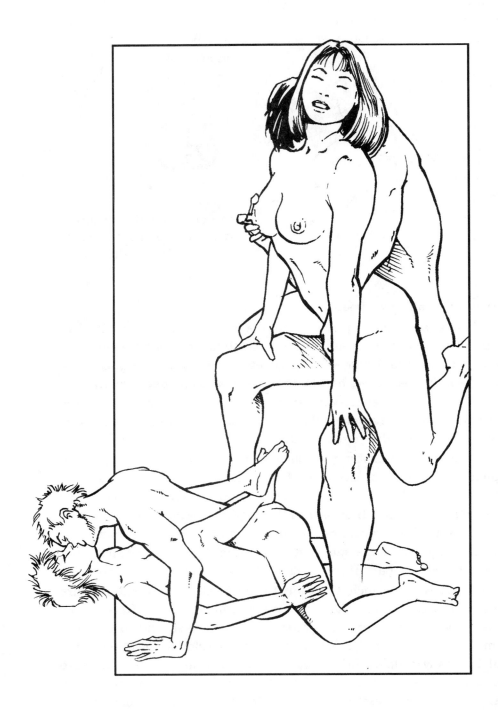

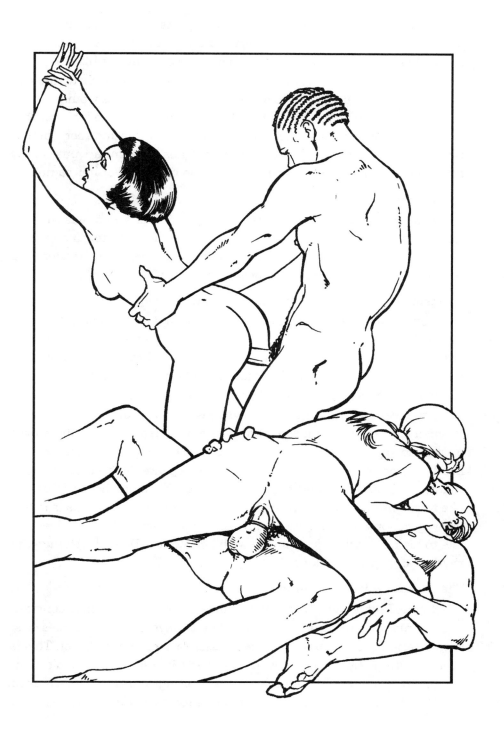

positions as being "advanced" or "for experts"—as if the missionary position is for losers. This is like criticizing a woman who is wearing a classic black dress and pearls for being unadventurous or plain.)

Deeper thrusting offers its own advantages: 1.) Deep thrusting can position a man's pubic bone to make better contact with a woman's clitoris; 2.) Deeper thrusting may allow the penis to pull on the labia minora (inner lips) longer with each stroke, providing more indirect stimulation to the clitoris; and 3.) As she approaches orgasm, a woman may find it pleasurable to have a penis filling the back part of her vagina.

Learning with His Fingers

A good way for a man to learn about his partner's vagina is with his fingers as well as with his penis. This will give him a better understanding of what needs to be done with his penis. (As one female reader says, "It wouldn't hurt for women to know this about themselves.")

Battering Ram or Pleasure Wand? Mosh Pit or Symphony?

Some men use a penis as a battering ram, believing women enjoy being slammed during intercourse. Other men, perhaps a bit more sensitive or experienced, realize there are different thrusting rhythms that can help make intercourse feel more symphonic than Screamo. Maybe she will like it slow at the start but strong at the end.

An excellent way to find out what works best during intercourse is when the woman is on top. That way a man can feel how she moves up and down on his penis and what parts of her vagina she focuses the head on. Does she move up and down on it repeatedly, or does she keep the penis deep inside and rub her clitoris on his pubic bone? Does she like to rub her breasts or clitoris with her fingers while a penis is inside her vagina, or would this be an unwelcome distraction? Where does she like to look, and what does she do with her mouth? Does she change the rhythm and speed, or does she keep it constant?

The Tantric Police Talk Thrust

Some Tantric and Oriental sex masters caution against constant deep thrusting during intercourse. They believe the vagina does best with a ratio of five to nine shallow thrusts to every deep thrust. This is an interesting observation, given how the Oriental masters don't allow women to be monks or to enter business meetings unless it's to bring tea. But they have no shortage of suggestions for pleasing women sexually.

If you are following the nine-shallow-for-every-one-deep thrust dictum, gradually increase the ratio to two deep for every four shallow, or live dangerously and go for one shallow to one deep.

Mixing up the thrusting between shallow and deep can be fun to experiment with. But if your partner starts threatening you with grief if you don't knock off the shallow stuff, you can safely assume she wasn't an Asian princess in a past life.

Intercourse as Your Private Language

Most couples have a variety of thrusting modes—hot and furious, fun and playful, giggly, tearful, passionate, powerful, passive, and maybe even angry. This becomes part of the private language that lovers share. So if you are feeling terminally reflective, you might think of intercourse as two separate acts: the thrusting part and the orgasm part. If the sole purpose of thrusting is to achieve orgasm, then intercourse might not have much emotional depth to it. That's because it is during the thrusting part of intercourse (before orgasm) when feelings of love, friendship and gratitude are often shared.

When a Penis Pops Out

During orgasm, the vagina can sometimes contract enough to expel a penis. When asked about this, most women advise, "Push it back in!"

Intercourse Without Thrusting

Some couples don't thrust during intercourse, but move their entire bodies in sync. Or the man might do a circular motion with his penis or pelvic bone grinding against the woman's genitals. Some couples stay really still during intercourse and try to coordinate their breathing. One partner breathes in at the moment the other breathes out.

Another way of enjoying intercourse without thrusting is to play "squeezing genitals." When the male squeezes his erect penis it momentarily changes diameter, and when the woman squeezes her vagina it hugs the penis—sometimes snugly and with memorable results.

Riding High

Each year a new book comes out that promises to reinvent the wheel sexually. One book talked about a radical "new" way of having intercourse. The couple starts by assuming the missionary position with the man on top. Right before the thrusting begins, Mr. Top makes a quick shift toward the head of the bed, like the Cowboys used to do at the line

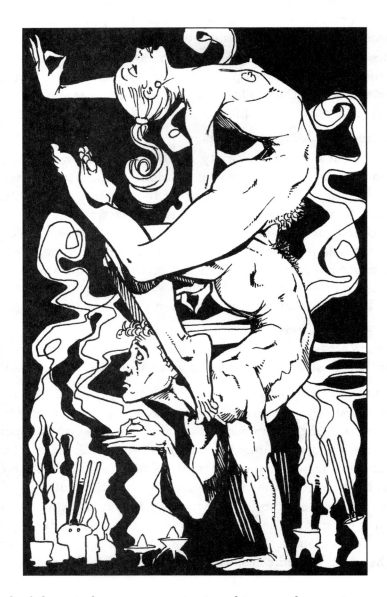

You don't have to be a yoga master to achieve peak experiences with breathing instead of thrusting. You don't even need to meditate or stand on your head. Just be in sync with each other, with one partner breathing in while the other breathes out.

of scrimmage before the set call, back when they were America's team and Tom Landry was coach. (Landry was one of the all-time greats.)

During the quick shift, the male pushes his entire body a couple of inches forward over the head of the woman. This puts him in the position of being able to say, "Honey, your roots are showing something awful," or "Time for a new weave." This new position also brings the man's penis in more direct contact with the woman's clitoris, assuming it doesn't cause his penis to snap off between the down-and-set-calls.

There is no in-out thrusting in this form of intercourse. The couple simply moves their hips back and forth in synchrony. This intercourse position attempts to maximize clitoral stimulation. Men who are sensitive lovers figured this one out long ago, although an occasional man may have had the knowledge forced upon him by a rambunctious lover who rode so low that she made him wonder if his penis would survive the night. Her riding low is the equivalent of his riding high.

Nasty Reflections—Gonzo Porn at Home!

Watching your genitals during intercourse can be an awesome way to pass time. There are positions that work well for this. A good-sized hand mirror can offer a nice view of genital play. Try using the magnifying side of the mirror. It will make you look huge! (A woman reader comments: "That's a frightening thought.")

Some couples use a phone instead of a mirror. They take a video of themselves when having intercourse and can watch it on a laptop or a desktop with a bigger display.

Kissing during Intercourse?

There's nothing nicer than kissing passionately when your genitals are locked in a loving embrace, but this isn't possible for some couples. If a woman is 5'1" and her partner is 6'4", there is no way her tongue is going to play inside his mouth when they are having intercourse.

This is one of the reasons why it is impossible to make recommendations regarding intercourse positions. Different couples come in different sizes. Some positions will feel better for lovers who are relatively the same height and of proportional weight, while those positions might be a disaster when a partner is really short and the other is really tall.

Certain positions will feel better or worse depending on the size and angle of your genitals, and some positions that feel best during the first part of a woman's menstrual cycle might not be the best during the later part of her cycle. And that's just physical differences. You also need to factor in each partner's psychological needs.

Intercourse When Standing?

To get an idea of how seldom couples have intercourse while standing, you might do a search of websites where amateur couples post clips of themselves having sex. The only time couples have intercourse while standing is when it's rear entry and the woman is able to lean forward on a piece of furniture or some sort of railing.

One of the problems with intercourse while standing and being face-to-face is that it can feel like a workout at the gym. Trying to thrust while bending your knees into a good angle can be tiring. Leaning against a wall can help, and some women say it works best for them if they can keep one leg firmly planted on the ground while tucking the other around a partner's waist. That way, they don't have to worry about a partner dropping them, and having the other leg up can improve the angle and amount of stimulation. He can help her hold it up.

In the Shower

You'd think that having intercourse in the shower would be as easy as shampooing your hair. Not so. While taking showers with a lover can be fun and incredibly sexy, having intercourse in the shower is a different story. The first concern is slipping, so if you're going to have intercourse in the shower, make sure you've got a non-slip shower mat or put down gripper fishies. You'll definitely want to install grab bars. Shower grab bars are easy to find and they aren't terribly expensive, but reviewers usually don't rate them for their sex worthiness.

Although water is wet, it washes away natural lubrication. So keep the stream of water away from your genitals. As for using sex lube, one little drop of silicone-based sex lube on the shower floor can make it treacherously slick, as in one thrust shy of a fractured femur. If you are using silicone lube, it is wise to apply it on before you get into the shower and while standing over a towel.

As for what position to use for shower sex, some couples find rear entry with the woman leaning forward can be the most practical. This is where the gripper bars begin to shine. Or you might consider doing what most couples do: enjoy showering together before or after you have intercourse in some other part of the house.

Signaling

Sex seldom works well when one partner is too passive or inhibited to let the other know what feels good and what doesn't. Fortunately, signaling during intercourse doesn't need to include words, because hands on a partner's hips or rear end can be great rudders. Try to work out a shared language that's based on signals that are easily understood.

How Women Have Orgasms during Intercourse

Women who have orgasms during intercourse seldom come by thrusting alone.

"I come faster sometimes when he's inside me, but I always have to rub my clit to climax." *female age 25*

"I rarely have orgasms with intercourse, unless I'm playing with myself at the time. The best way for me is oral sex or using a vibrator." *female age 36*

"I don't usually have orgasms during intercourse. In a very open relationship, I can have an orgasm after intercourse by manually stimulating my clitoris or by rubbing myself on his flaccid penis." *female age 26*

"I usually have them with intercourse if my husband is rubbing my clitoris or using a vibrator while he is thrusting. Sometimes when I am really excited, I can have one just with thrusting."
female age 35

More than 80% of the women from our sex survey who have orgasms during intercourse need to have their clitoris rubbed with fingers, by adding a vibrator, or by rubbing their clitoris on his pubic bone.

When Is Intercourse a Success?

Most people assume intercourse is a success if you give each other orgasms and a failure if you don't. Hardly. A woman can love the feelings she gets from intercourse, both emotional and physical, but still not have orgasms from it.

Intercourse needs to convey feelings between partners that are too primal for words alone. These feelings rest on the boundary between body and soul and are transmitted from one person to another in many different ways. If orgasm is part of that process, fine, but having an orgasm is no guarantee that anything special has taken place.

When is intercourse a success? When it leaves you feeling more solid, less grumpy, more able to face the day, and less afraid of the world when it's an overwhelming place. Intercourse is a success when it makes you feel more together and secure. It's a success when it's fun or satisfying and leaves you with a smile.

Intercourse is a failure when you wake up at three or four in the morning, look at the person who you had intercourse with and think "I wish I were home in my own bed, alone." This can be a particularly nasty dilemma if you are married or living together. Intercourse that conveys less pleasure than when someone leaves you a free hour on a parking meter is not necessarily worth having.

After Intercourse—The Drip Factor

Unless a guy is wearing a condom or pulls out and ejaculates to the side, he usually leaves semen inside a woman's vagina during intercourse. So where does the ejaculate go?

"Runs down your leg," says one female reader. "It usually drips out," replies another. "Like water in a cup that's turned upside down," says a third.

This might not be a problem if you are going to sleep, except for the wet spot on the mattress, but what if you had intercourse in the morning or at lunchtime?

"You can usually get it out in the shower" was one response, while another woman said, "Not true. It tends to drain out at its own pace, and all the showering in the world isn't going to hasten it along."

What if you already took a shower or don't want to take a shower just then?

"Sometimes I'll wear a panty liner," said one woman, "but it's not worth a tampon."

All of the women said they know of other women who douche right after intercourse even when they have sex at bedtime. Most thought this was silly and unnecessary. As one woman said,

"It's not dirty; I put the stuff in my mouth!" Another woman said, "I don't have sex with a man unless I really care about him. I find the occasional dripping to be a sweet and sometimes exciting reminder that he's been here."

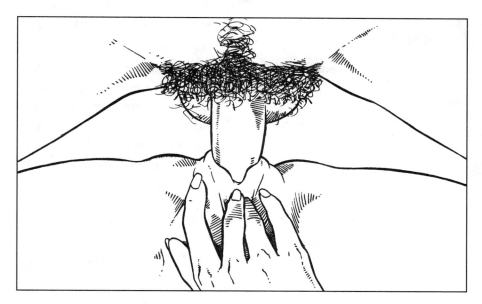

Of the five-thousand women who have taken our sex survey, the vast majority either need finger stimulation on their clit or they grind their clitoris into the pubic bone of their partner in order to have orgasms during intercourse. Few have orgasms from thrusting alone.

Top Dog

It has been said that people who always need to be on top during intercourse are insecure, while people who have it more together are happy to switch off. If this is true, then intercourse is no different from life in general. What's probably more true is the couple has tried it both ways and likes it better with one or the other of them on top. Also, feminists claim that intercourse follows a prostitute model of sex— once the male comes, the sex is over. If that's true in your relationship, work on finding ways to help the woman get her fair share of the pleasure.

Staying Inside After He Comes

Staying inside your lover after the thrusting is done can sometimes feel magical. Since most men lose their erections after coming, the two of you need to keep the fading member in while getting comfortable enough to stay in each other's arms. Some couples like to fall asleep this way. However, this is one of the downsides of using a condom. A man who is wearing a condom needs to pull out soon after he's come. Otherwise he might leave the condom inside his partner.

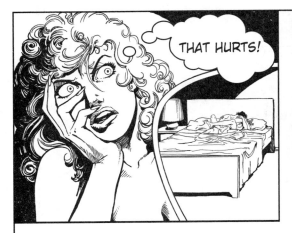

THAT HURTS!

This is what hurts when we have sex.

Women readers say men don't realize how much sex can hurt. They think porn is partly to blame, because women in porn never have pain. And when they do, the men get off on it. So here are some conversation starters for couples.

—Check any boxes that apply—

☐ If my vagina were ready for your penis the minute you get hard, we'd dispense with the kissing and conversation. Oh wait, what kissing and conversation?

☐ I would never use sandpaper on the head of your penis. But that's how it can feel when you randomly rub my clitoris.

☐ Nipples get hard from pain as well as pleasure. There are times when you grab my breasts and it causes a jolt of pain.

☐ Have you ever sucked on something the size of your penis for ten minutes without getting a sore jaw?

☐ I would like it if we could change positions ☐ more often or ☐ less often than we currently do.

☐ Many women say they have experienced pain or discomfort during anal sex. I feel the same way.

☐ If you want to get kinky, let's talk about it and explore it. But when you randomly slap my butt, it hurts!

☐ If I didn't like it the last ten times...

☐ I'll bet no one has ever hit the back of your throat with an erect penis. Yet you want to stick your penis down my throat?

☐ A facial? What if I collected your semen and dripped it in your eyes or smeared it on your face and chest?

☐ Has anyone tried to sneak a penis up your ass when you were having sex? I'll be happy to buy a dildo so you can experience what that feels like.

☐ It would be more exciting for me if you were ☐ more or ☐ less take-charge in bed.

☐ There's a difference between being assertive and having rough sex. If I want rough sex, I'll ask you for it.

☐ Please don't assume it feels good just because you saw it on Pornhub or read it online. Talk to me about it first.

☐ What if I rammed a finger up your butt every time you rammed a finger into my vagina?

☐ If you'll wait for me to tell you when I am ready for you to
_____
it will be more fun for both us.

☐ _____
_____

☐ _____
_____

If you experience pain every time you have sex, please see
Chapter 48: *Damn That Hurts! When Sex Is Painful.*

When a Man Can't Orgasm during Intercourse

Men who have trouble coming tend to pump faster during intercourse, hoping this will provide extra stimulation to help them ejaculate. This is a bad idea. The rapid thrusting desensitizes the penis, and it's possible his partner won't be able to walk right for a few days afterward. For more information, see Chapter 46: *Delayed Ejaculation.*

Passive Intercourse vs. Masturbation

Let's say a woman wakes up at 5:00 a.m., horny as heck, and would like to have intercourse. Her partner is not a morning person and is pretty much comatose until noon. Assuming he's not an early-morning grouch, he might allow her to stimulate his penis to a point of erection, or maybe he's already got an early-morning (REM-state) hard-on. The couple can then have intercourse in a position where he can be passive while she is active, or she massages her clitoris while his penis is inside of her. In a sense, she is using his penis as a dildo.

Or let's say it's nearly midnight and this woman's partner is feeling sexually amped, but she is dead to the world. She doesn't mind if he uses her vagina for intercourse, but doesn't want to have to fake being into it. So she allows him to have rear-entry intercourse.

Why didn't the horny partner just masturbate instead of bothering the one who is zoned out? Sometimes a partner honestly doesn't mind being "used" for sex as long as he or she isn't expected to get all turned on. He or she might even enjoy the other's pleasure. *As for having sex with a partner who is passed out or not able to give consent, this would be sexual assault.*

What's the Frequency, Dan?

When it comes to how often couples have intercourse, people who ask, "What's normal?" usually aren't asking the right question. If you are in a relationship, a better question is, "Do we have intercourse as often as each of us likes?" and "Do we have intercourse more often than one or both of us likes?" That's because what matters is what feels best for you—whether it's three times a day or three times a decade.

"Vaginal Wind"

When you ask women what's your most embarrassing moment during sex, many will say it's when they've had a vaginal fart. The official term for this is "vaginal flatulence," although this type of acoustical

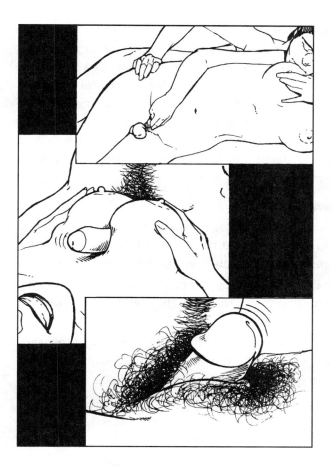

Alternatives to Penis-Inside-of-Vagina

From top down: intercourse between the thighs; intercourse between the breasts; and femoral intercourse, which is where the penis slides between the lips or labia without going into the vagina.

event is more commonly known as a queef, beaver burp, muff music, or a fanny fart when the woman is British.

Regarding the physics, think of the vagina as a bagpipe between a woman' legs. Air can collect in the vagina during intercourse and then belch out. This can also happen during exercise or yoga as well as during sex. The medical term for when sex is not involved is "vaginal wind."

Some women can produce vaginal flatulence on command, with the adeptness of middle schoolers in a burping contest. Because there is no way a woman can contract the opening of her vagina to modulate the outflow of air, vaginal flatulence will sound more like a fog horn or tuba than a tea kettle. Unlike gas coming from the rear end, vaginal flatulence shouldn't smell because the vagina is simply spitting out air that's accumulated inside of it rather than acting as a portal for foul winds. If vaginal flatulence smells or huts, consult with a gynecologist.

Pillow Power during Intercourse

Never underestimate the power of a pillow under the small of the back or rear end of the partner who is on the bottom. Changing the angle of the hips can change a person's experience of intercourse. If you like intercourse from the rear, keep a lookout for the perfect bigger pillow that will provide support and raise the woman's rear end to an angle that is comfortable and inviting. You might try bolsters and different kinds of cushions, including wedges with waterproof covers made specifically for sex.

Doing It in Different Environments

If intercourse is seeming a bit stale, it might help to scout out new locations. While it never hurts to try a resort on a tropical island or a four-star hotel in Europe, most of us will need to aim more modestly:

The Kitchen: Always a fine place for intercourse until you have children. After the kids reach school age, the kitchen is once again game for an occasional nooner.

The Yard: It's a shame to spend all that effort making the grass grow and never have sex on it—although local ordinances may prohibit using your yard for doing more with a weiner than barbecuing it.

In Front of the Fireplace: There's nothing like doing it in front of the fireplace, until you get wet pine instead of seasoned oak and a slew of hissing, burning embers showers your naked bodies.

In Water: Hot tubs, bathtubs, pools, and other bodies of water can be great places for people to do all sorts of nasty things. But intercourse in water washes away natural lubrication. Another solution is to bury the penis inside the vagina while both sets of organs are outside the water and decrease the length of each thrust once you are submerged.

Sex at the Office: A reader who is a commercial-real-estate agent has keys to some of the finest high-rise buildings. When he and his GF want a dramatic change of scenery, they visit the upper floors.

Candlelight: The candle excels at creating erotic ambiance. Make sure the wax doesn't drip on your carpet. (According to a reader who has been there: fold a paper towel a few times and place it over the cooled wax on the carpet. Then put a warm to hot iron on top of the paper towel. It will melt the wax into the towel.) As for stains from wet spots on lighter colored carpets, blame them on the family dog.

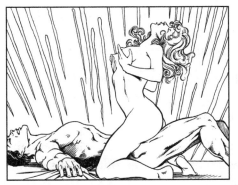

Warning! Fun But Be Smart About It
Intercourse injuries can cause a penis to forever bend in a strange way. Most of these injuries occur when a woman is on top and, strangely enough, when a man is having an affair with someone other than his primary partner. The woman should be well-lubricated and avoid or going too high and then exuberantly slamming down on her partner's penis on the downstroke. Putting a pillow under the man's butt can help make his pelvic bone more accessible so a woman can enjoy grinding against his pelvic bone for extra stim instead of using his penis like a pogo stick. She can also try squeezing his penis with her vagina, like when she is peeing and tries to stop the flow.

Intercourse Odds'N'Ends

Some couples enjoy using a vibrator during intercourse. This can work in any number of positions, or you can get artsy and try doing it like the couple in Chapter 29: *Oscillator, Generator, Vibrator, Dildo.*

A woman who is on top and facing a man's feet can watch his penis go in and out of her vagina, especially with a mirror or she can videotape it with her phone.

Rear-entry positions allow the head of the penis to focus on different parts of the vagina than missionary positions. Rear entry also provides extra padding, which can be welcome if you are really bony.

Rather than thrusting, some couples find that rocking back and forth with a penis inside to be a pleasant alternative.

Rather than inserting the penis inside a vagina, some couples enjoy a lubricated penis moving between her labia, like a hot dog going back and forth through a bun. The ridge around the head of the penis glides back and forth over the clitoris (aka "femoral intercourse).

In the highly recommended book *Tricks - More Than 125 Ways to Make Good Sex Better,* author Jay Wiseman suggests that the man lies on his back and the woman places a pair of her panties over his penis.

The penis sticks through a leg hole, with the panties draping down over his testicles and between his legs. The couple has intercourse with the woman on top. The material might stimulate him with each stroke.

☻ Some couples find a well-trimmed and freshly bathed big toe to be a fun penis substitute. Also, a heel that's jiggled back and forth can provide a solid way to stimulate a woman's genitals.

☻ There are couples who like to bite each other's shoulders or run their teeth along each other's skin while having intercourse. This works best when the skin is well-lubricated.

☻ Some lovers prefer the feeling of intercourse after a woman has had an orgasm rather than before.

☻ Women might not lubricate very well for the first couple of months following pregnancy, especially when while nursing.

☻ Extra lubrication may be necessary if the woman is using drugs such as antihistamines, alcohol, or pot, or if the man is wearing a condom.

☻ Some couples take an intercourse break to have oral sex; some do oral sex afterward.

☻ Why not try feeding each other while having intercourse? That's what nature created papaya for.

☻ Some couples enjoy a finger, thumb, vibrator, or butt plug on or in each other's anus during intercourse.

☻ Most sex stores sell vibrating cock rings that fit over a man's penis and provide extra stimulation to the woman's clitoris when she rubs up against his pubic bone. There are also small vibrators in harnesses that can be strapped over the clitoris to use during intercourse.

☻ Positions where you are sitting upright might allow more blood to pool in your pelvic regions, which could help some men get better erections and women receive more vaginal engorgement. These include positions where the man sits on a chair and the woman sits in his lap, wrapping her legs around his waist, or where he sits in the chair and she sits on his lap but is facing away from him.

Betty On Intercourse

What better way to wind down a chapter on intercourse than with a few passages from Betty Dodson's book *Sex for One?* These refer to what transpired during Ms. Dodson's sex groups for women.

On Pretending You're a Guy during Intercourse "One amusing and informative exercise was called 'Running a Sexual Encounter.' It involved reversing sex roles with the women on top. We made believe that our clitorises were penetrating imaginary lovers, and we had to do all the thrusting. I would set the egg timer for three minutes, a little longer than the Kinsey national average. As the fucking began, I would participate and at the same time comment on everyone's technique. 'Keep your arms straight; don't crush your lover. You're too high up; your clitoris just fell out. Don't stop moving, you'll lose your erection. Don't move so fast; you'll come too soon. And don't forget to whisper sweet things in your lover's ear between all those passionate kisses.'

"Watching the egg timer, I coordinated my theatrical orgasm with the ding of the bell, frantically thrusting for the last ten seconds. Then, falling flat on my imaginary lover, I muttered, 'Was it good for you?' and promptly began snoring loudly. It was always hysterically funny. Panting and exhausted, the women all exclaimed, 'How do men do it?' Complaints included tired arms, lower-back pain, and stiff hip joints. Most of the women had fallen out long before the bell went off. After that, there was always more empathy for men, and the women showed an increased interest in other positions for lovemaking."

Odds & Ends "Some of the women talked about experiencing pain with deep thrusting intercourse, while others claimed to want a hard fuck. In my youth, I'd confused hard pounding intercourse with passion, and experienced internal soreness afterward.... While I enjoyed a strong fuck when we were two equal energies in sync, I also loved the slow intense fuck."

"Another problem the women complained of was lack of lubrication and the pain of dry intercourse. Some women felt inadequate if they weren't wet with passion. My experience varied;

sometimes I lubricated when I wasn't even thinking about sex. Other times I could be dry even though I felt sexually aroused..."

On Orgasms "Some women had good orgasms with oral sex but not with intercourse. Others could come with intercourse but couldn't get off alone. Still others were having orgasms with themselves but not with a partner. All of the orgasmic women agreed on one thing: Their experiences of orgasm varied greatly from one orgasm to the next."

—From *Sex for One* by Betty Dodson, Harmony Books.

Readers' Comments

What are some of your favorite intercourse positions?

"My favorite position is doggy style, with me on my hands and knees, and him behind me. I like this best for two reasons: my vagina is tighter this way, and I can easily rub my clitoris and have an orgasm. I also love to sit on a guy while he is sitting up. This just feels wonderful. Our bodies are so close." *female 26*

"Good old missionary, with me on the bottom and him on top!" *female age 32*

"One of my favorite positions is sitting in his lap in a chair. He can kiss my neck or armpits, which drives me nuts, and I can move freely. If we are on the bed, I can also lie back and touch my clit if I want." *female age 38*

"My favorite position is sitting on top of him. That way I can stroke my clitoris or I can watch him do it." *female age 43*

"I like it best when we're doing it doggy style and I hold the vibrator and rub my clit with it. The sensation is wonderful!" *female age 25*

"I enjoy having him on top but recently discovered that if we lie on our sides with me in front and I throw my upper leg over his, he can enter me from behind and it's very exciting." *female 45*

"I like to be on my back with my legs up while he is on his knees entering me and rubbing my clitoris. We started using this position when I was pregnant and I still like it best." *female 35*

"I like to bend over a table and have my partner insert his penis from behind. We get great penetration this way, and he is also able to hit something in there that makes me feel really good!"

female age 34

What do you like the most, and least, about intercourse?

"Worst part: the big wet spot. Best part: making the big wet spot."

female age 27

"It is wonderful when we first start having intercourse and I love the cuddling after. I don't like how, if you don't clean up afterward, the ejaculate runs out of you (sometimes cold) and drips down your butt onto the sheets." *female age 30*

"I like it when he first inserts his penis into my vagina the best. The thing I like least about sex is having to really work for a long time to get him to orgasm when he's had too much to drink." *female age 34*

"I like the beginning the most and orgasm, of course. If somebody takes too long, the middle gets dull." *female age 25*

"The first moments of penetration are the best. The wet spot on the bed, the worst." *female age 44*

"The part I like best is when my man spends a long time getting me hot until I want him so badly I can't wait and he finally sinks his penis into me. It's such a relief to finally be joined together. I like it least when he enters too soon and comes too fast and says, 'I'm sorry' when I had my hopes up for more."

female age 38

"I love feeling him on top of me, kissing and caressing, and I love the feeling of his penis inside me. The part I don't like is the mess." *female age 35*

Top Notch Resources: It's explicit and excellent, showing real-life couples: Jamye Waxman's *101 Positions for Lovers* from Adam and Eve.

Fun, funny and perceptive—Sadie Allison's *Ride 'Em Cowgirl! Sex Position Secrets For Better Bucking*, Tickle Kitty.

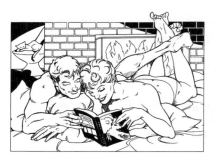

Dear Dr. Paul,

My new boyfriend is wonderful and I really want to have sex with him. But he's huge-porn sized and then some. I'm only 5' 2" and I'm worried he won't fit. I've had intercourse with other guys, with no problem, but he's bigger than the biggest. Do you have any advice?

Bambi

Dear Bambi,

Yes, I have advice.

One of the dumbest things people tell women with partners who are really big is "a baby can pass through your vagina…" Seriously? Have you ever heard a woman in labor who's trying to push a baby through her vagina? Intercourse isn't supposed to be like that.

As for your height and weight, I'm not so sure that's a factor. I interviewed a woman who is as petite as can be. Her husband's penis is in the 98th percentile for size, and she's never had any problem with intercourse. But another woman who is 5' 10" might have trouble with a penis that's even average size. So you can't predict.

I am assuming you have had a recent exam and have talked to a gynecologist about this. If there is a source of pain that is independent of your partner's penis, it is essential you resolve it first. Then I would suggest you and Thor call it quits on any attempts at intercourse for the next month or two. There are lots of ways you can please each other sexually besides intercourse. The illustration on page 269 shows how you get him off orally without dislocating your jaw.

Also learn to give him handjobs that are beyond anything he's ever experienced before. Do a browser search for "erotic massage." As for fitting his penis into your vagina, consider working on some or all of the following during your vacation from attempts at having intercourse:

1. Have your partner squirt a generous amount of sex lube on his fingertips. He can gently clasp the outer lips of your genitals between his thumb and forefinger and do a small circular massage on one area at a time. Tell him what feels good and what doesn't. He should massage as deeply as is comfortable for you, then move to an adjoining spot. His goal is not to stretch the skin, but to get the blood circulating deep

inside of the folds. He should do your entire genitals, including the outer lips and inner lips. (Guys of all sizes can do this kind of massage!)

2. When you are highly aroused, he can gently insert a well-lubricated finger into your vagina and rest it there. If it feels okay, he might insert a second finger and eventually a third. Breathe deep and work on relaxing your vagina when his fingers are in. He or you should then try stimulating your clitoris while his fingers are still inside your vagina. Having an orgasm with his fingers inside of you can help train your vagina to allow a penis that's bigger than it's used to.

3. If it's comfortable, the two of you can practice what midwives and obstetricians call "perineal massage." He inserts a well-lubricated thumb into the opening of your highly aroused vagina and rests it there. His forefinger should be on the outside, resting on the skin that's between your vulva and anus. He then clasps the tissue that's between his thumb and forefinger and massages it as well as gently pushing down. This stimulates the part of your vagina that stretches wider when you have intercourse. The ceiling of a vagina doesn't stretch very much, as the pubic bone is right above it. It's the part that's next to your bum that stretches. (Do a browser search for "perineal massage.")

The two of you should do steps 1 to 3 at least a couple of times a week until the floor of your vagina can more easily relax.

4. You might also try what's called "femoral intercourse," but it isn't intercourse at all. It is where your partner lies on his back and you lube up his penis and the lips of your vulva. You then straddle him and ride back and forth along the length of his well-lubed penis as it is lying against his belly. Think of your vulva as being like a hotdog bun, and his penis is like a Ballpark Frank. You slide up and down the length of the dog, enjoying the sensations without him trying to steal home. Be sure to use birth control. His penis is not going into your vagina, but he's going to ejaculate near the opening of your vagina and that's reason enough to call out the contraceptives. (You can also do femoral intercourse with him on top or from behind.) Since you are in complete control, it can be helpful if you learn to give yourself orgasms this way, or at least enjoy the sensations.

5. Consider purchasing two or three dildos that range in size from small to large. Start by lubing up your vagina and the smallest dildo.

Once you become comfortable inserting the dildo and moving it around inside your vagina, try the next size. But never move up to the next bigger size until you are completely comfortable with the current one. This should be done over several weeks and not all in one night. Try having an orgasm with the dildos inside your vagina.

6. Once you are comfortable with these steps, have your partner rest the head of his well-lubed penis against the opening of your vagina, but to go no farther. A day or two later, have him move in about a quarter-of-an-inch if it is comfortable for you. Try another quarter of an inch as long you feel comfortable with it. Stop if you feel pain.

As for intercourse positions, you'll want to be really conservative. Stay with the classic missionary position where you are on your back and your legs are slightly spread. Avoid rear-entry positions and stay away from anything where your legs are flexed. Flexing your knees will compress or shorten the available thrusting space in your vagina. Also, having an orgasm before intercourse help to relax your vagina.

To prevent pain that's associated with deep-thrusting, your BF can put his fist or a gasket around the base of his penis. This can shorten the plunging depth. (To make a gasket, cut an inch or two off the end of a masturbation sleeve called The Maven.)

If none of this helps, you might try finding a physical therapist who specializes in pelvic pain, or accept the fact that his penis isn't going to fit. Learn to have great sex by getting each other off in other ways besides intercourse. You might end up having a better sex life than a lot of couples who can have intercourse.

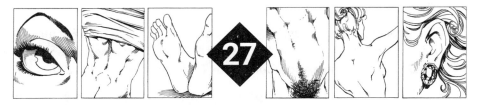

Surfing the Crimson Wave
From Period Gear to Period Sex

There aren't many men who have had to ask a friend to check the back of their pants because they were afraid period blood was soaking through. And no guy has ever had to change a pad or tampon during a five-minute break between classes—all while acting like nothing is up so they didn't have to risk being ridiculed for having their period.

But instead of being thankful about not having periods, guys sometimes behave like dorks when it comes to menstruation. Perhaps this is the price we pay for sending young men out of the room during discussions about menstruation. We turn a fact of life into a mystery.

Another fact of life is that once you are in a relationship, periods impact both of you. That's why this chapter was written—to help explain the nuts and bolts of menstruation to men and to help encourage discussions between partners about everything from back aches and cramps to period flow and period sex.

Nearly 20% of the Women You Know Are Having a Period Right Now

At this moment, nearly 20% of all non-pregnant women between the ages of 15 and 50 are having their periods. That's one-in-five. When you put it in that perspective, it's hard to understand why anyone would think there's something unusual or embarrassing about periods. It's also important to know that a woman's intellectual or job performance is not affected by her menstrual cycle. Plenty of women have won Olympic medals and recorded platinum songs while having periods.

The Pad and Tampon Wars

Two young boys walk into a pharmacy one day, pick out a box of tampons, and proceed to the checkout counter. The man at the counter asks the older boy, "Son, how old are you?"

"Eight," the boy replies.

The man continues, "Do you know what these are used for?"

"Not exactly," the boy says. "But they aren't for me. They're for him. He's my brother. He's four. We saw on TV that if you use these you would be able to swim and ride a bike. Right now he can't do either."

Over the years, advertising for period gear has not been the smartest. For instance, here's a dreadful Kotex ad from seventy years ago:

Mothers—Why get all involved trying to explain the facts of menstruation to your little girls when there's a simple, easy way to do this dreaded task? Let the new booklet "As One Girl To Another" do this job for you! It will spare you a session that may only end in confusion, and embarrassment.

Fortunately, advertising for pads and tampons has not been all bad. As you can see from the story about the boy wanting to get tampons for his younger brother, period-gear advertising has helped put to rest the long held notion that women's bodies are weaker than men's because they have periods:

Every Day of the Month Is a Day of Freedom. —*Tampax, 1936*

Don't Give Up Athletics Any Day of the Month. —*Tampax, 1939*

Why let trying days of the month rule your life? You don't need time-out... That is, if you choose Kotex sanitary napkins.
                                                            —*Kotex, 1942*

Long before feminism, ads for period gear were telling women their bodies and brains were not inferior to men's as long as they bought the right pad or tampon.

From Evil Spirits to Modern Science

Blood has freaked people out since the beginning of time. We see it as a sign of injury or disease. So instead of viewing menstrual flow as being normal and natural, period blood has often been interpreted as a sign that something wong was going on inside of a woman's body. Aristotle said periods were a sign that women's bodies were not fully developed, because if they had been, women would have started to produce semen during puberty instead of blood. In some cultures, menstruation was thought to be the work of spirits, and there must have been times when women wondered if spirits hadn't taken over their bodies during their periods. Some still do.

cervix. The percent of blood in menstrual flow can range from very little to around 70%, depending on what day during a woman's cycle it is. This can also vary from woman to woman and from cycle to cycle, as can the thickness of the flow.

Some men and women believe that period flow is caused by the walls of the vagina shedding. This is not correct. Vaginal secretions can contribute to period flow, but the vagina is by no means the source of period flow. This is why it's safe to have period sex as long as a woman feels like it and does not have a blood borne disease.

Period Facts

👁 Women are told that the normal time for a cycle is 28 days, with the duration of bleeding from 4 to 6 days. That would be fine if one size fit all, but for many women cycles range from 21 to 32 days. The time between periods can be the same from cycle to cycle, or it can be all over the place. The duration of bleeding can vary as well.

👁 The total amount of flow during an average period is about 1/4 of a cup or 4 to 6 tablespoons. This is way less than most people think. However, women don't calculate period flow with tablespoons or cups. They usually quantify their menstrual bleeding with how many tampons or pads they use.

👁 Period cramps are related to labor pains. Both are mediated by prostaglandins. Inflammation can make them worse, which is why anti-inflammatories such as aspirin, ibuprofen or naproxen can help with cramps. The trick is in taking them a day or two before you think your cramps will begin. Birth-control pills can also help decrease cramping.

👁 Orgasms can help relieve cramps and period pain. They pump pain relievers into the body and the contractions can help push accumulated fluids out of the uterus. Still, can you imagine a mother telling her daughter, "Honey, if you're having cramps, why not masturbate?"

👁 The faster period blood drips out, the more red it's going to be. The slower it drips out, the darker it might be. That's because when period blood flows more slowly, it spends a longer time in the upper part of the vagina and becomes oxidized, which can result in its turning brownish. The reason why period blood often looks brown on pads is because it has mixed with oxygen and has oxidized. When period blood comes out really slowly, it can look like a dark, tar-like paste.

The book's gyno consultant said that when there's heavy flow, she likes to see clotting, because it means the body is working to decrease the amount of bleeding. It concerns her when there's a lot of bright red blood that is thin like Koolaid and has no clots in it. As a woman gets older, "she'll start to shed tissue from the lining that looks like 'strings' of tissue."

After a woman turns 40 or so, the volume of flow might increase, but for only 1 to 3 days rather than the whole time. There might be more clumps, as well.

If you are concerned about any of this beyond the basic annoyance that it has to happen to you, be sure to ask a healthcare provider!

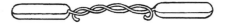

Some of the Things Girls Want to Know about Periods

Girls in their teens want to know how to control the flow, how to make cramps and backaches disappear, how to get stains out of their underwear, pajamas and sheets, how to predict when their periods will arrive and to know how heavy they will be. They want to know how to carry period gear inconspicuously and how to deal with embarrassing moments when boys find out they are having their period.

When girls get older and become sexually active, they might want to know more about period sex, and no matter how young or old they are, women frequently wonder "Why does this just happen to us and not guys?" Women also wonder why they're the ones who have to pay the cost of period gear, a financial burden that few guys appreciate until they become the fathers of teenage daughters.

Positive Things about Periods

Periods give girls a chance to share information about their bodies at a time when parents still refer to female genitals as "down there" and a lot of teenage girls don't even know what their clitoris is. Sharing experiences about periods can also be a source of bonding, not to mention an outlet for personal horror stories like when the hottest guy on the planet got behind you in the checkout line after you had just put a gigantic box of Kotex on the conveyer belt.

Period Parties & "You Are Becoming a Woman"

A lot of mothers today are framing a girl's first period as an important milestone in a girl's life. Some moms take their daughters out to a special lunch or dinner, and some even have parties—which might be a bit much as far as some daughters are concerned. But if parents feel the need to mortify their kid with a cake and party to celebrate their daughter's first period, at least it's a step in the right direction.

As for the cake itself, do you stay with a classic white cake or do you make a bold statement and go with a red velvet? What color frosting do you use, and do you decorate it with marzipan pads and tampons?

As for saying that a girl has "become a woman" after her first period, that seems to be stretching it a bit when you consider how early girls are having their periods. To think that an 11- or 12-year-old girl in Western culture has reached womanhood begs a reality check. A girl's first period marks an important biological passage, but it's more reasonable to think of her high-school graduation as a transition into womanhood.

One of the most significant passages a first period marks is it allows a girl to enter into the same "club" that her mom, friends and older sisters are in. This can be empowering and socially important. Some girls who have their first period later than their friends feel left out of this "club" and can't wait to join it—until they start having their periods.

For First-Time Tampon Users

"I didn't realize the cardboard was supposed to come out (while the cotton wad stays in). It was a rather uncomfortable first hour, 'til I finally asked a girlfriend 'What the hell?'"*female age 28*

"I mostly use pads, but they used to get stuck in my pubic hair. OUCH! Tampons are only useful for pools and hot tubs, otherwise it feels really weird walking around feeling like you have a soft dick stuck in you all day." *female age 21 [The soft dick feeling could be happening because she isn't pushing the tampon in far enough.]*

"Pads were so horrid, even though I used them for many years. They were just so gross, it felt like wearing a diaper, but I could never get the hang of applicator tampons, so I just used pads.

When I got to college we got a free trial pack of OB applicator-less tampons and I fell in love instantly and have never looked back!" *female age 20*

"I hated pads because I felt gooey and gross when I wore them. The blood never absorbs like the commercials say it does. I hurt the first couple of times I put a tampon in, and had to force it, but eventually that stopped and I didn't have a problem any-more." *female age 21*

"I never had a problem using tampons, and I hate it when my pubic hair gets stuck to the bloody pad. YUCK. So I'm a tampon girl—though I have to use the slim kind, as the larger ones hurt."
female age 20

A number of female readers have reported strange or painful expe-riences when they first tried using a tampon, including trying to pull out the tampon while it was still dry. This probably resulted from wearing a higher absorbency tampon than was needed and the tampon ended up sticking to the sides of their vagina. Tampons come in a couple of absor-bencies. While guys might think "Get the biggest and baddest tampon you possibly can," it' best not to use a tampon that is more absorbent than you need. And always be sure to read the directions, especially about how often to change them.

When a Woman Drops a Tampon

Researchers did a study where a woman "accidentally" dropped either a tampon that was still in its wrapper or a hair clip on the ground. They asked people who viewed the woman dropping the objects what they thought about her. When she dropped a tampon, the woman was considered to be less competent and less likeable than when she dropped the hair clip. It's not like she dropped a used tampon, not that it should matter. To this day, people still have issues with periods. (What do you think the response would have been if she had dropped a condom?)

Cycle-Related Breast Tenderness

Some women's breasts get really sore when they are having their period. Other women experience breast soreness at a different time, like when they are ovulating. Period-related breast soreness can be slight, or it can be so extreme that just driving over speed bumps can hurt. Some women say their breasts will feel like they are bruised. Both breasts can become tender, or just one. Breast tenderness can be helped by taking birth-control pills, or it can be caused by taking birth-control pills. Some women find that anti-inflammatories such as aspirin, ibuprofen or naproxen are helpful. Talk to your gynecologist about it.

Breasts can also become sensitive in a way that welcomes kisses and caresses during certain times of the month. So if you are in a relationship, breast tenderness is important to talk about.

Tips for Having Period Sex!

Some couples prefer not to have period sex. But for those who do, here are some tips and suggestions:

Some couples say the flow feels better than store-bought lube. Others need to add store-bought lube for period sex. That's because a woman's estrogen level tanks during her period, which can result in less natural lubrication.

A woman's cervix drops when she's having her period, so you might find certain positions are better for period sex. Explore and see what feels best for you.

Some women get extra-horny during their periods. This might have to do with a change in hormones, or perhaps they feel more relaxed since it's harder to get pregnant. Menstrual swelling can also help some women have a really nice orgasm.

Some couples are cool being coated with period flow; others act like they've arrived at a crime scene. You can vary your flow exposure with the following:

Use a Softcup or Flex Disc that catches the flow as it drips from the cervix and can't be felt during sex.

Put a towel down to catch the flow, or have shower sex.

If intercourse during periods isn't for you, you can always get each other off by hand, with a vibrator or dildo. Orgasms can help ease period pain.

👓 Anal sex can be an option if both of you enjoy it, but it's hard to think that a woman who enjoys anal sex would have a problem with vaginal sex while she's on her period.

👓 DO NOT wear a tampon during intercourse!

Tips for receiving oral sex while on your period:

👓 Use a Softcup, Flex Disc, Menstrual Cup or Diaphragm. These will collect the flow so it doesn't run through a vagina. Some women get a diaphragm for the sole purpose of having period sex. While menstrual cups like the Diva Cup are great for oral sex, they aren't good for intercourse because they sit in the vaginal canal.

👓 Splash some water into your vagina, then insert a tampon before a partner goes down on you. The tampon will catch most of the flow. If intercourse follows, be sure to take the tampon out first.

👓 Cover the outside of a woman's genitals with a barrier or plastic wrap. A little lube between plastic wrap and her genitals might help.

👓 Some guys like going down, period flow and all.

Reader Comments about Period Sex

"I enjoy it but it tends to gross me out. It's different, more sensitive and I tend to orgasm faster." *female age 32*

"Period sex helps with cramping. I feel fat and ugly but know that when I cum my cramps will feel much much better/be gone." *female age 27*

"I prefer not to, because it's messy, and I can smell the blood, which I really don't like." *female age 34*

"Period sex definitely feels different. It feels heavier, more solid, and the pleasure from penetration is usually heightened somewhat. I'm usually a bit hornier when I'm on my period. I love having sex in the shower—don't have to worry about cleanup!"

female age 23

"Period sex feels gross and nasty, too wet." *female age 19*

"I am always really horny when I am on my period, so I kind of enjoy it. However, I feel like ironically I dry out quicker." *fem 21*

"It kind of burns when I have period sex." *female age 31*

"I love having period sex even though it's kinda gross. It's way different. It just feels much better." *female age 25*

You can get pregnant from period sex, although the chances are often lower than at other times. You can get sexually transmitted infections like hepatitis or HIV from period blood if a woman has those infections, even if she shows no symptoms.

Period Gear That Works for Intercourse

The Softcup and Flex Disc are period flow collection devices that a woman inserts with her fingers into the back of her vagina. They collect period flow as it drips from the cervix so it doesn't go through the vagina. Unlike menstrual cups and tampons, the Softcup and Flex Disc can be a good choice for intercourse during periods because they don't intrude into the vaginal canal.

Menstrual Cups—A Cross between a Diaphragm and A Shot Glass

A menstrual cup is a soft, flexible container made of silicone rubber or latex that is inserted into the vagina to collect period flow. Once it's in place, it forms a seal that allows it to collect the blood. It looks a bit like a small, upside-down funnel, although the stem is not hollow and the body of the cup is more rounded than a funnel. Menstrual cups should not be used for intercourse, but they will keep period flow out of the vagina for oral sex. There are a number of different brands of menstrual cups. Each has a slightly different length, softness and stem.

A lot of women who are devoted users say they originally thought the concept of a menstrual cup was gross or disgusting. But they experienced so many advantages in using menstrual cups that they wouldn't think of going back to pads or tampons. According to users, here are some of the advantages:

☻ Unlike a tampon, which absorbs the natural secretions of the vagina in addition to period flow, a menstrual cup collects only period flow. As a result, it won't dry out a vagina.

👓 A lot of users don't get the kind of leaking that they do with tampons. With less leaking, the chances are lower that a woman's underwear will be stained.

👓 Some cup users say they experience less cramping than when they used tampons, and no more late-night runs to the store to buy tampons or pads.

Making Your Own Custom Pads

It's fairly easy to sew custom period pads. They look great and help save landfill space. There are a number of websites that have patterns and show how to make pads. Enter "period gear" in the search box at www.Guide2Getting.com.

Period Suppression

Period suppression refers to a woman preventing her period from happening by ditching the placebo week of birth-control pills or keeping her NuvaRing in for all four weeks instead of for just three. (You should never attempt this without first discussing it with your gynecologist. It will work with only certain pills or other hormonal methods and there might be health concerns that could make it a bad idea.) The hormone-releasing IUD can also cause a decrease in a woman's periods.

There is still a lot of debate about the safety of period suppression. There are theories that nature never intended women to constantly have monthly periods because women were pregnant so often or were nursing infants. The reasoning goes that having as many periods as women do today is not good for you. Other theories claim that a monthly fluctuation in hormones that happens with periods is good for a woman's body and is one of the reasons why women outlive men by five years or so. There are also concerns about the impact of period suppression on bone health, which could vary from woman to woman.

While menstrual suppression appears to be safe, we don't have the kind of long-term studies yet to help seal the deal.

Tipped Uterus Considerations

Some women with a tipped uterus experience period pain more as a back ache than a pain in their abdomen. They may have diarrhea during their periods which is caused by a release of prostaglandins. They might know when their period is coming if they start having loose stools.

PMS

PMS is short for pre-menstrual syndrome. It refers to period-related mood fluctuations. To this day, PMS remains such a loosely defined concept that in addition to women, most men qualify as having it.

During World War II, when the bulk of American man went to war, millions of women manned the nation's industrial-war machine. Our female-dominated workforce turned out an armada of planes, tanks, ships, and guns that was unprecedented in history. It wasn't until the men returned from war and needed their jobs back that the myth of women's so-called hormonal instability began to rear its head. This corresponded to our society's need to get women out of the workplace and back into the home.

An entire PMS industry sprung up during the 1990s that attempted to turn hormonal mood fluctuations into a disease. This helped fuel the notion that women as a group are flakier than men. Just as flaky, absolutely; flakier, no. While period-related mood fluctuations can definitely result in mood swings, this usually doesn't make a woman emotionally unstable unless she's emotionally fragile to begin with. Studies show that men have as many monthly mood swings as women, but there's no psychiatric diagnosis for that. Something that might help women with severe period related mood swings is birth-control pills and dietary changes. However, some women find that the pill creates mood swings or makes them worse. It depends on the pill and the woman.

Getting The Red Out—Removing Period Blood

If you've been having periods for a few years and haven't stained a whole bunch of things, consider getting treatment for an obsessive-compulsive disorder. If you do a browser search on how to remove blood stains, you'll find a lot of disagreement. One reason is because the percent of blood in period flow can be high or low, depending on where a woman is in her cycle. So something that might work for period-related stains one day might not work the next.

It's always best to treat stains that have blood in them as soon as possible. If you can, try hitting a new stain with a wad of saliva and blotting it up (do not rub, as it will rupture the blood cells and make the stain worse). Better yet, if there's some contact-lens saline solution handy, try that, or mix 1 cup of salt in 2 quarts of cold water. Soak the garment in that. Never treat fresh blood stains with hot water.

A lot of women say that hydrogen peroxide can be helpful for fresh stains that haven't been set or gone through the washing machine. However, hydrogen peroxide can make the fabric weaker. That's why hydrogen peroxide is not a product of first choice on delicate fabrics, unless you were hoping for crotchless panties.

Blood stains can become really nasty when the hemoglobin in the blood mixes with oxygen in the air. This binds the stain to the fabric. Since hemoglobin is made up of iron, what you might be dealing with in a blood stain is a rust stain. The folks at Tide suggest using rust remover if the usual removal techniques fail. Carefully apply Whink Rust Remover or another liquid rust remover following the instructions on the package. Then rinse the fabric in 1 quart of water to which 3 table-spoons of baking soda have been added. Air dry and repeat if necessary.

A lot of women have specific panties for periods, which could have been underwear they really liked but ended up with stains that wouldn't come out. Others wear dark underwear that won't show stains, and some get Walmart specials to wear when they are having their periods.

A Brief History of the Tampon

The modern tampon was born in the late 1920s or early 1930s. It was called an "internal sanitary napkin." It did not have an applicator or a string. It was wrapped in gauze, which formed a tail that a woman pulled on to remove the tampon.

Another early tampon was called Paz. In 1936, the Tambrands company bought the Paz renamed it Tampax, which was the first tampon with an applicator. (The very first tampon was called FAX. The name Tampax covered all three bases: Tam+Paz+Fax.)

An early problem with using tampons is they required women to touch their genitals. There were widespread fears that this would lead to wanton immorality. There were also fears that tampons would devir-ginize teenage girls. As late as the early 1990s, Tampax ran ads to help dispel this fear.

A Brief History of the Pad

Kotex had its origins during World War I. Since cotton was in short supply, companies started to make bandages from cellulose. Army nurses found that the cellulose bandaging made an excellent substitute for the menstrual rags that they wore. It was cheap, absorbent, and they could throw it away.

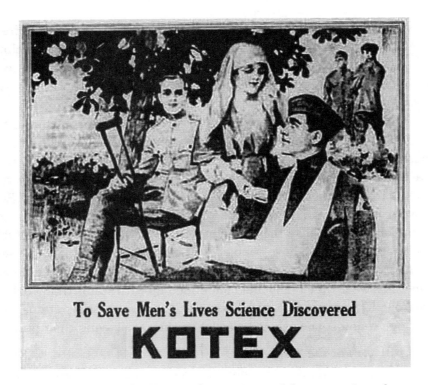

This 1920 prototype of a Kotex ad was rejected for magazine placement because it contained too many men in a product that was for women. (Notice how the object the nurse is handing the soldier is about the size of a Kotex and is almost in the line of sight of where a sanitary napkin is worn.)

As soon as the war was over, Kimberly-Clark, the company that made the bandages, looked opportunity in the crotch and created Kotex, which stood for KOtten-Like-TEXture. They hoped that by using a cryptic name such as "Kotex," women would be able to buy the product without the embarrassment of male clerks knowing what it was.

Another challenge for Kotex was to create an ad for their new product that magazines in the early 1920s would run. This was advertising for a product that went between a woman's legs at a time when su1h an item was still new and possibly scandalous.

As for the reference to "science" in the ad above, there is a similarity with the way we sell products today by claiming they were "Developed by NASA."

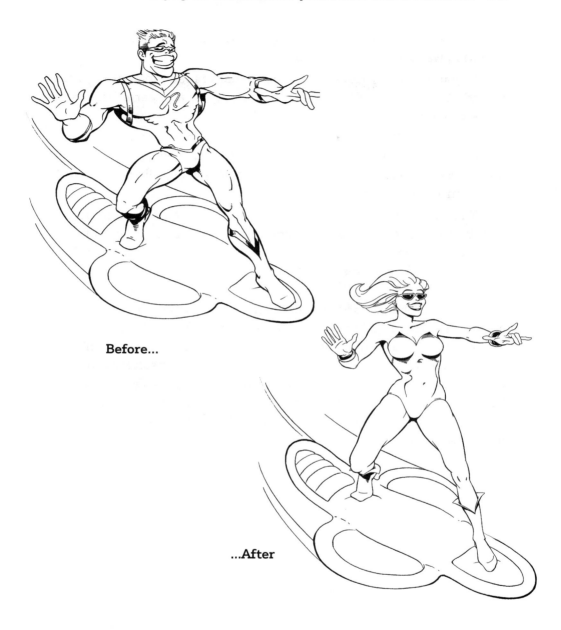

Before...

...After

Before the last edition of The Guide, Captain Menstruation was a guy.
He was a parody about the ridiculousness of period gear ads showing pads
with wings flying through the air. But women said he was a little creepy
and they felt it would be more empowering if Captain Menstruation were a
woman. So Daerick gave the Captain a sex change.

Recommended: Be sure to check out the amazing *Museum of Menstruation* website: www.mum.org.

If you are doing research on menstrual products patented in the United States from 1854 to 1921, read a copy of a paper of the same name by Laura K. Kidd and Jane Farrel-Beck.

While the following book title is a tad on the academic side, it could be the most spot-on period book to date: *Girls in Power: Gender, Body, and Menstruation in Adolescence* by Laura Fingerson, Albany, New York, State University of New York Press.

The classic period book *Are You There God? It's Me, Margaret* by Judy Bloom has sold roughly 8 million copies since it was first published in 1972. It continues to sell more than 100,000 copies each year. This makes it one of the best-selling books of all time.

A Special Thanks to Maureen Whelihan, MD, gynecological goddess, and to Rear Admiral Anne Schuchat, MD, from the Center for Disease Control and Nina Bender at Whitehall Laboratories. Also, thanks to Harry Finley at the *Museum of Menstruation* for consultation on the history of sanitary napkins and tampons, and to Jane Farrel-Beck for being so generous with photocopies of her articles! The original negative of the 1920s Kotex ad belongs to the Wisconsin Historical Society, used with thanks.

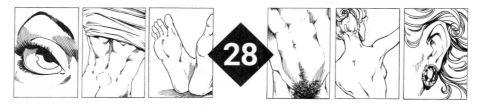

Playing with Yourself

Masturbation has fallen on hard times.

I honestly thought it couldn't get any worse than when we had to deal with the ridiculous No-Fap movement that was using warmed over pseudoscience to make young men feel bad about jerking off. But then, a college newspaper reporter who was interviewing me last year said there are a lot of young women who aren't comfortable with the idea of women masturbating. In disbelief, I checked with sex educators at other colleges around the country. They confirmed that a lot of young women feel it's "nasty" or wrong for women to masturbate.

It seems that the billions of dollars our government has spent on abstinence-only sex education has achieved one of its primary goals—to make young women feel shame about their genitals and wrong for doing what people do when they have a healthy sex drive.

I'm not saying that a woman should or shouldn't masturbate. But for young women to assume it's nasty for them to masturbate implies that they shouldn't be enjoying one of Mother Nature's greatest gifts to humankind. Compared to partner sex, masturbation is totally under your control and a woman doesn't need to shave, shower, and worry about which bra and thong to wear. Better yet, no woman has ever gotten pregnant or contracted a sexually transmitted infection from taking matters into her own hands.

Also, masturbation is one of the best ways there is for a woman to learn about her own body. How are guys supposed to know how to get a woman off when she hasn't learned how to get herself off? There is no medical reason why you shouldn't masturbate. It's your hand and your pants; if you want to stick one into the other, it's totally up to you.

Masturbation Over the Lifespan

As teenagers, most of us felt certain that masturbation was an adolescent thing, something people get over when they become adults. That never happened.

There are times when people masturbate a lot, and times when they hardly do it at all; times when it feels great, and times when it's a letdown. During those times when the world doesn't seem like such a nice place, masturbation can usually be counted on to help take some of the edge off. It also helps ease the transition between wakefulness and sleep. And contrary to what you might think, it can play an important role in relationships even when the sex between you and your partner is wonderful.

Some people find their bodies work better if they have an orgasm every day or two, with masturbation being a natural way to help this happen. Sometimes, you might find you get into a certain state of mind where you need to masturbate to relax enough to get your work done.

Vital Statistics on Fapping

The following was told to Harry Maurer by a young woman for his book *Sex: An Oral History*, Viking Press:

> "My mother has a vibrator that my father gave her one year. When I used to come home from college, I knew where she kept the vibrator, and I knew they never used it, so I would put it into my room and use it for the vacation. One summer I came home and it wasn't there. I was going crazy, I'm really a vibrator addict. Finally I was just so horny I said, 'OK, Mom, sit down. Where's the vibrator?' She's like, 'What!' I said 'Look, here's the deal. I've been stealing your vibrator for three years, and I need it now.' She was blown away, but she goes into her room, comes back with the vibrator, and says, 'By the way, have you ever used the jet in the hot tub?' "

According to just about everyone who has ever researched the subject, somewhere between 80% and 95% of men eventually masturbate and between 50% and 85% of women do it.

Contrary to what you might think, people don't masturbate any less as they get older. Many people who are married or deeply involved in a sexual relationship still get themselves off by hand. Masturbation doesn't decrease a person's desire for shared sex. For some people, it increases it. They masturbate more when they are in a relationship.

How often do people masturbate? It varies from a couple of times a day to never. As for the number of orgasms per effort, researcher Thore Langfeldt interviewed children in Norway from kindergarten through high school. He found younger boys and girls could give themselves multiple orgasms when they masturbated. But as they got older, the boys started reporting fewer orgasms per attempt, while the girls reported more. This is a trend that continued with increased age and experience.

What the Sandman Knows about Masturbation

According to the Sandman, the most common time when people masturbate is at night before they go to sleep or before taking a nap.

Sometimes it feels good to masturbate after a workout. Plenty of people masturbate during a study break or when they have to spend long hours doing a paper or a project. It helps them to refocus. Some people masturbate before a date so they will be more intellectually present. Women sometimes masturbate during their periods to help relieve cramping, or before intercourse to help it feel better, and a lot of women masturbate after intercourse. Some people wake up feeling horny. They might masturbate early in the morning, before having their Corn Flakes®.

Seriously Twisted Lunacy from Kellogg's of Battle Creek

Kellogg's Corn Flakes were created to give children more stamina so they wouldn't want to masturbate. John Harvey Kellogg, M.D., founder of the flake, believed that masturbation was "more immoral" than adultery. He called masturbation the "most heinous, revolting, and unnatural vice."(In case you think that was then and this is now, we now have the "No-Fapp" movement, which is every bit as strange as Dr. Kellogg.)

Kellogg proposed a six-point program for every American male that included taking cold enemas every day and wearing a wet girdle to bed at night to help prevent masturbation. His advice for parents whose children were caught masturbating included bandaging the genitals, covering them with cages and tying the child's hands together.

Dr. Kellogg, who was a prominent physician, recommended circumcision without anesthesia for boys who masturbated. He believed the pain would be a helpful punishment. Any foreskin was left should be sewn shut over the glans of the penis to keep the young man from having erections.

Kellogg was an interesting guy.

Dr. Kellogg's cereal is still known as "Kellogg's of Battle Creek."

Battle Creek was the name of his mental asylum, where he served his special cold cereals to help keep the inmates from masturbating. The finest medical minds of the day couldn't quite agree on the specific horrors that masturbation would cause. Some claimed it caused a man to become feeble, lackluster, feminized, impotent and to have underdeveloped genitals. Others claimed it had the opposite effect, turning young men into sex fiends who would have uncontrolled eruptions of lust and would blow the family fortune on prostitutes. Ads in popular papers promised to cure "the excesses of youth" and "underdeveloped genitals," which were what happened if you masturbated.

To keep Dr. Kellogg spinning in his grave, you might occasionally masturbate while eating a bowl of Kellogg's Corn Flakes.

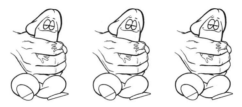

Wanking Protocol for When You Have A Roommate

Even if they're not particularly horny, a lot of people masturbate in bed at night to help turn their brains off. But good luck if you have a roommate. Most people would find it less embarrassing to be walked in on while they are having sex with a partner than when they are masturbating. And firing up a 30-amp vibrator or humping your teddy bear until his stuffing starts to explode could be a thing of the past.

The usual solution for masturbating when you have a roommate is to wait quietly until your roommate is making sleeping noises. This is not as easy as it sounds, since your roommate is probably waiting for you to make sleeping noises as well. Fortunately, there are common-sense solutions they usually don't tell you about at your college orientation.

First, pull out your copy of *The Guide* and open this part of the book. Say to your roommate, "I wonder if we should talk about this?" Of course, there are roommate situations where you'd rather be anally penetrated by a herd of buffaloes than talk about masturbation. But let's say your roommate is reasonable and has the same needs you do.

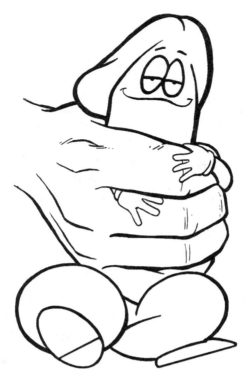

Here are some options to consider, or you can suggest some on your own. Some roommates are comfortable only adopting the first solution, others are fine with whipping it out together. It just depends.

😎 Agree to share with each other your class and work schedules, and agree to text your roommate if there are any changes, especially if a class was cancelled and you're returning early. A quick text, call or a long, loud series of knocks on the door accompanied by a verbal warning such as, "I can come back in ten minutes" shows consideration.

😎 If you are leaving and won't be right back, you agree to tell your roommate, "I'll be gone for at least ??? minutes." Don't come back before then unless it's totally necessary, in which case you'll knock loudly and wait to hear "Come in" before coming in.

😎 You agree that after the lights are out, it's fine for either of you to masturbate as long as you are reasonable about it. While it's usually impossible to be totally silent, you don't need to moan and snort or have porn blaring. (Even when you're using earbuds, porn can be annoying and distracting to roommates.)

☻ You agree it's okay to rub one out first thing in the morning while you are still in bed to help to tame a raging A.M. erection or to relieve a case of sunrise horniness.

☻ If one of you has a significant other at a different school or on another planet, you agree to work out times when the one with the distance relationship can be alone to chat or do whatever with his or her lover. That way, they can get themselves off to the sound of their lover's voice or from the phone between his or her legs. However, this is a privilege that a less-than-sensitive room-mate can easily abuse, so the one with the distance relationship needs to be fair, reasonable and not overdue it.

☻ You agree if one of you is seeing a person who is abstinence-only to the extreme or doesn't want to have sex yet, that upon returning from an evening with this person, you will provide he or she with at least fifteen minutes of alone time in addition to heartfelt condolences.

Two Things to Avoid

It's not a good idea to masturbate while wearing earbuds or noise-cancelling cans, as you won't be able to hear your roommate's warning knock or keys in the door.

And never, ever masturbate in a bathroom stall unless it's in your own dorm and it's well understood that everyone does it. The problem with jerking off in a rest room stall is that it could be against the law and you could get busted if there's a sting operation going on. It doesn't matter if you have the stall door locked and are being discreet.

And Finally...

Tissues and toilet paper are usually what guys masturbate into, although socks and dark-colored underwear are frequent standbyes. Do not leave your cum-soaked tissues or whatever sitting around.

For males who are wanking in the shower, don't leave a wad of your hair on the drain cover with chunks of clumpy spunk stuck to it. That's gross. Also, it's better to use hair conditioner for lube than soap, because soap can make your urethra burn. Unfortunately, while hair conditioner may claim to add volume or thickness, your penis is not what they have in mind.

Men & Masturbation

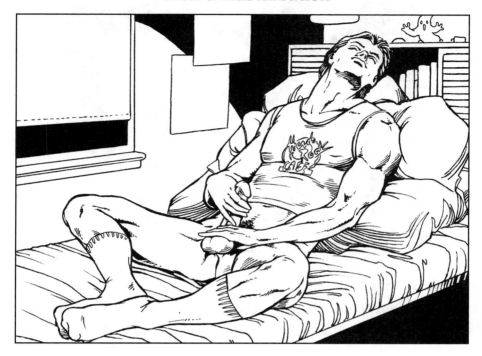

How Guys Learn to Masturbate

"When I was ten, an older friend showed me how to masturbate.
He had a full ejaculation, but nothing came out of my penis.
Time was the answer to that problem." *male age 45*

Males often learn to masturbate from friends, porn or a big brother.
Or they learn on their own. That's because a teenager has to be pretty
numb to miss the connection between soaping his penis in the shower
and the nice feelings that result. Also, when lying on a mattress with a
hard-on, most guys will eventually hump or rub. More than other human
organs, the penis pleads to be yanked, stroked and squeezed. (Anyone
who has raised a daughter in a non-repressive environment might disagree, saying that girls can give their clitorises a pretty good work out.)

If they haven't seen porn before having their first ejaculation,
some guys will experience concern or terror the first time they produce
semen, e.g., "Oh no, I broke something!" accompanied by promises to
never do it again, until the next day.

Today's pre-teen males who are raised on porn might have the
opposite concern, "Mine doesn't squirt, what's with that?"

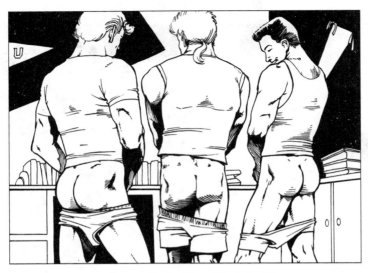

Lo and behold, a Circle Jerk!

The Group Thing

> "I can understand all sorts of things about guys' sexuality except why they jerk off together. It seems gay. Why do they do it?"
>
> *female age 23*

First, let's consider boys and then men. Boys need little encouragement to take their pants off and explore. Getting naked can be so exciting that they can get hard-ons from that alone. It's also natural for boys to share experiences with each other, whether it's checking out an abandoned house or showing what you do with your dick. Then comes the teenage years and beyond.

> "When we became teens, some of us boys would get together for a masturbation meeting in the tree house, but it was more the thrill of something exciting and forbidden than anything else."
>
> *male age 26*

Lots of men will say, "I never jerked off with another guy when I was a kid and have no desire to now." Others will say, "Sure, that's how we did it." There might be games connected with this, like who shoots the farthest or who comes the fastest (it's interesting how priorities change as you get older). Some young men feel excluded until they have been allowed to beat off with members of the local gang.

The urge to masturbate together seems to peak before high-school and drops off after that. However, there are some adult males who are straight and who enjoy the companionship. This isn't as much of a contradiction as it seems. Straight men enjoy watching other men ejaculate in porn, and some guys enjoy spanking it with their friends. Consider the following answers to a survey in the newsletter *Sex & Health*:

> "While partying with fraternity brothers, someone suggested a contest to see who could ejaculate the farthest. Each of the five of us took our turn in a tiled shower room. Surprisingly, the least endowed among us won!"

> "Sometimes when I'm camping with my friends and our girlfriends are otherwise occupied, we get to joking about sex. We soon get so aroused that when one of us whips it out to pee, we start joking and the others whip theirs out, too. Then we just start stroking ourselves and talking about our favorite techniques. We don't touch each other, but we do comment on each other's members and may cheer one another on to climax. We're all good friends and have become closer sharing our sexuality this way."

Sex & Health had a large male readership, with 95% of the men identifying as totally straight. Most were married and many had children. Still, a number reported fantasizing about masturbating with other men, e.g., "Although I'm happily married with two children, I do sometimes fantasize about masturbating with friends. I've thought about asking one friend in particular, but I haven't had the nerve." Is this because of hidden bisexuality in the men with this fantasy, or is it something special about masturbation that puts it into a no man's land when men who are into women do it together? We don't have the research to tell us very much about this.

Guy Tricks —"First, Nuke a Jar of Miracle Whip, Then..."

> "I made a false pussy from a bicycle tire inner tube and it worked quite well. I have also used banana peels, watermelons, and a hole in a piece of wood." *male age 42*

Most men use their hands to jerk off with. Most do it dry, especially guys who have their foreskins. But some men who are circumcised like to add lubrication which includes saliva, soap, Vaseline, vegetable oil, coconut oil, baby oil, baby oil gel, and anything else under the sun that can make their penis slick. A lot of men masturbate in the shower. Hair conditioner works well for lube. If you must use soap, start each stroke by grabbing your penis around the base and pulling outward only. Soap is not a friend of the peehole.

Another way that men sometimes masturbate is by lubricating the inside of a condom with a water-based lube and pump away. A variation of this is to lube up the inside of a Baggie or plastic bag and put it between your pillows or mattress and box springs. You then get on your knees and hump the bag. Be careful not to get your mattress pregnant.

As for banana peels, if you are having trouble with the peel falling apart and condoms are plentiful, try putting a condom over the peel. You can also heat it in a microwave for a few seconds, but be careful: microwaves heat unevenly.

Foreskin Tricks for Men Who Are Intact

Some men will fill a turkey baster with warm water, then pull their foreskin over the head of their penis and crimp it with their fingers over the end of the turkey baster. As they gently squeeze the end of the turkey baster, the warm water fills their foreskin and causes it to balloon out. As they let go of the bulb, the baster sucks up the water. They keep repeating until they come. Another method is to keep the foreskin retracted and pull it down toward the scrotum. This will cause it to become taut. Keep repeating until you come (via JackinWorld.com).

Rushin' Roulette

Men tend to rush themselves when they are masturbating. There are reasons for this.

🕶 To get to the heavy-duty pleasure part as soon as possible.

🕶 Lack of privacy. The last thing most guys want is for someone to walk in on them, so they try to come quickly and quietly.

🕶 If a guy takes a really long shower, everybody knows what he is doing. The extra speed also helps him finish before the hot water runs out.

Learning to Live in the Zone of Subtle Sensation

Taking extra time when masturbating might help a man learn about subtle sensations that he won't notice if he's always red-lining it. If he slows down as ejaculation approaches, he might discover a rush of feelings in his stomach, bladder, or rectum. Instead of going for the big squirt, he might try to back off, teaching himself how to live in the zone of subtle sensation. Pre-squirt feelings can be intense and last for long periods of time without becoming an actual ejaculation. Learning to stay with these feelings might help a man experience deeper levels of intimacy when he is with a partner.

Instead of reaching for his crotch each time he masturbates, a man might start by touching or massaging other parts of his body: scalp, face, neck, shoulders, chest, hands, feet, etc. This can be a way of reminding himself that sex is a full-body activity rather than something that just happens between his legs. (One female reader says this section should have been written for women as well as men.)

Taking a Vacation from Porn

An entire generation of young men have now grown up masturbating to the most explicit porn in the history of humankind rather than jerking off to their own sex fantasies. In fact, we don't know if young men who have been watching porn since middle school even have their own sex fantasies that haven't been shaped or influenced porn.

No one knows if there is anything about this that is good or bad, but it would be nice if we weren't letting the producers of porn influence every aspect of sexuality today. So why not try giving porn a rest for a month or two if you can, and enjoy jerking off to the images, fantasies and sexual scenarios that are your mind's own creations.

Possible Intercourse Spoilers

Grip of Death: Guys tend to grip themselves tightly when masturbating. Yet few vaginas come close to generating this kind of squeezing action. This might be why some men have more intense orgasms when they masturbate than during intercourse. Try masturbating with a lighter grip, at least occasionally.

Face Down: It has been said that men who always masturbate face down can have trouble reaching an orgasm when trying to have sex with women. If you masturbate face down and are having these kinds of problems, try to limit your jerking off to sunny side up.

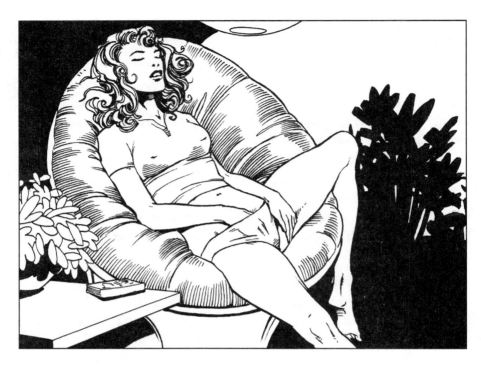

How Girls Learn To Masturbate

"It was my freshman year of high school. I was kissing this guy and was getting really turned on. He put his hand on my inner thigh and I was going crazy! This was my first heavy petting session. I didn't quite know what to make of it. When I got home, I went to the bathroom. My underwear was very wet. I went to touch myself and BAM!—instant orgasm! My very first. I've never had it that easy since." *female age 27*

"When I was young, climbing a flagpole always brought on such intense tingling feelings that I was only able to hold on tight and my legs would clamp around the pole. When the feelings subsided enough, I would resume climbing." *female age 37*

"When I had my first orgasm I kept saying, 'Oh my God!' over and over. I was really shocked because I didn't know I could do that to myself!" *female age 25*

It is every bit as normal and natural for girls and women to mastur-bate as it is for boys and men. But girls don't do "show and tell" nearly as often as boys, so they tend to learn about masturbation on their own or by reading about it. Some learn by watching women do it in porn. Some learn by putting a pillow between their legs or by leaning up against the washing machine when it's on the spin cycle. It might also happen when they have a sex dream—the sensation is still alive in their genitals when they wake up and all they need to do is reach down and rub. One woman learned to masturbate by pushing a sanitary napkin against her genitals; another by stroking the shaft of her clitoris with a pencil.

The possibilities for discovering how to masturbate are too numerous to name, but here are some of the ways women readers say they do it now:

"Bathtub, vibrator, boyfriend's fingers (my own don't work). Electric toothbrush handle, my ex-husband's hammer (the handle), even celery once." *female age 26*

"I get the most intense orgasm by leaning on a hard surface like a counter and wiggling around till I come. I also use a dildo, and I use my fingers to massage my labia and clit, occasionally fingering my vagina." *female age 37*

"Occasionally I use my hands, but usually I use a running faucet before I take my bath." *female age 19*

"I rub my clit in a circular motion with my fingers or use a trusty old vibrator. I've tried putting things inside my vagina, but so far that's been a very neutral experience—I need my lover's hand or torso to be attached to what's going inside. Sometimes I gently rub my chest as I masturbate, or run a soft piece of cloth over my nipples." *female age 47*

"I use my Hitachi magic wand because I am an impatient person." *female age 28*

"I use my fingers, one or two fingers, and sometimes all. I also use a dildo, a pillow, the edge of the bed, a chair..." *female age 22*

"I do it while reading a book or having a fantasy. Usually I stimulate my clit directly with one or more fingers. Only rarely do I put anything inside my vagina, although I do like the feel of a tampon. I also like anal stimulation. That will make an orgasm more intense and more diffused." *female age 36*

"I start with my fingers, move to a magic wand and/or a dildo."
female age 46

"I'll use my hands. I lay on my stomach and rub my labia majora with the thumb-sides of my hands. Or I'll use a high powered vibrator. And I'll often combine the two. I'll rub my labia while a vibrator is against my clit." *female age 25*

"I use a finger, then fingers." *female age 49*

"I do it with a rabbit style vibrator, often in combination with ben wa balls." *female age 31*

"My hands or a shower head with a sock tied onto it to make the water flow in a single stream when I lie under it." *female age 26*

Additional Ways

Some women can have an orgasm by doing stomach crunches (mini sit-ups). Others get off by humping pillows or water bottles, swinging on swings, tugging on underwear, rubbing up against things, and riding a bike down bumpy roads. Some like to stimulate their anus, either by putting pressure on it or by sticking a finger or butt plug inside of it. Some use the handles on hair brushes, some do it while looking in mirrors, others get turned on by wearing their boyfriend's shirt or underwear. Fill in your own blanks. Some prefer to masturbate with their fingers over their underwear while others love to reach inside. Some squeeze their lips or labia together or push against their genitals in ways that create pressure rather than penetration. A woman who has responsive nipples may make nipple stimulation part of her masturbation. It would require a database to list all of the ways that women masturbate. (See pages 188-191 for nine finger techniques alone.)

Straight to an Orgasm, or Making a Night of It?

"In my younger years, it usually took an hour or so before I had an orgasm. Now, if I'm especially hot, five minutes with a vibrator can do it, or about fifteen to twenty minutes by hand. Sometimes I like to keep things slow; I prolong it by starting and stopping. Other times, I just want to get off as fast as I can. Sometimes I masturbate, but not to orgasm. It feels good and relaxes me without wanting to come." *female age 47*

One woman might masturbate on and off for an entire evening, reaching between her legs while reading a book or surfing the Internet. Another woman might masturbate with the sole purpose of reaching orgasm, going from beginning to end without pause.

That's one of the really nice things about masturbation—especially women's masturbation. There are no rules for how it needs to be.

Women, Masturbation & Intercourse

Far more men than women have orgasms from intercourse. A woman is much more likely to have an orgasm from masturbation than intercourse. Combine the two, and voila! The vast majority of women who have orgasms during intercourse need extra clitoral stimulation while their partner is thrusting. They will usually do this with their fingers or by grinding their clitoris into a partner's pubic bone. A vibrator can also be thrown into the mix.

It's not unusual for a woman to masturbate before intercourse to help her genitals get more into it, or after intercourse. It is unfortunate that women often hide this and assume their partners wouldn't want to know. It seems like a sign of a good relationship when a woman feels free to finish what we aren't able to, or when we help her get started and she takes it from there.

Tennis Elbow? Say It Ain't So!

Tennis elbow is a form of tendonitis. A female physician suspects that some of her patients with tennis elbow did not get their tendonitis from playing tennis, but from the number-one repetitive finger motion that women do: masturbation.

If you are a woman who is experiencing tendonitis or repetitive-stress syndrome in the arm you masturbate with, try using a vibrator for instead of your fingers and see if the problem doesn't improve. Ditto for males who routinely masturbate their female partners.

Men who get tennis elbow or tendonitis in the arm they masturbate with might try switching methods, unless they are ambidexterous, then just switch arms. They might try using a masturbation sleeve or sex toy they can thrust into with their hips instead of using their arm.

Squeezing Your Thighs Together

A woman who contributes to the women's section at JackinWorld suggests women can teach themselves to come by squeezing their thighs together. She says to masturbate as you normally would, but press your thighs together when you start to have an orgasm. After a few weeks of doing this, masturbate to the point where you almost have an orgasm, but pull your fingers away at the last minute and try to finesse yourself into orgasm by squeezing your thighs together. Start with the thigh-squeezing action a little earlier each time. Some women might prefer doing this while wearing tight jeans on so they get an assist from the seam in front.

Women and Their Horses

There can be a special relationship between a woman and her horse that isn't kinky or weird. It's simply powerful. A number of women report having orgasms when horseback riding.

> "My first orgasm? I was riding my horse and I felt a strange sort of pleasure between my legs. I felt like I wanted it to stop so I could concentrate on my riding, but it felt so good." *female 18*

> "I was standing in the barn with my horse when I had a spontaneous orgasm. I gushed and everyone laughed at me for peeing in my pants. I was fourteen or so. I didn't discover masturbation until I was twenty, and then I thought orgasm was so incredible, I wanted one every day." *female age 37*

> "My first orgasm ever was when I was riding a horse. I thought I was perverted and never told anyone. Then at a slumber party one of my close friends who also horseback rides admitted that she'd had a similar experience." *female age 18*

Giving Girl-Masturbation a Name

There are numerous slang terms for male masturbation. This is not the case with female masturbation (Diddle? Jill off? She Bop? These are not universal terms). Since women don't usually masturbate together, they haven't needed to establish slang to convey what they are doing.

The Limitations of a One-Grip Rhythm (Applies to All Sexes)

If you always use the exact same touch and rhythm when you masturbate, you might be teaching your body to expect that and only that. Given how it's difficult for someone else to do you in precisely the same way that you do yourself, you might consider occasionally mixing it up.

Quiz Based on Your Sex Survey Responses

"Have you ever needed to masturbate while away from home?"

Guess which answers are men's and which are women's.

a. "I have done so occasionally in the car, while driving. Tricky, but doable." *age 37*

b. "I would pretty much masturbate anywhere if I could. I know it sounds silly, but when I am on the beach or catching a killer wave I get kind of horny." *age 23*

c. "Yes. Although never at my current job, I have masturbated at work." *age 26*

d. "Yes. I've masturbated driving in my car; the urge was just too great and I had to deal with it right then." *age 36*

e. "It has happened. I feel pressure like I'll go nuts if I don't get relief, and I'll sneak off." *age 38*

f. "Except for when I was on a long vacation, I've always been able to wait until I got home." *age 26*

g. "One time I was driving and I had a terrible urge, so I brought myself to orgasm. I've also done it at work once." *age 43*

h. "I was once on a long-distance bus trip and a teenage boy was next to me. I don't remember why, but I got very aroused, so I put my coat over me and masturbated while he slept." *age 45*

i. "While my partner lived in a different city, I would masturbate all the time. I would lock myself in the bathroom and put my feet on the wall while sitting on the toilet, with my legs bent and above my head. It was most satisfying this way." *age 37*

j. "I was using the computer at my brother's house when no one was home. While online, I was chatting to someone who was so hot that I had to masturbate to release enough tension so I could keep chatting." *age 27*

ANSWERS: *a. female   b. female   c. female   d. female   e. female   f. male*
g. female   h. female   i. female   j. female   Darned stereotypes.

Random Comments from Women Survey Takers

"My ex understood that sometimes he needed to just be still inside me while I rubbed my clit. He'd even let me sit on him and essentially masturbate while he talked dirty and touched the rest of my body." *female age 39*

"I masturbate more often when I'm in a relationship. I think about the sex we've had, and I get turned on thinking of my partner."
female age 22

"I don't really masturbate, unless my partner is watching."
female age 40

"When I'm in a relationship, I masturbate less, much less. I just can't seem to please myself like someone else can." *female age 30*

"I can go months without masturbating at all, other times it's daily."
female age 38

"I use the middle finger of my right hand. I use the same finger for touchpad or trackpoints on laptop keyboards. We girls at work used to smile at each other like partners in crime when we noticed that another girl used the middle finger for the trackball rather than her thumb like the guys. I loved my Blackberry with that vibrating track ball, I wish, Blackberry kept the concept."
female age 37

"I use one or two fingers rubbing clit over undies. Weirdly enough, I almost never come from external clitoral stimulation with a partner. I'm pretty trained to only like the levels of pressure and stimulation I can provide." *female age 22*

"I have toys that I enjoy; however, I prefer clitoral stimulation by my hands. I am a visual person; therefore, fantasy and a vivid imagination are essential...being able to access both are key. If I can't focus on a fantasy, my go-to is *Gaspar Noe's Love*. Specifically, the threesome scene." *female age 39*

A Warning About Bagging, which is a form of erotic asphyxiation. It's when a man masturbates while choking himself. There is no safe way to do this/ A number of men die each year while bagging. Bagging is discussed on pages 493-494.

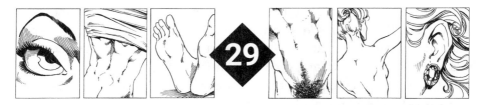

Oscillator, Generator, Vibrator & Dildo

It used to be "sex toy" meant a vibrator. Vibrators were one of the first electric machines created back in the 1800s. They have been a hit ever since. Newer sex toys include sleeves for male masturbation, harnesses, dildos in countless shapes and materials, toys for anal sex, nipple clamps and accessories for BDSM.

While sex toy manufacturers will call this blasphemy, there are lots of people who don't use sex toys and still have wonderfully fun sex lives. Plenty of women prefer their fingers to vibrators, and the absolute best sex toys are those that tap into your imagination rather than your pocketbook. So instead of being a fluff piece in favor of sex toys, this chapter looks at what might and might not make a toy sexy. It covers sex toy safety and sex toy use in relationships, and what to do when a partner might feel threatened by your vibrator or dildo.

Sex Toy Strategy, Part 1

Before investing in the latest sex toy or getting your hopes up that the hype is real, why not think about what it is you want a sex toy to do for you? If you are trying to get a sex toy for a partner, what are some of the things that turn him or her on? If your gift doesn't resonate with a lover's fantasies, it will end up being just another buzzing piece of plastic or whatever without any sexual oomph.

Ask yourself, "Would my partner prefer flowers and the latest book by her favorite author?" "Would he like it better if I got him a new computer gizmo or brake cable for his mountain bike rather than this strange looking sex toy that he's supposed to stick up his ass?"

Let's say you are a woman who is trying to rev up her partner's interest. You could always buy him the latest vagina-like sex toy that promises to make real-life pussies obsolete. Forget that it might feel like the vagina of a dead woman, or that most of the 5 star reviews were posted by the company that makes the product.

Over the years we have tried a $1200 sex-toy device that had nothing on a $30 vibrator. We also tried a $600 male masturbating device that made you appreciate how good your own hand feels. Just because it's supposed to be great doesn't mean it's great for you or your partner. One solution is to shop at sex toy stores with high ethics. One such store is called "A Woman's Touch" in the Midwest. It's run by a physician and a social worker. There are other stores as well where the staff truly cares about your pleasure and can competently advise you.

Sex Toy Strategy, Part 2

You might find that the perfect sex toy for your lover is one that you use on yourself. Perhaps he'll be turned on by watching you use it. Or make a deal with your partner: she selects a toy for you to use on her, and you select a toy for her to use on you. Then go shopping together. Using toys in this way helps you reveal new things about yourself to your partner, and vice versa. Sex can get boring when you think you know all there is to know about the person you are sleeping with.

And why not search for some cool videos that the two of you could watch? Check out sites where the staff reviews the videos and only carries what they consider to be the best. There's also a world of erotic books and literature that you and your partner can read together or to each other. Collections of short stories by competent writers abound. A collection of erotic short stories might be the best sex toy ever.

Beware the Phthalates

Not long ago, Greenpeace issued a warning that sex toys put off a dangerous class of chemicals known as "phthalates." Did Greenpeace fear that schools of dildo-using dolphins were in danger? No. They were worried about humans. Very worried. Phthalates have been linked to liver damage, kidney damage, lung damage, and damage to the developing testes in the fetus. Phthalates are added to plastics to increase their flexibility. They are used to create favorite sex-toy materials such as Cyberskin, Softskin and Futurotic. Phathalates put the jelly in jelly rubber sex toys.

Hard plastic toys usually do not contain phthalates, nor do 100% silicone toys or dildos made of glass or steel. The trouble with silicone is that it doesn't need to be 100% silicone to be called silicone. So you are at the mercy of the seller. As for the "quick fix" of putting a condom

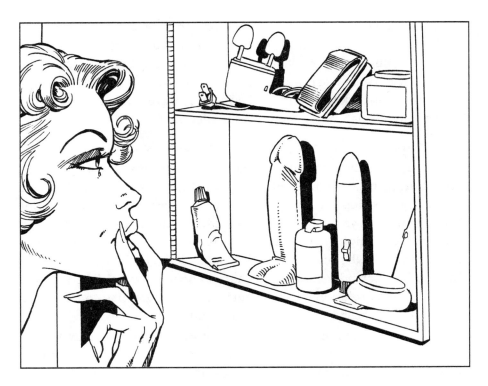

between you and your phthalate-containing sex toy, the amount of phthalates in sex toys has been described by researchers as being so high as to be "off the charts." A condom may decrease exposure, but...

Creative & Low Cost

There are plenty of great sex toy substitutes that cost hardly any-thing. For instance, you can make coupons for your partner. Each lists a special thing you are willing to do, from giving your partner a full-body massage to things that can't be printed in a family resource like the *Guide To Getting It On*. Your partner gives you the coupon when she wants you to do what it describes. (Author Laura Corn's *101 Nights of Great Sex* is built around this concept.)

Another idea is for each of you to describe a scene that is a per-sonal turn-on. Shop for props to make the scene happen. For instance, if one of you has the fantasy of being stopped and frisked by an offi-cer in uniform, you can go to a used-clothing store and buy the perfect uniform for acting out the scene, perhaps including handcuffs. If the fantasy concerns a visit to the doctor, shop at a medical supply house.

If you don't like that idea, try surprising your partner with a sex toy that's found at your local pet store. When your lover comes home, you can be standing there naked with your new dog collar around your neck; hand her the leash and say, "I'm yours for the night!" Attach a bow to the collar like they do at the fancy pet groomers and hope she didn't bring her parents home for a surprise visit.

Penis Casting Kits, Especially for Deployments & Skyping

Consider making a mold and stunning sculpture of your partner's penis! During this magnificent and often hilarious sex-toy adventure, you will be creating an exact replica of your partner's penis. Imagine his excitement if you use the finished casting of his penis on yourself, or the fun you might have using it on him! (As for putting it on your desk at work, maybe that's not such a good idea. Then again...) It's also something to consider if your partner is about to be deployed, or you have a distance relationship. Showing him what you like to do with it can add some pizzaz to your Skype calls and Snapchats.

You can find kits that are specially designed to mold and make castings of the penis or breasts at www.artmolds.biz (.biz not .com). Under "Lifecasting Kits" look for the "Intimate Kit" and "My Breast Friends" or "Full Torso" kits. The penis kit even includes skin and hair release cream, which could be the most important part!

Oscillators, Generators,Vibrators and Dildos

Some people claim the light bulb is the most important electrical invention of the last 130 years; others say it's the vibrator. The rest of this chapter is about vibrators and dildos. Its emphasis is on the use of these devices by couples as opposed to individuals, although many people use them for solo sex. (Because a lot is written in this chapter about vibrators, please don't view this as an endorsement for them. Fingers usually work just fine, and a lot of women prefer them.)

If what you want is a vibrator, dildo or butt plug, reputable sex-toy stores can be a helpful resource.

Confusing Vibrators with Dildos

People often confuse the vibrator with the dildo, which is like confusing a rhino with a giraffe. Both are native to the bush, but that's where the similarities end.

Vibrators are valued for their buzzing properties and are usually rested on the surface of the genitals rather than placed inside them, although there are newer "rabbit" hybrids that can do double duty.

Dildos are penis-shaped and are used as such. Most don't vibrate, but are made to be kept inside the vagina to give a feeling of fullness or to be thrust in and out. Women can also slide them up and down between their labia, which can be good for whatever ails them.

People often think of the common battery-operated plastic vibrator as a dildo. While some women use them as dildos, the vibrating part is usually located on the tip, which means a woman can't insert it deeply inside her vagina and expect it to keep her clitoris happy. These are also made of hard plastic. Some of them don't pack much of a wallop compared to the more adequately appointed AC models. Most of these novelty devices aren't in the same league as a well-made dildo or vibrator, although highly devoted users will disagree.

Some Men Worry

Most guys have no problem with a partner who uses sex toys; many find the situation a turn-on. However, some males worry their lover will prefer the vibrator or dildo to them. Some believe it means they aren't hung well enough or can't deliver the goods. This isn't necessarily true.

Some men are particularly confused when their partner says she loves having intercourse with them, but prefers a dildo that's bigger than they are. A reason for this is a woman totally controls the dildo play, so she can maneuver the dildo exactly where she wants it. Sex with a partner is more athletic and more random, so she may prefer a penis that isn't as big as her dildo for actual lovemaking. Some women also like to use a dildo during intercourse in addition to having a partner's penis inside. And plenty of women like to use a vibrator during intercourse.

If he is a considerate, caring, real flesh-and-blood guy, most women will still want a real-life partner regardless of how often they fire up their vibrator or pull out their dildo. It's hard to have a meaningful conversation with a dildo, and no vibrator has ever played catch with the kids or gotten up in the middle of the night to change the baby. Also, you can't cuddle up next to sex toys after you have an orgasm—not that you can with all men, either.

In purchasing a new vibrator or dildo, a woman who is in a relationship should consider making her partner part of the selection process. This way, her partner won't feel left out, resentful, or inadequate. Perhaps it might not hurt to show him this chapter, which encourages men to take pride in a woman's sex toys. It might also help to let him know that women who buy vibrators and dildos are often extremely happy with their flesh and blood sex partners.

Making Friends with Your Lover's Toys

There's no point in feeling at odds with your partner's vibrator or dildo. If you are a man and your partner orders a new sex toy, ask her to show you how she uses it. Hold her tight while she's getting herself off with it. If she has a vibrator, why not let her use it on you? Men might like the feel of a vibrator on their perineum (space behind their scrotum) better than on their penis.

Ask your partner if she'd like to use her vibrator during intercourse. Some couples find the vibrations during intercourse are sensational. You might also combine vibrator play with oral sex. The man pushes a small battery-operated vibrator against the bottom of his tongue while the tip of his tongue is touching his partner's clitoris. Or you can place a dildo in her vagina while planting wet kisses on her clitoris. With enough of feedback and a willingness to explore, you and a partner can have lots of fun with a vibrator and dildo.

Vibrator Details

Coil vs. Wand: When it comes to vibrators that plug into the wall, there are two different types: wandlike vibrators with longer bodies and large heads, and coil vibrators with compact heads. Each type delivers a unique sensation. Coil vibrators are smaller and very quiet. Their sensations tend to be more localized. Wand vibrators are bigger and make a distinct humming noise. Newer models are rechargeable and will hum for up to an hour per charge. Some come with two heads instead of one.

Between the Lips vs. On the Clit: Women who use vibrators with a large head, such as the Magic Wand, often prefer to place the head between their labia near to the opening of their vagina as opposed to higher up on their clitoris. This helps vibrate the structures inside their pelvis and saves the glans of the clitoris from stimulation that is painful or numbing.

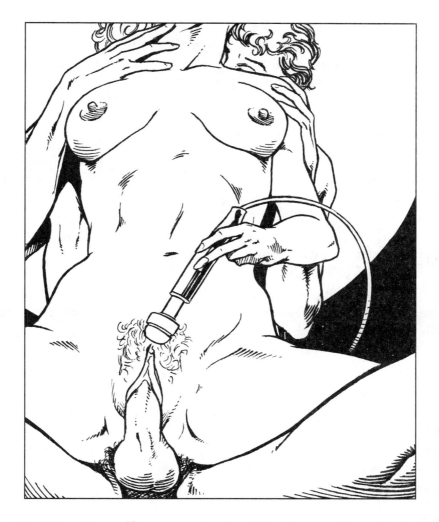

First-Time Users: If you are new to a vibrator, use it on the lowest speed while you learn to navigate the head around your pubic bone. Some new users have bruised their pubic bones by placing the head of a vibrator on a bony pelvis.

Sensation Types and Levels: Different types of vibrators produce different kinds of sensation. Some rumble and others hum. Some women will like the sensation full blast; others like to muffle the vibrator with a towel or even a pillow. Some hold the vibrator in a way that allows their fingers to transfer the vibrations.

Hands: Some vibrators strap on the back of your hand. Your fingers deliver the vibrations. These are fun, but they can numb out your hand.

Finger Vibrators: There are tiny vibrators that fit on your finger. They are incredibly small and almost unnoticeable.

No Hands: Some women rest a vibrator between their legs so they can use their hands for other things such as holding a book, playing with their breasts if they enjoy breast stimulation, touching a partner's body, or channel surfing. There are harnesses which can hold the head of a vibrator snugly between your legs.

Joni's Butterfly: This is a small vibrator with straps that hold it in place. It can be worn during intercourse, at work, in the library, during a lecture, at church to help you stay awake during the sermon, on a date, or anywhere a woman wants to get a private buzz in a public place.

Positions: Unlike men, vibrators are meant to be abused. Try different positions with it on top of you, you on top of it, and as you lie on your side.

Vibrator Vacations: People sometimes worry a woman will become used to the vibrator and want only that. If you are concerned, take vibrator vacations for one week every month.

Attachments: There are a number of vibrator attachments for both coil and wand vibrators. Do a browser search to see the possibilities.

Our Gynecology Consultant offers a vibrator solution that won't break the bank: "My new favorite item is a vibrating toothbrush. The vibration is a perfect frequency for clitoral stimulation. I remind my patients not to use the bristle side but the back side of the bristles. It travels great, is inexpensive, and doesn't threaten a man's masculinity..." [The disposable, battery-powered toothbrush is from a well-known Oral hygiene company. It has bright, multi-colored bristles that Pulsate, and is less than $10 USD for a twin pack wherever toothbrushes are sold!]

Vibrators and Airport Security

When viewed through X-ray, vibrators can resemble detonating devices on bombs. Airport security will make you open up purses, briefcases and suitcases that have vibrators in them. Resist informing them about what your vibrator does and doesn't detonate.

Dildos

Vibrators have become so socially acceptable that even Walmart and Target display them, although the boxes show women using them on their necks or calves. With dildos, there are fewer options for subterfuge and denial. And if people hear a woman say the word "dildo" in a public place, they are more likely to think that she is referring to a former lover or a politician than to an object that gives her pleasure.

After reading the next couple of pages, you won't be left in the dark about dildos, even if people often use them in the dark.

Dildo vs. Penis

Since the human penis is anchored to the male crotch, it imposes limitations upon a woman's sexual pleasure that the dildo does not. A penis can't be radically flipped upside down without requiring a trip to the hospital for the man whose body it was attached to. The male penis isn't always hard when a woman wants it hard, nor for as long as she might desire. And a penis is not like a car that can be traded in. Even if her partner's penis might not be the best size and shape for her, a married woman is pretty well glued to it till death or divorce. Fortunately a woman needn't ditch the man she loves because she prefers an SUV-type penis when nature gave him a Mini Cooper. She can purchase a dildo instead.

Dildos are made from a large variety of materials, including jade, acrylic, alabaster, latex, leather, glass, brass and wood. However, the most highly regarded dildo material is usually silicone. Silicone has a soft but firm texture with a smooth surface that is durable and easy to clean, although it doesn't stand up to cuts too well. The silicone material also warms up rather nicely, which is an added plus unless you like cold things in your vagina.

Since there is a fair amount of craftsmanship involved in producing a high-quality dildo, be sure to purchase dildos from places that carry only proven products and take pride in pleasing their customers. Check how long they've been in business and how well they support their products.

Getting the Right Size Dildo

The most important consideration in sizing a dildo is width or girth. One strategy for determining which width is best for you is suggested by the women at Good Vibrations. They say to buy different-sized zucchinis, carrots or cucumbers that have an inviting girth. Steam or nuke them for just a few seconds so they won't be cold, wash them, and put condoms over them. Add lubricant and try them in your vagina. Use a vegetable peeler to fine tune the girth. When one feels just right, cut it in two and measure the diameter, which will most likely be somewhere between one and two inches. If the dildo is for your own private play and you are the one who will be inserting it, order one that has the perfect sized width. However, if a partner will be doing the inserting, consider getting a dildo with a slightly smaller diameter. That's because a partner won't be as precise as you are, so a little room for forgiveness can be a godsend.

As for length, a four- to five-inch-long dildo should be just right if you plan to keep it stationary inside your vagina, while six to eight inches might be easier to handle if you like thrusting.

Dildos are a bit like purses: some women have one favorite dildo; others have dildos of different shapes and sizes for every day of the week. Expect to pay from $50 to $150 for a good-quality silicone dildo. Rubber dildos have tiny divots in the surface which make them next to impossible to keep clean. You should always use a condom over them.

Shape and Lubrication

With dildos, there are plenty of variations within a basic theme. Some dildos are made to look like penises, complete with veins and testicles. Some look like dolphins or bears, and some have ridges. Dildos also have different-sized heads. With a bit of effort, you are likely to find the dildo of your dreams.

No matter how wet you might be, consider lubricating the dildo and yourself, adding more as you go. If it's a silicone dildo, don't use silicone-based lube. It will cause your dildo to have a meltdown.

Stationary vs. Movement and Possible Layering

Women don't necessarily use dildos for thrusting in and out. A woman might like a dildo to be stationary inside her vagina while she uses her fingers or a vibrator on her clitoris. The dildo provides extra fullness that can amplify the sensations in her clitoris. Or she might like to have a dildo in her vagina as a partner gives her oral sex or stimulates her anus. Some women like having a dildo in their vagina at the same time a partner thrusts during intercourse, or a woman might enjoy running the dildo up and down between her labia. And she might like the feeling of a dildo up her butt, but for that, she will need a dildo with a flared end so it won't accidentally get sucked up into her rectum.

Cleaning & Other Facts of Dildo Life

Dildos should be washed and dried after each use. If not properly cleaned, the porous surface of some dildos will grow microorganisms that are best not introduced or reintroduced into your body. If you are sharing sex toys, sterilize your dildo with hydrogen peroxide or a light bleach solution (nine parts water to one part bleach).

If you use the dildo in your bum, be sure to wash it with soap and water before putting it into a vagina. Better yet, slap a condom on it before it goes up anyone's rear. People who enjoy both anal and vaginal penetration are wise to have dedicated dildos for each orifice.

Dildo Harnesses: Dildos with a flared base can be worn in a harness which makes them appear like erect penises. With enough skill and effort, the person wearing the harness can penetrate a partner. However, the dildo isn't connected to the wearer's nervous system like a flesh-and-blood penis and she can't feel what the dildo is feeling. Still, plenty of straight and lesbian couples enjoy using a dildo in a harness. The best harnesses are made of leather or nylon webbing. Harness construction and fastener application can be tricky; be sure to research the do's and don'ts of dildo-harness buying and wearing.

Also, there are dildo harnesses that fit on the thigh. Users of these marvel at the utility and claim the human penis should have been attached to the thigh of the male instead of between his legs. There is even a dildo mounted on a beach ball that the aerobically-inclined can bounce up and down on, as well as dildo harnesses that go on the chin.

Dildo Harnesses for Inner Wear: Let's say you're trying to take the boredom out of shopping at the supermarket. You can do it with your favorite dildo inside your vagina and no one will ever know unless you want them to. That's because there are dildo harnesses that hold the dildo inside a woman's vagina so it won't pop out.

Doubles? A double dildo can be hand held or worn in a harness, with one end going up the wearer's vagina and the other end sticking out in front like a penis. There are some highly-rated double dildos that have different lengths and shapes. Do some research before buying.

Double Penetration: Some women like to be penetrated in both the vagina and rectum at the same time. In lieu of finding a second male for a threesome, try a dildo in one end and a partner in the other. Or a partner and dildo in the same orifice if you like double vaginal penetration.

Beware Of Gumby-Like Dildos: These are embedded with wire. If the wire separates, it will puncture the walls your vagina or rectum.

Suction Cups: There are dildos with suction cups on the bottom so the woman can move her entire body up and down. These can also be stuck on the wall in your dorm room for decoration.

Dildos for Pegging: Good Vibrations says that about half of the dildo harnesses they sell are to straight couples where the woman wears the dildo for anal intercourse in her male partner's rear end.

Man Toys

We have tested a few masturbation sleeves and other toys. Few come close to using your hand and a few cents worth of lotion (or just your hand if you are intact). As for the vagina substitute that's shaped like an oversized flashlight, sticking your penis into cold mud would have been more fun and less of a hassle to clean up. But these man toys sell incredibly well and thousands of men enjoy using them.

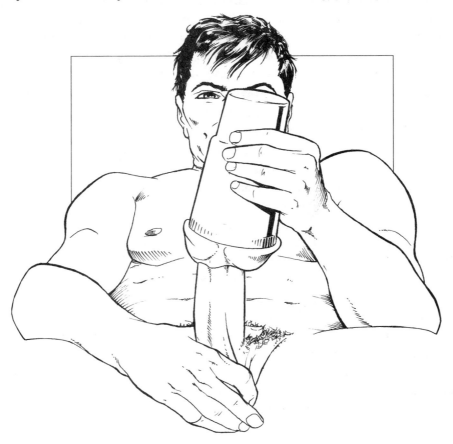

Up Your Bum — Anal Sex

"I grew up in the country. We had neighbors, Amos Wheat-ley and his wife. One night while washing dishes, Mrs. Wheat-ley told my mother that she let Amos 'use the other hole.' Then they had a baby girl, and I heard my father comment that Amos must have got it right at least once. Sometime later, Amos, who was uneasy about the expense of having a new baby, told my father he'd rather have had a team of horses. My father said, 'Isn't that expecting rather a lot of Mrs. Wheatley?' "

—The recollections of a very old woman, as told to Julia Hutton in her *Good Sex: Real Stories from Real People,* Cleis Press.

Some couples would rather drink goat sweat than try anal sex; others enjoy an occasional rear-end soiree. Whether you are straight, gay or somewhere in between, the chances are good that at some point in your life you might try anal sex. Please be aware this Guide couldn't care less whether you do or don't practice anal sex, but it does have a few suggestions in case curiosity nips you in the rear.

For those of you who have been watching a lot of porn—where a woman's rectum has become the new vagina—consider the responses about anal sex from thousands of sexually-amped people who have taken our sex survey. Less than 10% of the straight couples have anal intercourse on a regular basis. And "on a regular basis" might be once or twice a month, if that. Most of the women described anal sex as the most painful sexual experience they've ever had. However, some have their strongest orgasms when anal stimulation is part of the mix, and some men find a finger on the prostate to be a welcome sensation.

In Butt Play, What's Good for the Goose...

It's only fair that if a guy wants to stick his penis up a woman's rear end, she should be able to stick something of comparable size up his. Plus, it should help him become a more sensitive anal lover.

Vegetables aren't a good idea; you don't want a vegetable breaking off inside your partner's rectum. Use a dedicated anal toy or butt plug. These have special flared bases so you don't end up in a hospital emergency room needing their help to surgically remove a lost toy.

Anal Massage

If someone says they had sex last night, we assume they had vaginal intercourse. When you add the modifier "anal" in front of the word sex, we assume it was a penis up a partner's bum. Yet one of the nicest forms of anal pleasure comes from anal massage, where a penis is not inserted into the anus.

The anus is alive with nerve endings. A well-lubed finger or thumb massaging the anal opening can bring enjoyable waves of pleasure.

"I hate admitting this, but I like it when Dave wets one of his fingers and slides it into my anus. It is a huge turn-on, and there are times when it makes me orgasm. The only problem is pulling it out. It always hurts coming out and usually throws off my bowel movements for the next few hours. It feels like I have to go...." *female age 26*

"When Erica is all worked up, she sometimes likes me to massage her anus. When I slip a lubricated finger inside her, it is often the thing that puts her over the edge. If I have a finger inside her vagina and one in her anus, she reacts very well to the sandwiching of the wall when I press the two together. Other times, she really hates it when I touch her there. I can never quite guess when it's going to be a green light." *male 25*

Why 'Rimming' Is Called Rimming

Rimming is when one partner licks his or her lover's anus. The reason it is called "rimming" is because most of the feel-good nerve endings in your rear end are located around the rim of your anus. So if becoming the receiver of a penis during anal sex is on your radar, it can help to learn how to enjoy the feeling of being rimmed. You might start with your own finger in the shower, and then graduate to a partner's lubricated finger or tongue. (If a partner is going to rim you with his tongue, it's a good idea to shower first, soaping and rinsing your butt crack twice. There is more on STIs and hepatitis later in this chapter.)

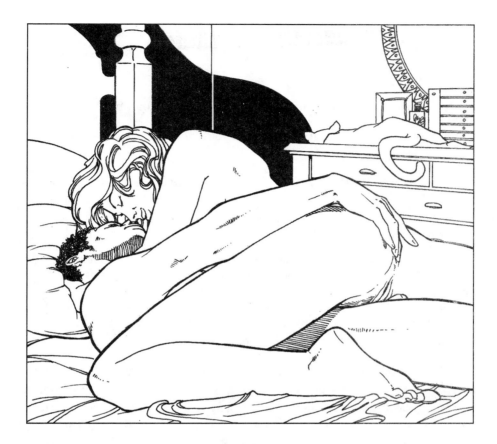

You'll be ahead of the game if you learn how to enjoy rimming for a few weeks before going any further. If you plan on having anal sex that isn't among the most painful sexual experiences you've ever had, proceeding slowly should be one of your priorities. And the last thing you want to do is have anal sex the way they show in porn.

People Have Anal Sex Because...

Some people like anal sex because it's forbidden. Some men have anal sex as a way of getting work in the entertainment industry. Some women have anal sex who would like a partner's penis inside of their vagina but can't because of chronic pain. But the most obvious reason why people have anal sex more than once is because they enjoy it.

> "Anal sex helps me feel a whole different part of my vagina and vulva. The fact that it is so tight and kind of nasty is a turn-on to me too." *female age 23*

"My wife asks for anal intercourse on occasion, usually late at night when she is very aroused and her inhibitions are down."

male age 41

"I've tried it with different guys, taking it slow and doing all of the right things. It still feels weird and uncomfortable." *fem 29*

"I can come from anal intercourse, but not from vaginal intercourse." *female age 32*

"Both of us like it. I will sometimes put a finger in her anus while we are having intercourse. It's very exciting for her, and I can feel my penis through the wall, which I find to be very erotic." *male age 39*

"Its not a pleasant experience unless there's little movement, and I only enjoy it knowing that he's happy." *female age 22*

"A lot of guys want to do anal; it's annoying at times. I don't find it painful really, but it's uncomfortable and leaves me sore so not something I really do often." *female age 24*

Occasionally, a women will say the only reason they have anal sex is to please a partner, but most women who have anal sex more than a few times do it because they like the way it feels. Some report getting an extra intense orgasm when they stimulate their clitoris at the same time they are having anal sex. Some find anal sex to be emotionally intense, as well.

Some men enjoy having their anus massaged or penetrated, and some have memorable orgasms when their prostate gland is being stimulated. Few women and men will have an orgasm from anal stimulation alone. It usually requires simultaneous clitoris or penis stimulation.

There are couple who have anal sex for birth control, such as in countries that take seriously the Catholic Church's opposition to contraception. Unfortunately, semen can run out of the anus and into the vagina which can result in pregnancy. Pregnancies from anal sex are common enough that the term "splash conception" is used to describe them. Perhaps this is how people with anal-retentive personalities are conceived.

Some women who want to remain virgins will try anal sex as an alternative to intercourse that involves the vagina.

Mother Nature & The Human Backside

When Big Mama Nature designed the female body she gave it a vagina that's rough, tough and durable. She made the walls of the vagina so they would stretch, swell, lubricate and straighten out at times of sexual excitement. This allows objects of desire to slide in and out with a fair amount of ease and enjoyment.

Nature was working from a different set of plans when she built the rectum. The rectum's main purpose is for elimination rather than romance. As a result, the walls of the rectum don't stretch and lubricate, although they fit objects that are larger than a lot of penises. There's also a curve in the rectum that the head of penis will collide into unless the person who is receiving anal intercourse knows how to get into a position that will help straighten it out.

The rectum includes a pair of pugnacious sphincter muscles that guard the gates of your anus. These muscular rings were designed to facilitate outgoing rather than incoming objects, although with enough effort, they can be taught to yield in either direction. The anal sphincters are two of the most important muscles in the human body if you plan on living and working in the vicinity of other human beings.

Reports that anal sex will damage the rectum are not backed up by science as long as you are using lots of lube, your sphincters are relaxed, and you aren't using crystal meth or things that might numb your bum.

A Brief Summary of the Structure & Function of the Human Rectum from the Time of Cro-Magnon Man Until the Founding of Ancient Greece

If you consider the history of the human rectum, say from the time of Cro-Magnon man until the founding of ancient Greece, its sole purpose was to hold things in. It wasn't until the ancient Greeks invented sodomy that our bums became multipurpose. (In giving credit where credit is due, the Old Testament had an interest in anal activity that possibly predated the Greeks. At the very least, one of the early Biblical plagues visited upon the Egyptians apparently included hemorrhoids.)

Thanks to the inventiveness of the ancient Greeks, we now have things in our lives like politicians, lawyers, doctors and anal sex. The only one of these that should never cause you pain is anal sex. If it does, you are doing it wrong.

The key to pleasurable anal sex is training the anal sphincter muscles to open for incoming objects. One set of these muscles is under conscious control. It's what people use to maintain their dignity when waiting to use the bathroom. The second set of sphincters is a total free agent. It automatically closes whenever something pushes against it. To have comfortable anal sex, the second set of sphincters must be taught how to relax when you ask.

Popular Culture Historical Note: When Jack Morin published the first edition of his book titled *Anal Pleasure and Health*, it was such a taboo subject that few bookstores would stock it. Now, a few decades later, Jack's book has been joined by several others. It's no longer unusual to see butt-sex books on bookstore shelves.

Four Key Elements

There were originally three keys to anal insertion: relaxation, feedback and lube. The difference between anal pleasure and pain is having generous amounts of all three. Trust has now been added to the mix.

Even the toughest of condoms can tear if the anus isn't relaxed. So the goal is to be turned on and relaxed as opposed to turned on and tense. And it's difficult to be turned on and relaxed if you don't trust your partner.

The Right Chemistry

"I truly hated anal sex the two times I had tried it before. But I agreed to do it with my new boyfriend, and it feels incredible with him! Am I weird, or are there any other women who enjoy anal sex?" *female age 28*

We posted this reader's question on our sex survey and found a surprising number of women who said they'd had a similar experience. Many said the keys for them were feeling totally relaxed with their partner and being exceptionally horny.

Even a finger on your anus can be annoying if trust and arousal are missing, while a reasonably-sized penis can feel fine when you are relaxed and ready.

(*This chapter has been written as if the male is doing the inserting. This was only done to keep you from gagging on too many pronouns. For instance, pegging is the insertion of a dildo into a male's butt by a female partner. It may not be as popular as blogging, but it's not uncommon.*)

Learning the Difference between 'It Feels Strange' and 'Pain'

When experimenting with anal play, you'll want to learn the difference between sensations that are unusual or strange versus those that are painful. When you or a partner first start groping inside your anus, it will probably feel strange. With time and experience, the initial strange feeling can evolve into sexual pleasure. Or, it might continue to feel strange. You never know how your brain will translate the sensations until you are in the throes of sexual passion and desire.

If the sensations are painful as opposed to strange, back off and try to figure out what's causing the pain. Don't explore again until you have come up with ways to prevent the pain. There should be no pain in anal sex. Strange, yes. Pain, no.

Nail Alert

When it comes to the rectum, jagged finger nails are weapons of mass destruction. Make sure your fingernails are trimmed *and filed,* and your hands are washed. (Trimming without filing can still leave nasty edges.)

Practice and Preparation—By Yourself First

The best way to prepare for anal sex is in the shower, for a couple of weeks before you try it with a partner. Get used to the feel of your finger on your anus. Over time, try inserting your finger up your bum. Its job is to provide you with information about the geology of your anus. With each successive shower, you will learn more, and you will hopefully be teaching your anal sphincters to relax.

Another thing you might try is to masturbate while you have an anal toy or finger in your rear. This will help you get used to new sensations that involve both your front and rear, or two parts of the nervous system instead of one. Then, you might try having a partner give you oral sex while he has a lubricated finger pushing against your anus, or inside of it.

Practice and Preparation—With a Partner

Psychologist Jack Morin suggested the following technique for teaching your rectum to relax: each night for a week or two, one partner lubes up a clean finger and gently inserts it in the other partner's rear, pushing very softly and slowly. This should encourage trust and relaxation.

Rectal expert Erik Mainard—known as the Avatar of Ass—encourages a gentle massage of the anus and suggests angling the finger slightly upward toward the tailbone, since that is how the rectum curves. He says to push in slowly and only as the resistance eases. This should feel good for the receiver; otherwise the person who is inserting the finger is rushing it or violating your comfort zone, in addition to violating your anus.

One way to help relax the anal area is for the receiver to push down as though she were trying to move her bowels. In addition to relaxing the sphincters, this adds a bit of suspense to the exercise. Another trick is for the person to try clamping their anus tightly shut while their partner gently pushes against it. After about 20 to 30 seconds of trying to clamp it shut, it will automatically start to relax and a partner should be able to ease a well lubricated finger into it.

However, anal purists say that with the help of a patient, caring partner and a great deal of lube, one needn't trick the sphincters into relaxing. And even though only one partner might be inserting a penis, each should experiment with fingering the other's rear. This will help build knowledge, trust, and bum-bonding.

The receiver needs to feel comfortable with finger penetration before trying any unnatural acts. It is not until the sphincters learn to relax that anal sex will feel comfortable, and if it doesn't feel comfortable, you shouldn't be doing it. If there is any discomfort other than a feeling of fullness, which shouldn't be painful, spend an extra week doing the finger exercises or give up the concept of anal intercourse.

Swabbing the Decks of the Hershey Highway

Some people prefer to give themselves a quick enema or "short shot" with a bulb syringe before having anal sex. Others will equate this with removing the patina from the Statue of Liberty. Fortunately, the rectum is not usually a storage space for poop. It's more like the toll booth between the colon and the toilet. A good soaping in the shower should make most anuses sparkle.

If you decide to give yourself an enema, do it an hour or so before sex. A bulb syringe with water should do the trick. Follow the instructions on the box. Make sure the water is not too cold, unless you enjoy giving yourself cramps. Do not use a Fleet or Fleet-like enema for anal sex, as it contains a laxative. For more cleaning options, see *The Ulti-mate Guide to Anal Sex for Women, 2nd ed.*

What Porn Leaves Out

In *The Ultimate Guide to Anal Sex for Women*, Tristan Taormino warns that porn leaves out the most important parts of anal sex. When porn actors have anal sex, they use lots of preparation, lube, anal fore-play and sometimes drugs—none of which they show porn. So when you are watching porn classics such as *Bongwater Butt Babes, Anal Buffet* and anything with *Tushy* in the title, don't for a moment try to replicate it in real life.

Anal Intercourse

Assuming you've spent a few weeks teaching your anal sphincters to relax and you feel comfortable with a finger or sex toy massaging your anus and being inserted into it, consider moving forward with anal intercourse if that is your goal.

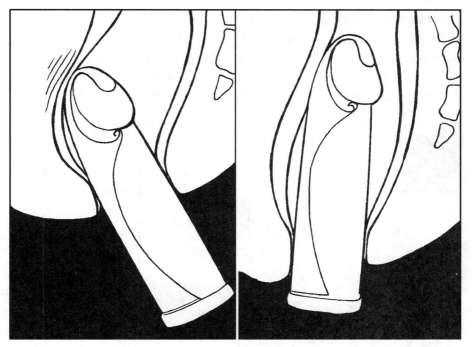

Unlike the vagina, the rectum curves. So you will want to experiment with positions that will help straighten out the rectal curves. Other-wise, a penis might rear-end the walls of the rectum.

Some people recommend that a woman has an orgasm before you try anal insertion. At the very least, she should be relaxed and highly aroused. As for who does what, the couple needs to decide if he will slowly push a well lubricated penis into her anus or if she will ease herself onto it. Also, using a condom is advisable, not only because it will help the penis glide in more easily, but it can protect her from getting an STI and him from getting a prostate infection. And clean up will be ten times easier.

In Slow—Out Slower

As one gay male writer says, when it comes to the anus, an inch can feel like a yard. So no matter what you are putting inside a rectum, it needs to go in slowly and come out slowly. While it's easy to appreciate that incoming objects need to be inserted slowly, this is even more true for things being pulled out of a rectum. It doesn't matter if it's a finger, penis or butt plug. Pull it out very slowly. Otherwise, extreme discomfort and possibly even damage might result.

Simultaneous Clit Play

Several women say that clitoral stimulation helps take anal sex from being nothing to write home about to something that can feel good. Talk about ways to give the clitoris plenty of attention while you are doing anal play, eg. stimulating it with your fingers or using a vibrator.

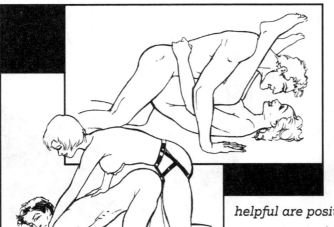

Positions for anal intercourse are the same as with vaginal intercourse. Some are more intimate and allow for the couple to kiss, while others provide better access to the clitoris or penis. Especially helpful are positions that allow the rectum to straighten. (Highly Recommended: "The Anal Sex Position Guide" by Tristan Taormino from Quiver.)

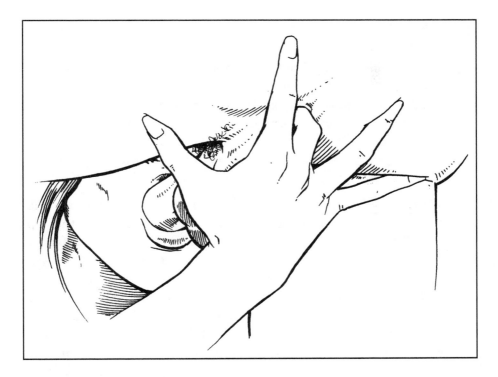

Anal Play Combined with Oral Sex

"I like to have my anus stimulated when I'm receiving oral sex.
I like to have one finger inserted, but it doesn't have to be very
far, just past the sphincter will do. And rather than sliding all
the way in and out, it is better if there is just a slight tugging
movement. It adds one more sensation to the myriad of sensations involved in oral sex." *female age 37*

"My boyfriend likes me to rub a finger on his anus while I give
him oral sex. Gentle pressure and a rotating finger add a lot to
his pleasure." *female age 23*

Some couples enjoy adding a finger or butt plug on or up the anus
during handjobs, oral sex and vaginal intercourse (see the illustration
below). Decide if you want the finger or toy to move in and out, or to
stay put to stimulate the prostate or give a sense of fullness.

Wearing a well-lubricated latex glove can help a finger glide nicely,
into a partner's anus and it will make clean up much easier.

Pegging or "Bend Over Boyfriend"

> "My boyfriend of five years actually made the suggestion that I penetrate him anally. I lubricated the finger with the shortest nail on it and slowly slid it into his anus. He enjoyed it so much that he asked for two fingers and then three. While doing this, I also alternated sucking and manually pumping his cock with my other hand. He had a mind-blowing orgasm. He tells me it's the kind you feel deep down to your toes.... I'm now looking for a strap-on that stimulates me as well as him!" *female age 40*

Some people believe only gay men enjoy anal stimulation. Yet straight men have rectums that are every bit as sensitive as those of gay men. While plenty of straight men would rather not have a dildo or butt plug up their rear, other guys enjoy the feeling. There have even been straight videos titled *Bend Over Boyfriend* and *Babes Ballin' Boys.*

As for penetrating male partners anally, fingers that are well lubricated work incredibly well. Some women will use a dildo. Some even wear a dildo harness and propel it with their hips. A dildo harness looks somewhat like an athletic supporter. It holds the dildo in the same position as a man's erect penis. This allows the woman to thrust in and out, more or less. Learning how to use a dildo in a harness is an acquired art that takes time, patience, and practice. (If a harness is what you'd like, there are different kinds of dildo harnesses, including some that strap to your thigh.)

When it comes to anal sexplay, a man's anal sphincters need just as much practice and preparation as a woman's.

Prostate Stimulation

The only time most straight men get anal stimulation is during a physical exam, and this is more like a drive-by than an attempt to provide pleasure. Men who are curious about feeling their own prostate and who have a finger as long as ET's can do so by inserting a finger up their anus. Pressing on the prostate will create a dull, subtle sensation in the penis. But for men with fingers that are normal sized, the physical contortions needed to reach their own prostate can ruin the moment. A man can purchase a sex toy that's made to help stimulate his prostate. For more on the prostate gland, see Chapter 10: *The Prostate & The Male Pelvic Underground.*

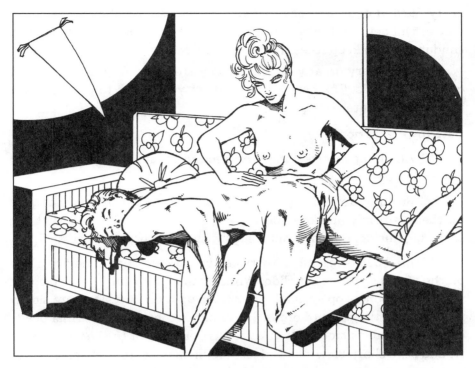

Using the index finger instead of the middle finger allows for a deeper probe. If you use a middle finger, the knuckles on the index and ring fingers act as governors. They prevent it from going very deep.

Butt Plugs

Butt plugs are dildo-like toys made specifically for the rear end. They are wide in the middle and have narrow bases that flare out to keep them from getting lost in the rectum. Butt plugs come in many different sizes, and some even vibrate. Because of their unique shape, butt plugs don't work well for thrusting. People use butt plugs to give their rear ends a feeling of fullness.

If you are looking for sex toys, do research on which ones are best for anal play. If the toys you are sticking up your rear end don't have a flared base, they need to have a butt-toy approved handle or string to pull the toy out with in case it disappears up your butt. This is a hazard that should not be taken lightly. Objects that are lost in the rectum often require Emergency Room assistance. If you plan to use a sex toy for both vaginal and anal recreation, get a separate toy for each port of entry. Having dedicated sex toys helps decrease the chance that fecal matter will get into the vagina. If a sex toy has a porous surface, use a condom on it to keep feces from collecting in it.

Sex toys vary greatly in price. Some are made from funky or dangerous materials. The best way to protect yourself is to purchase sex toys from a reputable source.

Butt Toy Precautions

Anything inserted into the rectum must be smooth with no points or ridges.

Rectums are hungry orifices. Make sure that anything that goes up them is firmly anchored on the outside of the body so it can't get sucked up inside. Dildos or butt plugs with flared bases are best.

Anal beads resemble worry beads, but each bead is held in place on the string so it doesn't slide. While anal beads can be used to count your worries on, people usually stick them up their butt. They are slowly pulled out at the point of orgasm to enhance the sensation. Anal beads can be as small as mothballs or as big as golf balls. If the beads are plastic and have sharp blow-mold edges, file them down first. Also, it is wise to encase anal beads in a condom before inserting. That's because they are very difficult to clean.

Wash anal sex toys with soap and hot water, and then disinfect them by boiling them or soak them in a 10% bleach solution for at least 20 minutes. If disinfecting a toy will damage it, then you shouldn't be using it for anal sex unless you can put a new condom over it each time.

Why Using Condoms Is So Important for Anal Sex

Few women understand that their chances of getting HIV from anal intercourse is 17 times greater than their chances of getting it from vaginal intercourse. Straight or gay, single or married, monogamous or orgy-inclined, it is best to use a condom when having anal intercourse. While avoiding HIV, AIDS and other sexually transmitted infections is the most important reason to use condoms during anal sex, there are other concerns as well.

Fluids deposited in the rectum are absorbed more easily into the body than fluids deposited in the vagina. So a woman's colon is going to slurp up male ejaculate that's been deposited in her rear end. How her immune system will respond is anyone's guess. If you put a condom on the penis, you've eliminated a potential source of concern. And both of our prostate consultants balk the thought of sticking an unbagged penis up a rectum, even if you are having sex with a wife of twenty years. That's because the same bacteria that are prevalent in the rectum can cause a prostate infection (prostatitis). They can also cause vaginal infections when a penis goes from an anus to a vagina.

No matter how hard you wash a penis after anal sex, bacteria-laden chunks of feces can remain inside the urinary opening. Using a condom will prevent this. If he is not using a condom for anal sex, a man should wash his penis well afterward and try to take a leak help flush out unwelcome bacteria. Here are three more things to consider:

👓 Don't used ribbed or studded condoms for anal sex. The extra friction from the ribbing on the surface is not helpful.

👓 Please read "Lubes for Anal Play" on pages 290 - 291.

👓 Some people have been trumpeting the value of the female condom for anal intercourse. Experienced users recommend that you take out the inner ring before inserting the female condom in the rectum. Plus, you can leave the female condom in your ass if you want to take an intermission or need to go shopping or something. However, using female condoms for anal sex has not received FDA sanction, so beware.

Rimming —Hepatitis and More

Rimming refers to when one partner sticks a tongue up or around the other's anus. Whether you are straight or gay, it's not a good idea to rim just anyone, as this can be a way of getting hepatitis, E. coli, salmonella, shigella, amoeba, giardia, and cryptosporidiosis.

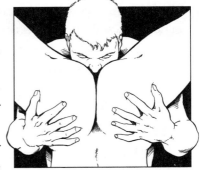

By the time a couple has been having sex with each other for a few years, they pretty much share the same anal and intestinal flora. So you probably won't get anything worse from licking your partner's anus than you would from licking your own. But in more casual relationships, you should definitely get a hepatitis vaccination and consider using a safe sex barrier between your mouth and a new partner's anus.

Double Penetration

"I have had anal sex intermittently. It's okay. I was double penetrated twice and *THAT* was the most incredible thing, but it was a dangerous science to get the positioning just right." *female 28*

See Chapter 41: Double Penetration for more information about DP.

Anal Fisting

Anal fisting involves sticking you fist up a partner's rectum. While it can be safely done between partners who are highly experienced, it can be dangerous if done by anyone else. There is a highly regarded book on the subject by Bert Herrman: *Trust: The Hand Book—A Guide to the Sensual and Spiritual Art of Handballing.* The subject is also covered in Tristan Taormino's *Ultimate Guide to Anal Sex, 2nd ed.*

It never hurts to check with a physician first, perhaps one who is recommended by your local gay and lesbian health center. Even if you are not gay, an LGBT center is more likely to know about the practice and will send you to a more fisting-friendly practitioner. There are also organized groups of fisters in large cities who offer talks and demonstrations.

When a Condom or Sex Toy Gets Lost in the Dungeon of Doom?

According to the excellent *Sex Disasters* by Charles Moser, M.D., a condom lost up your rectum can go farther up than your partner can reach with his or her fingers. Not to worry, it will most likely come out the next time you have a bowel movement. However, if you are concerned you will die from a condom up your crapper, visit an ER.

As for a sex toy lost up your bum, that is a different story. Do not try to reach up and grab it, as you are likely to shove it farther up. If you can't squat and push it out, seek medical attention. Depending on the object, this can be a very serious situation.

Precautions for Anal Sex—A Recap

Straight or gay, married or in transition, if you are doing anal intercourse, use a condom and LOTS of condom-friendly lube. Do not use lubes that numb your butt like *Anal Ease* and *Tushy Tamer Anal Desensitizing Cream.* This is the equivalent of unhooking the fire alarms in your home because you sometimes burn the toast. Don't use lube with sorbitol or glycerin (see page 291). Do not put anything up your rectum that has sharp edges or can break. Make sure that your nails

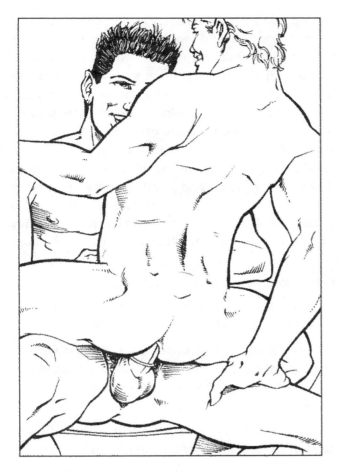

These lads want you to use condoms for anal sex even if you are married and straight as a road through Kansas.

are well-trimmed and filed. 😎 Use only sex toys that were designed for anal sex play. 😎 Make sure that anything about to go up your rectum is clean and well-lubricated. You may need to re-apply the lube often. That's because the rectum was designed to absorb fluids back into the body. 😎 Positions for anal intercourse are similar to those used with vaginal intercourse. Feedback is important. Discuss which positions and angles feel best. 😎 Remove anything you have placed in the rectum very slowly. This includes a penis. 😎 Don't stick a finger, penis or other object directly into a vagina when it's just been up an anus. Wash it first with soap and water. 😎 People who have anal intercourse should get a rectal swab done to check for sexually transmitted infections. 😎 Never, ever have anal sex unless your rectum is in 100% good health. Do not attempt anal sex if it is painful. 😎 Try not to hold your breath.

Breathing deeply will help you relax. 😎 Once you get a finger, penis, or sex toy inside your partner's rear end, don't start thrusting with it. Leave it in place and gently start making circular motions. If and when your partner wants you to start thrusting, pull out slowly and add more lube. Then start thrusting slowly. 😎 Using a latex glove helps fingers slide in more smoothly. Using a condom helps a penis slide in more smoothly. 😎 Don't have anal sex when you are drugged or drunk. Your rear end is more easily damaged by sloppy sex than other parts of your body. Anal sex requires that the driver as well as the passenger be alert and sober. 😎 If you have medical questions about anal sex but are not comfortable speaking to your healthcare provider, call an LGBT health center or national sex hot line. If they can't answer the question, they should be able to find you a healthcare provider who you will be comfortable speaking to.

Women's Comments about Anal Sex

"Best way to have anal sex with a partner? Me rubbing my clit with his finger or a small toy in/around my ass. *female age 39*

"If my partner hadn't already been experienced with it, it probably could have gone horribly wrong. My favorite is a finger in the ass while I touch my clit and finger myself with my partner sucking on my breasts." *female age 25*

"I like anal a few times a month. I have to be feeling clean and in the mood to cum hard as my orgasm is super intense." *female 39*

"It took practice but now I enjoy anal. Still can't just stuff a cock right in. The magic 'formula' if you will: oral, a bit of thrusting while stretching me out using fingers or a toy, then lots of lube and slow entry with a moment to let me adjust. Then I rub my clit while he fucks my ass and dear god I almost see stars when I cum!" *female age 39*

"Sometimes I masturbate using a dildo, sometimes a buttplug, sometimes both. Usually the dildo will make an appearance halfway in, but if I want the buttplug, it makes a very early appearance, sometimes even before I start touching my clitoris."*female 33*

"Sometimes I really want it and end up having insane orgasms with a little clitoral stimulation." *female age 32*

Sex Fantasies

Given how sex fantasies are nearly universal, it's surprising we tend to be embarrassed about them. But why bother fantasizing about things that everyone else approves of?

Some people have a single reliable sex fantasy that they return to time and again. Others have a toolbox of scenes, scenarios and images that help get them off. And some people, more women than men, report not having sex fantasies. However, they might have sensual fantasies that accomplish the same thing, but you'd never confuse them with porn. Their fantasies could be more like lying on a warm relaxing beach, or images of things that allow them to turn off the vigilant parts of their mind and become more at one with the sensations in their body.

Some sex fantasies are highly scripted, others are little more than collages or fleeting images. Some fantasies are hardcore, others are more sensual than sexual. Some begin with sexual imagery that evolves slowly. Most people find it difficult to masturbate without a sexual fantasy, and many people fantasize during intercourse.

The content of sex fantasies varies; some are sweet, kind and silly; others are weird, kinky and bizarre. Some are action-packed and exciting; others are quiet and etherial. Some sex fantasies are populated with past lovers, singers, people in uniforms, movie stars, teachers, priests, family members, total strangers and even furry friends from another species. One of the more popular sex fantasies involves things you've done sexually with your current or a past partner.

Fantasies get their fuel from the deepest recesses of our mind and they can often be shaped by the culture we were raised in. Fantasies allow us to be different from who we are in real life. We can be active or passive, devil or angel.

There's nothing that says an obsessively neat surgeon can't have a fantasy of being masturbated by a pair of smelly feet, or a faithful and loving wife can't have rough sex with her husband's best friend or be part of a threesome, which is one of the more common fantasies that women have. Or maybe she fantasies about something more tame, like having her back rubbed or being unconditionally loved.

Rape Fantasies

It's not unusual to have fantasies where sex is forced, nor is it unusual to fantasize about sex with people in uniform. Consider this passage from Betty Dodson's fine book, *Sex for One*, Harmony Books:

> "A friend who considered herself a radical feminist got concerned that her sexual imagery wasn't politically correct because it wasn't 'feminist oriented.' I assured her that all fantasies were okay. Lots of people imagine scenes they never want to experience. I also pointed out that we can become addicted to a fantasy like anything else, and suggested she experiment with new ones. One of her new assertive fantasies is about moving her clitoris in and out of her lover's soft wet mouth while he's tied down. Whenever she gets stuck or is in a hurry, she brings out her old fantasy of being raped by five Irish cops and always reaches orgasm quickly."

Being raped in fantasy can be a way to enjoy pleasure that would otherwise cause guilt. Sex that is out of your control keeps you from having to feel responsible for wanting it. It is also a way to feel sexually desired and valued, since the perpetrator would do anything to have you. If you ask most women who have rape fantasies to describe the man who is "raping" them, you'll find he's not what we picture when we think of a violent felon, unless the guy has been spending six hours a day in the prison weight room or reads slash fiction to his cellmates.

The perpetrators in many rape fantasies are actors, musicians or bodice-ripping hunks—someone who the woman might want to have sex with anyway. Often missing is the terror, violence, confusion, rage and disgust that makes rape RAPE. The woman is in control by virtue of who she has "raping" her or because she's the one scripting the scenario, while control is the last thing a woman who is being raped in real life has any of.

Even if the woman's rape fantasy involves her being degraded or humiliated, it doesn't make her fear men in real life like an actual rape often does. It doesn't make her afraid to go out of doors like having been raped in real life might. Then again...

Fantasies of Real Rape

When it comes to human sexuality, just when you think you know what you are talking about, someone will mercifully set you straight. When I did a post about rape fantasies for *Psychology Today*, several woman agreed that their "rape" fantasies had few similarities to rape in real life. But then, a reader made the following comment:

> "This does not apply to me, and I am a woman with rape fantasies. I think there is such a thing as a true 'rape fantasy,' and that is what I have. My rape fantasies involve scenes of violent and degrading sex torture committed by men who disgust me, like an overweight and dirty old man, or a socially awkward and unattractive geek who masterminded a plan to imprison me and torture me with strange machines."

> "For me, there is a strong humiliation-pleasure connection. My own fantasies disturb me and give me fear, but they are the only thing that works for me sexually. I can't get off without them."

This is an important reminder of how complex sexuality can be, and how complex our sexual fantasies can be.

Men's vs. Women's Sex Fantasies

Girls in our society are raised on videos and fashion images of attractive female models—attractive if you don't take into account the degree of Photoshopping it takes to make them look that way or how many meals these women barf up to stay slim, or how much silicone they have surgically packed into their chests. Add to this the influence of porn, and it's not like porn producers hire plus sized women.

As young women look at these images, they often think about other women's bodies, particularly the ideal woman whom they hope to someday become. Boys, on the other hand, have traditionally grown up fantasizing about doing things; for instance, being firemen, sports heroes, musicians, stuntmen and perhaps porn stars. Even when it comes to video games, boys are forever killing, bombing, shooting or building something. So boys' fantasies tend to be more about doing, while women's might be more a combination of doing as well as being admired for how they look.

Psychologist Karen Shanor believes that when women see an erect penis in their fantasies, they often relish it as a sign that the man finds them irresistible, as opposed to being in awe of the penis itself. She also says that when a woman walks into a formal affair like a prom, the first thing she often notices is how the other women look and how she feels in comparison. Men usually aren't concerned with how the other men look, unless they are actors or gay.

Shanor's theory does have its limitations. It doesn't explain why many women prefer the sexual touch and feel of a man's body. It doesn't explain why a lot of women enjoy the way a penis feels when it's inside of them, or why they might find a male's butt or shoulders to be sexy.

And when a woman is at a swim meet or water polo game, it's hard to believe her eyes don't stray to the front of the guys' Speedos, after checking out their butts and abs, of course.

Your Lover's Sex Fantasies

Every once in a while, one partner will tell the other about his or her private sex fantasy. Stranger things have happened. But don't expect to see the fantasy plastered on a billboard surrounded by neon lights. Most of us are a little embarrassed by our sexual fantasies, sometimes with good reason. As a result, we don't reveal our fantasies in a way that's particularly direct, nor should we.

So let's say you are a guy and your sweetheart casually or jokingly makes an off-the-cuff statement that she likes seeing guys in jock straps. Boom, ball's in your court. If you have half a brain, and not many of us do, you won't laugh and tell her how much better you feel in boxers than wearing some old athletic supporter. Instead, you will consider buying some new jocks, maybe in colors, maybe one with a cup, what the heck.

So there you are later that night, with your partner's warm familiar fingers slowly popping the buttons on your blue jeans and bingo, she discovers you are wearing a cool looking athletic supporter underneath! Before you know it, she's in sexual orbit and you are the happiest jock on your block! Or she might discover her fantasy was best when it was only imagined and that it loses it's erotic edge when acted out in reality. There are no guarantees.

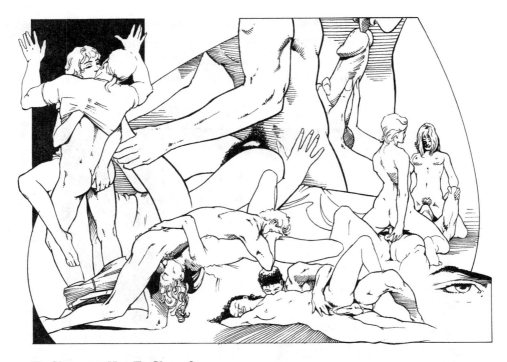

To Share or Not To Share?

People occasionally have sexual fantasies about someone other than their partner. Sometimes it is prudent not to share these fantasies, e.g., "The reason I got so hot is because I pretended you were Mike." Other times your partner might find these fantasies very arousing.

While it's great that you and your partner might be open to hearing each other's fantasies, this doesn't mean that you need to act them out. Sometimes you'll say, "That one doesn't work for me—let's look for something we can both get into!" When you do find the right fantasies that turn both of you on, acting them out together can be great fun.

Responsibility

Knowledge of your partner's fantasies is a trust that remains with you for life. This holds true even if you break up and find yourselves disliking each other. No one forced you to be in a relationship with the person, so don't go blabbing personal stuff just to be hurtful. In the long run, it reflects badly upon you. People who gossip about a current or former partner's sexuality are both shallow and deceitful. The laws of karma will someday haunt them, assuming there are laws of karma.

Readers' Comments about Their Sex Fantasies

"At work I daydream a lot about sex and what it would be like with certain people that I am especially attracted to. Since I am about to get married, I sometimes feel bad thinking of others, but as long as you don't act on it, you're pretty much okay." *female age 30*

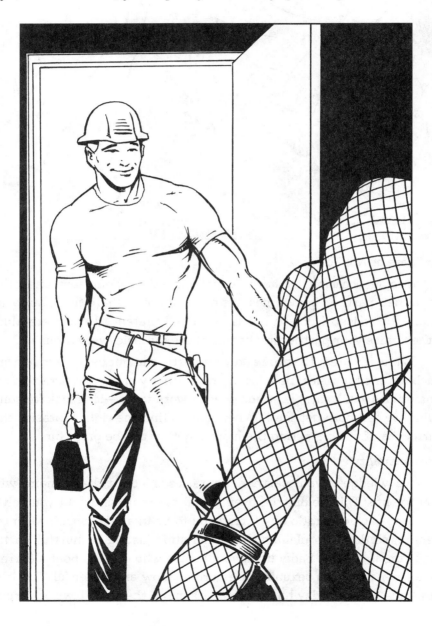

"As a working mother, I get sex and orgasms, but I rarely get romance, so that is what I fantasize about." *female age 36*

"I probably have similar fantasies to anyone who watches the Sci Fi channel too much." *male age 30*

"My fantasies always involve my current real life lover. We're making romantic love somewhere that is new to us—a beach, forest, remote island, in front of a fire in a cabin." *female age 34*

"My fantasies don't play a huge part in my life, except that I get confused why I have fantasies about other girls when I love penises and my boyfriend very much." *female age 23*

"I had always fantasized about my girlfriend being totally naked with her legs spread apart when I came into the room. One day she actually did this! It was awesome!" *male age 21*

"I don't have any clearly defined fantasy. They are more fleeting feelings and don't affect my life much." *female age 38*

"In my fantasies, I am always me, but not necessarily my biological sex or gender, rather like a body made out of my mind. As a teenager, I invented stories about a girl representing me. By completing quests, she earned magic to switch my bodily form. I think I stopped at about 16. By then the girl was made out of two women (one blonde, one red-haired), a young man and a mermaid. I've never told anyone, not because I feared judgment, but because it was mine alone." *female age 37*

"My husband and I have been married for 10 years and still love to act out our fantasies. Last month he was a customs agent and I was trying to sneak something across the border. After he completely searched me, I had to bribe him with sexual favors until he let me go. Later, I was a physician and he the reluctant patient." *female age 33*

"I'd love to see my girlfriend get it on with another woman and I know it would be a turn-on to see her get it on with another guy, but I don't know if I could keep from getting jealous." *male age 39*

"In general, I like to fantasize about money shots." *male age 32* *[Small wonder, this man said that when he masturbates, 99% of the time it is to porn.]*

"I have too many different sex fantasies to list and I tend to think about sex all day." *female age 32*

"My favorite fantasy is a threesome with another woman; I share my thoughts with my husband and we sometimes make fake plans how to organize it and what the person should look like." *female age 45*

"Mine is a threesome with two guys. I'd like to be double penetrated, but I'd have to trust the back door guy a bunch to not hurt me." *female age 39*

"Watching my husband have sex with another woman while a different women goes down on me! I think about it a lot when he goes down on me" *female age 28*

"I fantasize about BDSM a lot." *female age 20*

"Scenarios involving CFNM and small penis humiliation." *male age 31*

"I try to stick to memories of my girlfriend." *male age 29*

"I have fantasies about being forced to strip for examinations and being stripped searched." *male age 48*

Have you ever had homosexual fantasies?

"I used to fantasize about women all of the time. Finally, I decided to give it a try and had sex with one of my best female friends, who is mostly heterosexual. It was fun and every now and then we play with one another. I have never developed an emotional attachment to her or any other woman, and I no longer fantasize about women." *female age 26*

"I fantasize about being with another woman often, but I also fantasize about my boyfriend and Brad Pitt!" *female age 25*

"I am aroused by images of women with women; also by stories of multiple partners. On occasion, I use these fantasies to reach orgasm." *fem 32*

"I've had no fantasies or gay experiences, although I wonder sometimes if I could get turned on by another guy." *male age 30*

"I wonder if gay men fantasize about being with a straight man? *male 20*

Thanks to Wendy Maltz for her astute and thoughtful article *Women's Sexual Fantasies* by Wendy Maltz and Suzie Bossfrom in *Private Thoughts: Exploring the Power of Women's Sexual Fantasies*, Booksurge.

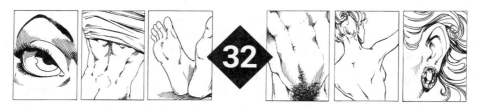

The Fairy Pornmother

Hello Sweeties! I'm the Fairy Pornmother. The author of the *Guide To Getting It On* asked me to provide you with some perspective on the porn industry, which I call Pornland.

Nobody in Pornland ever dreamed people would take porn seriously. I mean, look at my titties. Look at my waist. My lips are purrrrfect. (Both sets of them.) How many women really look like me or the other actresses in porn?

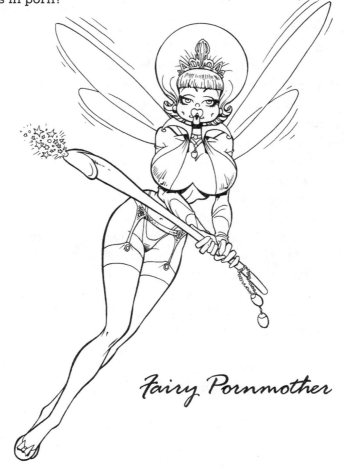

Fairy Pornmother

Nobody in Pornland ever thought 8- to 12-year-olds would start watching porn and it would become their only source of sex education. Now most middle schoolers think what we do is real! They think it's what they should do. They think guys can get hard on demand and stay hard for hours at a time like the men in Pornland. I'll bet you didn't know that two of my best actors ended up in the emergency room with doctors having to stick needles in their penises to help relieve the pressure. Porn actors take nearly toxic doses of boner drugs so they can have erections on demand, and sometimes their erections won't go down. (In Pornland, we call Viagra Vitamin D!)

People in porn excel at one thing: getting our freak on for the camera. We love it when you are watching us do things with our clothes off. But that's not making love and it should not be confused with it.

Have you ever seen any of us kiss for half an hour? Have you ever seen us give each other massages or laugh and tease? None of that works for the camera. No one who is horny wants to land on a website where porn actors are kissing. You'd hate us.

When's the last time you made love to someone whose crotch had makeup on it and a 400 watt spotlight shining between her legs? That's what we do in Pornland. We're an amusement park of excess. We exaggerate everything.

There are no A-cup breasts or five-inch penises in Pornland. They're forbidden. Our job is to create videos that will get you to click and stroke. That's our bread and butter. Even if you never pay us a single dollar, Pornland makes money each time you click. None of what we do is about sex in real life or making love.

I hire actresses who can convince you they're having orgasms when a man with a penis the size of a Pringle's can is pounding them in ways that would cause most women pain. I hire actresses who won't throw up when I tell them to suck on a penis that's just been up their rear end. I hire actresses who can have sex in positions that would make the joints of a yoga teacher explode.

I hire actresses who will do things that cam girls and prostitutes won't do. And I try to make you think it's normal, even if your wife or girlfriend won't do it either. For a lot of the girls who work in porn, it's their fifteen minutes of fame. It's about them getting to feel good about themselves because you're at home masturbating to them. And I don't want you to ever masturbate without watching porn. That would be a catastrophe as far as our business plan is concerned.

I understand that not all porn is from Pornland. There's amateur porn that people post online. But if homegrown porn doesn't look like what we produce here, you aren't going to watch it. You're not going to put up with some guy giving a woman oral sex for half an hour while she's laying there looking like she took a handful of tranquilizers because it feels so good. Who cares if he's rocking her world? It doesn't matter unless the camera can make it look like he's rocking her world.

Our job is to excite you without asking a thing of you. Good luck making that work in real life! But the truth is, very few of the actresses you watch in porn have sex this way in real life. One of my best actresses who you've watched faking orgasm after orgasm is not able to have orgasms during intercourse in real life. She needs to receive almost an hour of oral sex in order to come, and that's with her real life husband who's had to learn exactly how to stimulate her clitoris with his tongue.

So it's fine to enjoy porn, but remember it's not about making love and it's not about pleasing a partner. We don't care about that in Pornland.

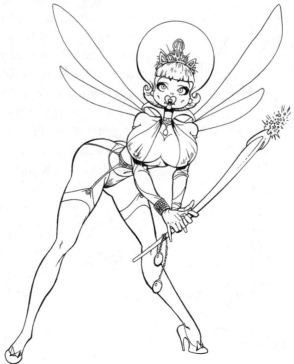

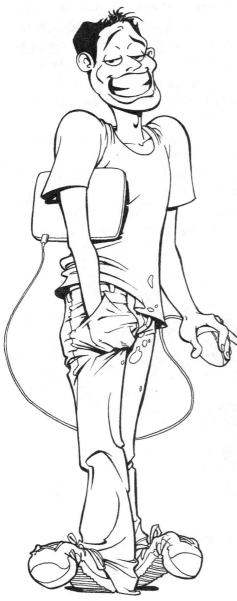

Porndoggie's
Dirty Dozen

People have been looking at porn since cavemen did the first chalk drawings of couples having sex. Fortunately, the technology has improved since then.

There is nothing wrong about enjoying porn, as long as you aren't doing it 24/7. If they had the choice, most people would rather be with a real-life lover or be able to watch porn with a real-life lover, except for Porndoggie who thinks that sex in porn is the best sex ever.

Here's Porndoggie's list of what he likes best about porn.

#1. Creampies and Money Shots (or 'Facials')

Porndoggie: *Creampies or facials, creampies or facials, I can't decide which represents a better use of a porn actor's talent.*

DEFINITION: The *creampie* has only been in porn for the past decade or so. It's where a man does a shallow ejaculation inside of a woman's vagina or anus, but quickly withdraws so the viewer can see his semen oozing out. The *facial* or *money shot* is when a porn actor pulls his penis from whatever part of an actress's body it's been in, aims it at her face, breasts or some other part of her body, and then strokes furiously until he ejaculates. Facials or money shots are the hallmark of modern porn. Almost 95% of mainstream porn movies include facials or shots of men coming on their partner's bodies.

ANALYSIS: Facials would rarely happen if it weren't for their popularity in porn, and creampies would almost never happen. We occasionally receive a sex survey from a woman who thinks it's hot when a guy ejaculates on her face or breasts. However, most women do not enjoy this. So do not assume your partner wants you to come on her face, breasts, belly, or back unless she asks. And do not get semen in her eyes. It will burn.

#2. Anal Sex and ATM

Porndoggie: *While I think ATM is the coolest thing since anal bleaching, nothing hits the spot like old fashioned anal sex.*

DEFINITION: ATM or *ass-to-mouth* is a recent addition to mainstream porn. It involves a porn actor pulling his penis from an actress's rectum and placing it directly into her mouth without washing it. It is referred to as ATM, A2M, or ATG (ass-to-gob) if you are British. Sometimes, the actor will pull his penis from the rectum of one actress and place it into the mouth of another actress, or he might do "ass-to-pussy."

ANALYSIS: Anal sex dates back to the time of the ancients, but pulling a penis out of a woman's ass and shoving it into her mouth is a recent invention. It's porn's way of going the extra degrading mile. How is it that a porn actress will never stick a finger or dildo up the ass of a male porn actor and put it straight into the male actor's mouth? Perhaps that's because most straight men would find this horrifying.

REAL LIFE: Anal sex requires trust, relaxation, lubrication, feedback, desire, and practice. None of these are ever shown in porn. If anal sex is something you both want to experiment with, then learn as much as you can about it first. Go slowly and cautiously. That way, your chances of it being an enjoyable experience will rise dramatically. But under no circumstances should you try to have anal sex like they show in porn.

#3. Women Always Want Sex!

Porndoggie: *The women in porn love sex more than other women. And they know that porn actors have the skills to please them.*

ANALYSIS: Sex in porn requires no intimacy and there's no investment in a relationship. There's no need to respect and treat a partner well. No one ever feels tired or just wants to cuddle.

REAL LIFE: Not all women want sex 24/7. For some, it's the non-sexual aspects of a relationship that help make sex feel special.

#4. No Time Wasted on Kissing

Porndoggie: *The reason women get tired of men is that men spend too much time trying to kiss them. Women want sex now.*

ANALYSIS: Porn defines women by their vaginas, with their rectums and breasts being other points of interest. There is no caressing, passionate kissing, or running your fingertips through your partner's hair.

REAL LIFE: There are times when a woman wants sex without delay. And many women wish their partners were more take-charge in bed. But that doesn't mean this is all they want. And many women prefer twenty minutes or more of kissing and other forms of sexplay before a penis is involved or before a man touches between their legs.

#5. You Never Need to Ask

Porndoggie: *Women like a confident man who doesn't need to ask.*

ANALYSIS: In porn, it's the man's job to magically know how to please a woman. "Asking" is relegated to the fringes of porn, such as when a submissive in BDSM says, "May I please lick the mistresses feet?"

REAL LIFE: In real life, a woman needs to let a man know if she wants to have sex. It's called consent. There's also a learning curve. In her book on sex, porn actress Nina Hartley says a millimeter can make all the difference when it comes to stimulating the clitoris. How would you know what feels best without asking and receiving feedback? No

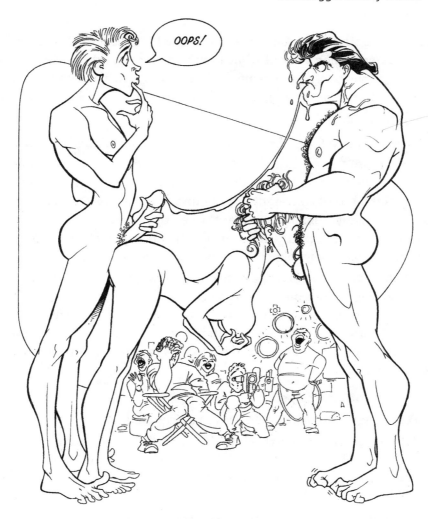

two women respond in the exact same way. Nor will a woman necessarily respond on Friday as she did on Monday. Asking and seeking feedback are the cornerstones of being a good lover, except in porn.

#6. You Get to Fuck a Woman's Face

Porndoggie: *Women enjoy a good face fucking.*

ANALYSIS: In porn, a man often grabs the sides of a porn actress's head and thrusts his penis as far as he can down her throat. There will often be a look of deadness or fear on the face of the porn actress.

REAL LIFE: Most women despise it when a man grabs their head and thrusts his penis down their throat. It feels like assault. They say it's far worse than going down on a man with smelly balls, which is number two on many women's list of what they don't like about oral sex. If you are lucky enough to be receiving oral sex, go out of your way to make sure your partner never gags or feels like she isn't in total control.

#7. Girl-on-Girl

Porndoggie: *What's better than watching a girl tongue another girl's pussy?*

ANALYSIS: In porn, the sex that women have with women is usually choreographed to fit a straight man's fantasy. (Lesbians with long nails, really?) Not many lesbians consider the sex that's shown in mainstream porn to be sex. And porn actresses usually end up sucking on a penis after they've had their token sex with another woman.

REAL LIFE: When women are having sex with women, they usually aren't doing it for the pleasure of men — except for drunk college girls who kiss and grope each other's breasts to up their status with college guys. If you are a woman who is interested in experimenting sexually with another woman, the sex that women have in straight porn is probably not your best guide.

#8. Pussies without Flaps

Porndoggie: *Women in porn have perfect pussies.*

ANALYSIS: Way more women want to be in porn than porn has room for. So porn producers are able to select women with smaller inner labia or women who have had labiaplasty. This has little to do with pleasure in real life, and everything to do with the camera.

REAL LIFE: Labia come in all shapes and sizes. Inner labia get thicker when a woman is sexually aroused. They also have nerves that can feel delightful sensations when they are gently caressed and tugged. While some men might prefer women with inner labia that are less pronounced, others might prefer women with labia that are larger. Most men are so happy to be having sex with a real life partner, a woman's labia are seldom a deal breaker.

#9. Men Have Man-Sized Meat

Porndoggie: *If you have to look at another guy's dick, it might as well be a decent size. And a thicker dick leaves a gaping hole in a woman's pussy or ass for the camera to look into.*

ANALYSIS: Porn actor penis size falls in the top 1% to 10% of all men, while the average penis is just under 5.5 inches long when erect, give or take. The thickness varies as well. So does the shape, head size, color, angle of erection, and number of visible veins on the shaft.

REAL LIFE SOLUTION: Most men who compare themselves to porn actors come up short. And most women who think their male partners should measure up to porn-actor dimensions will be disappointed.

#10. You Get to Call Women Bitches and Whores

Porndoggie: *Women like it when you talk dirty to them!*

ANALYSIS: Women often like it when a partner tells them how hot they look, how good the sex feels, that they give the best blowjobs ever, that their vaginas smell sweet, that they've got great legs or breasts, and that he'd die if he couldn't be with them. This is very different from calling them names.

REAL LIFE: There's a difference between talking dirty and being an asshole. Do not insult or demean your partner unless she tells you it turns her on.

#11. Women Always Come

Porndoggie: *Women really get off in porn. You can tell.*

ANALYSIS: A lot of women don't like porn because they can tell that porn actresses are usually faking that it feels good and faking orgasms. Rather than being about pleasure, everything a porn actress does is to provide the best camera angle and to fool the most people.

REAL LIFE: In real life, women often need a good deal of time and stimulation to orgasm. They also need to be highly aroused. None of this happens in porn. Most women in real life who have orgasms during intercourse either need to stimulate their clitoris with their fingers while a partner is thrusting, or they need to grind their clitoris against their lover's pelvic bone. Also, couples who are making love in real life like to hug and feel each other's skin. In porn, skin-to-skin contact gets in the way of the camera's view of the woman's crotch.

REAL LIFE SOLUTION: Make sex about pleasure instead of orgasms. Never ask your partner if she came as a way of reassuring yourself that you are good in bed. Realize there will be times when she is more aroused by your brushing her hair than by intercourse.

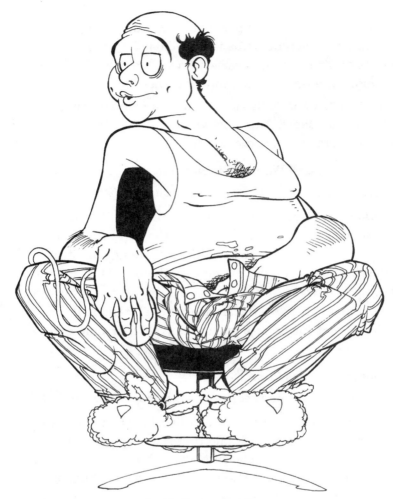

Porndoggie in Twenty-five Years

#12. You Can See Everything and It's Insanely Intense!

Porndoggie: *Not only do they have more kinds of sex in porn, but you get to see it all up close. Really up close.*

ANALYSIS: The only thing porn has to turn you on with besides the sound track is what you can see with your eyes on a flat screen. So everything about porn needs to push the visual limits. The more extreme, the better.

REAL LIFE: People usually don't make love with banks of lights on and with their faces staring into each other's crotches the entire time.

Wait—It's a Baker's Dozen!

#13. No Condoms, Diseases or Periods in Porn!

Porndoggie: *Porn actors don't need to worry about sexually transmitted infections. Plus they never get pregnant except for preggo porn and lactating porn, and the women don't have periods.*

ANALYSIS: According to a study in the *Journal of Sexually Transmitted Infections,* the incidence of chlamydia and gonorrhea among porn actors is much greater than in the general population. Female porn actors are more likely to have more reinfections than other women, which is a concern given how reinfections can impact a woman's reproductive system. The porn industry does not require porn actors to have tests for most sexually transmitted infections.

REAL LIFE: Porn actors, like anyone who is having casual sex, should be wearing condoms. They also need to be just as concerned about birth control as anyone else. A big advantage in staying at home and watching porn is you don't need to worry about pregnancy and getting STIs. As for periods, they are a normal, healthy part of life. Porndoggie should read Chapter 27: *Surfing the Crimson Wave.*

Final Porn Thoughts

Watching porn can be fun, instructive, and hot. It can be a way to treat yourself when your partner is having her night out with her friends, or when you don't have a partner and it's just you and your fist. It can also be helpful to watch porn with a lover and have her tell you what parts she likes and what parts she doesn't like. But try to keep it in perspective, because it really is a much different experience than what happens when you are making love in real life.

Most people understand that sex in porn starts at third base, while in real life, you seldom get to third base until you've spent lots of time on first and second. Except for Porndoggie.

Recommended: If you are looking for a smart and thoughtful way to enjoy porn, be sure to read Dr. David Ley's book titled *Ethical Porn for Dicks: A Man's Guide to Responsible Viewing Pleasure.* David has a great mind and a good perspective on life. I've often asked him for advice with the *Guide To Getting It On.*

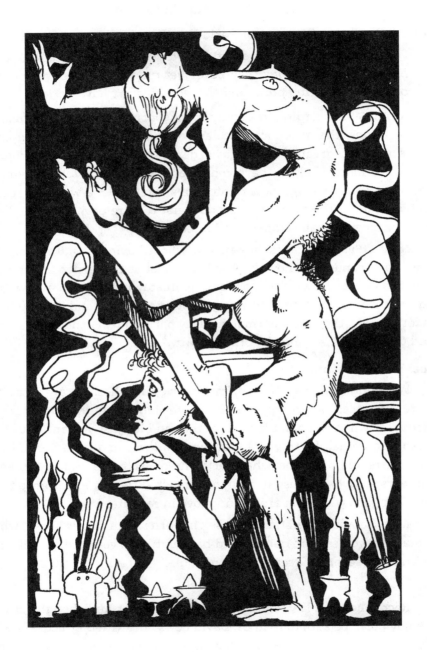

Tantra Porn

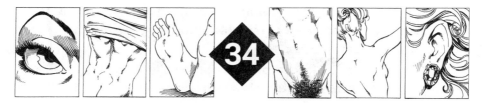

When Women Watch Porn

There are a lot of women who enjoy watching porn. Some like heterosexual porn, while others prefer different types of porn because, as one viewer stated, "Women in het porn are often portrayed as sex-crazed objects that exist for a man's pleasure."

There's also the long held view among women that it's okay for men to watch porn because that's what men do, but it's not okay for women. It's more acceptable for women to look at the Photoshopped spreads of anorexic models in women's magazines than to watch porn.

Whether you are a man or woman, it's totally okay to watch porn. But there can be interesting differences between men and women in the kind of porn they watch and how they watch it.

Differences in the Ways Men and Women's Brains Process Porn

Men's and women's brains are made up of the same structures. But there are times when men and women use these structures differently. Consider the way we interpret facial expressions and body language.

When a man sees the face of a porn actress, he might be focused on her eyes or mouth. But a woman might be more focused on the expression on the face of the porn actress. She might wonder why the porn actress has the expression of a woman who is faking enjoyment or is trying to hide feelings of discomfort or pain.

When a man sees a porn actress's body during a sex scene, he might be thinking how sexy it looks, while a woman who sees the exact same scene might be more focused on the porn actress's body language, and how it seems like she's not fully engaged or involved with her partner. So a man might be noticing one aspect of a sex scene, while a woman might be noticing another.

There are also social issues that could impact men and women differently. When a man sees a porn actor being sexually aggressive with a porn actress, he could be focusing on how good she says it feels while a woman might be reminded of the power imbalance between men and women when it comes to sex.

There can be other aspects of porn that men and women process differently. For instance, when there's a close up between a porn actress's legs, a female viewer might focus on the porn actress's anus and not be turned on by it. Perhaps that's because feces aren't attractive to most people, and anuses are the portal through which feces enter the world. A male viewer might see the same scene and want to put his penis up the porn actress's anus. (One of the greatest advances in the human life span didn't come from the invention of antibiotics, but from the creation of sewer systems in large cities where people live in close proximity. So if women's brains are wired to be more sensitive to hygiene issues, that might not be such a bad thing for society.)

There are also dedicated parts of our brains that process visual input. They help us to link what we see with what we feel. It could be that sex hormones impact these parts of our brains and influence how sexually aroused we become when we watch movies and videos. So some woman might find porn more arousing during ovulation when their sex hormones are at the highest levels.

What Women Who Like to Watch Gay Male Porn Have To Say

One of the world's most popular porn sites has begun releasing search engine data on the types of porn that male and female viewers watch. One of the most fascinating findings is the number of women who watch gay male porn. So researchers interviewed 275 women who like to watch gay male porn to find out why. The women's responses almost sound like a critique of what many women don't like about porn in general. Here's a summary of what they said:

The camera angles in straight porn are from the male partner's point of view. This forces viewers to have to look at sex from a man's perspective. Women have to deal with that often enough in real life. They say that gay porn is more from the perspective of both partners, so it's more comfortable for them to watch and enjoy.

In gay male porn, the man who is on the bottom (in the traditional woman's role) has an erection and gets to ejaculate. So he's not there solely for the pleasure of the guy on the top like women often are in straight porn. This makes it easier for women to enjoy what's being done to the guy on the bottom, because he's receiving as much pleasure as the man on top.

👓 When women watch straight porn, some feel they are supposed to identify with the porn actresses. But porn actresses are often faking it or doing things women find to be distasteful. When women are watching gay male porn, they can identify with whichever partner they want, or simply enjoy the men's bodies and not have to identify with either partner.

👓 The women said that straight porn usually just focuses on the penises of the male actors. So the men don't have much of a personality, and it's hard for women to feel turned on by them.

👓 Since both partners in gay porn are men, the more aggressive partner isn't automatically given that position because he's male. So it can be more fun for women to watch rough sex in gay male porn, because it's all about the sex and not about gender roles.

👓 The women who like seeing hot naked men said they get double their pleasure with gay male porn. And since there are no female actresses in gay male porn, the women don't need to feel jealous of their bodies.

From Our Sex Survey

In our own sex survey, we asked women: *Do you ever watch gay male porn? If so, what are some of the things you like about it when compared to heterosexual porn?* Here are the responses of the women who said they at least occasionally watch gay male porn.

> "I've watched a bit of it. I like that the men are usually very well built and seeing two sexy men going at it together is a huge turn on. It's still quite taboo, so it feels naughty watching it which adds to the eroticism. I also like watching anal sex."
>
> *female age 25*

> "Sometimes I'll chose gay porn over heterosexual porn. I like the penetration, the blow jobs, everything. I think it's awesome to see two people with similar body configuration know how to please each other." *female age 25*

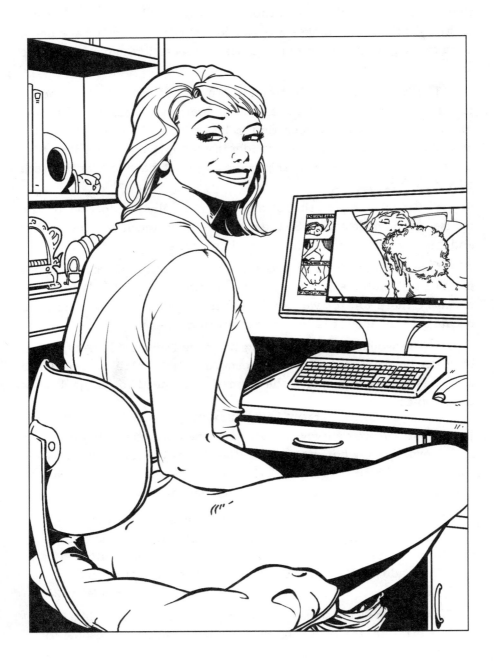

"I like seeing the two actors push each other around a little without feeling scared for the girl if it were straight porn." *female 23*

"It's not as 'fake' as heterosexual or lesbian porn." *female age 26*

"Two guys kissing is nicer plus maybe the more equal power balance is nice." *female age 26*

"I watched it as a teenager because it was arousing and didn't include women acting like children/teens for men." *female age 22*

"I like watching guys cum. Not necessarily gay guys, I just like watching them cum." *female age 50*

"I have a fetish for water sports, and it's more common in gay porn than straight. They also seem to be having a better time than in het porn." *female age 30*

"I like that it doesn't involve women being objectified. Even though it is for the male gaze, it feels less dirty to watch. I also like that you can see if all the performers are hard." *female 22*

"It was the first porn I ever saw, so it still gets me pretty turned on. Mostly I like the fact that there's no woman making fake sounds of arousal!" *female age 45*

"I watch some MMF bisexual porn and that's not too bad. There's something about two guys getting it on is so hot when it is not forced like it typically is in porn." *female age 22*

"I especially like the intensity of how the men react. In straight porn the men don't always react very audibly or expressively."
female age 46

"I like gay porn, but on mute or in brief GIF animations. The actors seem more equal (e.g. a bottom is a totally different empowered beast than most women in porn; there's less of the submissive porn chick shit that is depreciating to women); and I can relate to fucking men more than women. I also prefer M/M romance over heterosexual romance, even though my relationships are with men." *female age 37*

GIFs (MicroPorn) and Tumblr Blogs

Some women who watch porn prefer to watch brief video clips or animations called GIFs. These only last for a few seconds and keep repeating. These brief videos are often highly explicit, but since they only last for a few seconds before repeating, a woman can make sure that each frame turns her on. For instance, not many women are turned on by men coming on their faces or by men suddenly ramming their penises up women's rear ends. So women and couples can create their own GIFs that show only the parts of porn they find arousing.

This is where Tumblr comes into play. A number of couples have Tumblrs where they post images and GIFs of themselves having sex. The focus is often on men giving women sexual pleasure. Some sites have dozens of GIFs that a woman can visually immerse herself in, or she can keep watching a specific GIF while masturbating or getting herself in the mood for partner sex. Or a couple can watch them together.

Women-friendly Tumblr blogs are far outnumbered by Tumblrs with clips from mainstream porn. But with searching enough effort, Tumblr blogs can be a great source for women friendly porn. There are also websites that include women friendly porn.

Lesbian Porn

There is plenty of lesbian action in mainstream heterosexual porn. The only problem is that much of it has little to do with women giving women sexual pleasure. Instead, it's made to appeal to straight men. As a result, much of the lesbian porn isn't really lesbian porn, but the invention of the people who produce and direct straight male porn.

So if you are a woman who likes to watch lesbian porn, you already know that some sites claiming to have girl-on-girl action aren't the best, and you need to search for the sites that work for you.

A Big Thanks! to brain researcher Adam Safron and to Lucy Melville for her "Male gays in the female gaze: women who watch m/m pornography" in Porn Studies Vol 2, 2015.

How the Internet Killed the Plumber in Porn

There used to be a saying about porn and plumbers: "Porn paints an unrealistic picture of how quickly you can get a plumber to your house." Most people over the age of forty get the joke. Yet few teenagers understand what's funny about this, and it's not because they don't watch porn.

There's no room for fantasies or foreplay in today's mainstream porn. Instead, there's a nearly infinite supply of free videos with frame after frame of highly explicit sex. Today's porn viewers would click to another site if they had to watch a fully clothed woman pretending not to notice the bulge in her plumber's pants. Just like *Video Killed the Radio Star*— the Internet killed the plumber in porn.

Parents need to understand this because porn is how their children are learning about sex. Many of today's male college students tell us they saw their first porn between the ages of eight and twelve. Not only have parents been preempted from telling their children about the birds and the bees, but their kids are being sold on the idea that sex happens instantly, with no playfulness, discussion, or intimacy.

So it's important for parents to talk to their children about porn. That's because watching porn is a very different experience for children than watching movies or playing video games. Kids can usually understand that movies and video games are entertainment rather than actual fact. When children watch the Fast and Furious movies, they can tell there's a difference between the way the actors drive and how their parents drive in real life.

When kids are first watching shows where people are killed, they usually have parents or siblings to tell them "They're just actors, and that's not real blood." This is not the case with porn. There's no parent standing over the shoulder of an eight-year-old saying "Men don't usually ejaculate in women's faces" or "That woman isn't screaming in pain, although I would be if someone did that to me."

To children, porn seems like a documentary of how sex is supposed to be. So one of the first things parents need to tell their children from the time they enter middle school is "Porn is not real. Sex in porn is edited to make it look real, but sex happens differently in life." If your kid wants to continue the conversation, great. If not, leave it until next time when you tell them the same thing again. And if your child stares at you blankly or nervously dismisses you by saying "I know that!" nod in quiet agreement, but don't let that dissuade you from bringing it up at another time.

Parents should explain that sex in real life is usually part of a relationship or a friendship. Tell them sex is just as much about hugging, kissing, back rubs and giggling as it is about anything that's going on between their legs. And you cannot remind children enough about the importance of conversation, kindness, romance and respect when it comes to sex. These are qualities they seldom see in porn.

Never ask your children if they watch porn; this will cause unnecessary embarrassment and denials. Just say "A lot of people watch porn, and they don't realize that sex in porn is way different than sex in real life." By not shaming your kids or lecturing them, you are letting them know it's okay to talk to you about sex.

Porn actresses often make being degraded look sexy. They also make it appear that women have a voracious appetite for sex the moment a man wants it, without conversation, consent or condoms. Women in porn do whatever the men want, no matter how bizarre.

In today's middle-schools and high-schools, there is often pressure for girls to act like porn stars, and it's not unusual for girls to send boys naked pics. Talk to your teens about how the quest for popularity and the desire to be wanted is fraught with as many perils as rewards. Help them to form a strategy for reaching their social goals without having to sext their way to the front of the line.

Plenty of boys watch porn on their phones during class or at lunch, and too many of their conversations with girls are straight from the pages of porn. Most teachers and administrators turn a blind eye or offer hollow reprimands. It has become too prevalent for the schools to police. If your daughter feels uncomfortable about the conversations at school, don't assume she's being overly sensitive or that it's the usual boy boasting that's gone on since time began. It's different now. And tell your sons not to watch porn at school or to use language that's sexually disrespectful.

Parents should also be aware of how often Viagra is used in porn. This allows males in today's porn to achieve hydraulic perfection. There isn't any failure, hesitation, or "Oops..." So parents should let their children know that sex in real life is full of awkward and imperfect moments, that a sense of humor is what makes sex and relationships work, and that people with average-sized body parts don't get cast in porn. In our sex survey of more than 10,000 men and women, few have complained about the size, appearance or function of their partner's genitals. Yet from watching porn, you would think that's the only thing that matters.

Also, remind your children that it's perfectly normal to have sexual feelings, but that there's no rush to have sex or to even think about it if they don't want to. Try to be a nonjudgmental voice of moderation in a world that is far more sexualized for children than most parents know.

Hysteria about Sexual Predators Online

Much of what parents hear regarding their kids and the Internet focuses on sexual predators. Yet your teenage daughter is at much greater risk from the influence of the fry cook who she works with at Burger King than she is online. And if your child is going to be molested, in 9-out-of-10 cases it will be done by someone you personally know. You have more to fear from your relatives, baby sitter, neighbors, or the people you might be dating. Far less than 1-in-100 cases of child abuse happen through a predator on the Internet.

As for risk reduction, my wife worked in the juvenile-justice system with teenagers. She'll tell you about a problem that is a million times more immediate for most kids than weirdness on the Internet. It's when teenage girls go to the beach, river, park, or to some unknown house with boys and get high on alcohol and prescription drugs. She's seen case after case of this, and she says the number of young girls who are in trouble with alcohol has skyrocketed. These are girls with good grades from good homes who get into cars with guys who they've never met. So if you are trying to get your harm-reduction priorities straight, drinking and drugs should be at the top of the list.

This doesn't mean you shouldn't be hyper-vigilant about what your kids do on the Internet. It just means that if you are concerned about harm reduction, there are bigger fish to fry in most kid's lives than what they face online.

Sexting, "Send Me a Hot Pic," and Dic Pics

Consider the following words from the mom of a teenage boy. She has full access to his texts and emails. She says all he has to do is text "send me a pic" and "he gets a picture of a girl topless or holding a teddy bear over her breasts, and he'll be like, 'Mom, can you believe this? I just asked her for a pic, and look what she sent.'"

As for your teenage sons, let them know there are district attorneys who are not what we would call enlightened, especially if the dad of the daughter who ends up with your son's penis on her phone contacts the police, or someone finds the naked pic of an underage girl on your son's phone. If someone sends a naked pic of a classmate who is under 18 to your child, tell him to delete it immediately and to never, ever resend it.

Porn in Perspective

Once your kids get to be preteens, you are not going to stop them from seeing porn. Most teenage boys (as well as their fathers) masturbate while watching porn or soon after. Porn is as much a part of male masturbation as tissue and lotion. This is not going to change, and parents shouldn't try to shame their children. Instead, they need to help educate them that sex in porn is as different from sex in real life as the freighters in Star Trek are from airplanes today.

Also be aware that millions of girls and women enjoy watching porn. The porn they watch might sometimes appear more realistic, like on some of the Tumblr blogs where real life couples post pics and videos of themselves having sex. Or maybe they will watch GIF animations, where the action is repeated and there is less chance of the woman being degraded. But the idea that it's just men and boys who watch porn is not correct.

A final thing to keep in mind is that while sex in the movies and on television is seldom as explicit as porn, it often gives the idea that sex happens magically or automatically, just like porn does. Let your kids know that having a satisfying sexual relationship takes way more work in real life than they usually show on TV.

LGBT NOTE: The Internet can be a lifesaver for the isolated gay or transgender teen. There are wonderful resources for LGBT youth online, and while gay and transgender porn is as unrealistic as straight porn, it can be an important validator that it's okay "to be different."

Bye Bye V-Card—Losing Your Virginity

There is more information in this chapter than you probably need if it's your first time. The trouble in leaving out parts is while they may not apply to you, they might be important for someone else.

Keep in mind that couples can become VERY pregnant from their first time, even if they are doing it when a woman is having her period. For a brief legal reminder: If you are under 18, you may be breaking some of your state's laws if you have sex. And regardless of your age, please read Chapter 18: *Consent.* Now, for the fun part.

The Importance of Having a Good First Time

When people have a lousy first time, it tends to negatively color the sex they will be having for the next few years. It's as if the bar gets set so low they don't expect sex to be any better. So taking charge of your first time and trying to make it a good experience is in your best interest for now and for the years to come.

The Realities of a Girl's First Time vs A Boy's First Time

Here are some things that would be good to discuss with your partner before the two of you have intercourse:

By the time most boys lose their virginity, they've had a few years of masturbating under their belt. Most will know what an orgasm feels like. Girls, on the other hand, aren't encouraged to explore their bodies. Few girls will have masturbated before their first time, so not many will know what an orgasm is. Nor will their bodies have experienced anything inside of it. A tampon, maybe, but the chances are good partner's penis will feel different than a tampon; and hopefully it won't have a string attached.

What this means is that unless a girl has a favorite dildo, her vagina will undergo more changes during her first time than her partner's penis will. This doesn't need to be a negative, it's just different.

Another thing is that for most guys, the only love-making education they've had is from watching porn. Porn actors will be the first to tell you that porn was never meant to be used for sex education or as a model for having sex, whether it's your first time or not. Porn never shows couples talking about what they want to do. It never shows them discussing what feels good and what doesn't. Most of the guys in porn take boner drugs and the women do things for the camera that they don't necessarily do at home. Everything is magic in porn and everyone pretends to have great sex all of the time.

Couples in real life spend way more time kissing and caressing before they have intercourse than porn actors do. Real-life couples can enjoy each other's bodies from head to toe instead of focusing on each other's genitals. And the last thing a first-time couple should ever attempt is a hard pounding fuck like they do in porn. Easy does it is the way to go. You've got plenty of years ahead to have sex like a porn star, assuming you would want to. For now it's about being tender and loving.

Preparing Ahead for a Most-Excellent Journey

> "It was very hard to do, but I waited until I was 18 to have inter-course. It was with a guy who cared deeply about me, which made my first experience very fun and comfortable." *female 36*

Most people's first time is unplanned and more awkward than it needs to be. Hopefully, you will make it a time you can remember with fondness—the beginning of a most excellent journey.

In Addition to This Chapter

If you'd like more information about intercourse, check out Chapter 26: *Intercourse—Horizontal Jogging.* But for your first time, you'll want to keep it simple because there are different priorities. Reading this Guide's chapters on romance, kissing, handjobs, finger fucking, and oral sex will put you years ahead of the game.

Who To Do It With Your First Time

Not many of us are still with the person who we lost our virginity to. While we might have been in love with them at the time, our perspectives and romantic interests will often change.

> "I would have waited until I was in college. I would have saved myself years of painful, uncomfortable, inexperienced and hurried sex. And while it just felt good to be close to the guy, I realize that I haven't thought of him in years. Girls, you ain't missing nothing!" *female age 32*

Think about the difference between a crush and a friend. A friend usually has to earn your trust and respect, while a crush automatically gets it because of the way he or she looks or acts. The chances are good you will still have your friends in a year's time, but you will probably have blown through your current crush and you might even gag at the mere thought of the person.

This isn't to say you should ruin a good friendship by having sex with a friend instead of with a romantic interest. But worse things have happened. At least try to make sure your first lovemaking partner is someone who has the qualities of a friend, and he or she is not someone who pressured you to have intercourse.

Doing It Sober

Please, don't do it your first time drunk or stoned. While this is often how it happens, every survey on first-time intercourse is chuck full of sad stories from virgins who did it drunk. Couples who do it sober will often have a better and more satisfying time.

Advice for Girls

This part of the chapter is written mostly for women. (Hopefully, guys will read it as well.) One of the keys to having good sex is knowing your body well enough to be able to say "That feels good" or "Let's try something else" in a way that a lover can understand. This is a skill that can take years to perfect. Women who have had sex countless times keep discovering new things about their bodies. So consider yourself at the start of an exciting journey that will last for much of your life.

Girls who masturbate might have a bit of an advantage their first time, but if you haven't masturbated before, not to worry. Do try to feel inside your vagina before you have intercourse for your first time. Wash your hands and get some water-based sex lube or use your own spit. Saliva is water-based and can work well if you don't have sex lube.

When you've got at least a half-hour to yourself (good luck!), or when you are tucked under the covers in bed, start exploring up and down your body with your fingertips. Spend some extra time on your neck and chest and on the area from your navel to your knees. If it makes it more fun, pretend it's a partner's fingers instead of your own. Once your fingers have explored up and down your body for at least ten or fifteen minutes, you might start to focus on the area between your legs. Let your fingertips glide up and down and around your genitals.

While one hand is exploring between your legs, there's nothing that says your other hand has to be tied to your side. At the very least, see what it's like resting it on one of your breasts. When you think it's time to venture inside, get a finger good and wet. Slowly inch it inside your vagina. The emphasis should be on "slowly." You want to feel what your finger is feeling, as well as what your vagina is feeling.

At this point, some girls will want to put their finger in farther; others might be feeling a little overwhelmed, especially if they've been raised in a household that was not safe or supportive of their sexual growth. If you are in the "go for it!" group, let your finger keep going. Remember to be asking yourself what your vagina is feeling. If you are so inclined, you might try adding a second finger. Given how penises are wider than a single finger, two fingers is a nice goal.

If you are in the group who is starting to feel like enough is enough, then this is a good place to stop. Just letting yourself go this far is a really important step. If you can, try to go a bit farther next time, but don't be discouraged if you hit a personal wall. Maybe it would be easier to ask a partner to explore you with his fingers, but only if he knows the difference between exploring with his fingers and his penis!

Don't assume your partner is going to have a clue where the opening of your vagina is. Whether he's your first partner or tenth, be ready to help guide his penis in, unless you don't mind if it accidentally ends up in your belly button or rear end. So if and when you feel ready, you might practice guiding a tampon or small tube-like vibrator or dildo into your vagina when you are lying on your back. Also practice doing this when you are squatting, as if you were in a girl-on-top position.

If all of this seems overwhelming, maybe it's not the right time in your life to be having intercourse. There are other ways you and a partner can enjoy yourselves sexually without a penis going in your vagina.

The Importance of Feeling Sexually Aroused

A lot of guys would be happy if a partner grabbed their penis and started playing with it. But women don't always do as well with surprise dives for their crotch. Women's genitals do way better if they are highly aroused before a partner touches them.

When a woman is aroused, her genitals expand as much as a penis does. This includes blood flowing into the area around the vagina so it straightens out and puffs up more. This will help make it ready for an incoming penis and it will help intercourse feel better.

Being aroused changes how contact with your clitoris will feel. Touching or kissing a clitoris might be painful if a woman isn't aroused, but it can feel exquisite after she becomes highly aroused. It can take twenty minutes or more of kissing and caressing before a partner should reach between a woman's legs. That's way more time than they show in porn, and it's usually way more time than it takes a guy to get hard.

Hymens Don't Pop

Most women who have taken our sex survey did not experience bleeding during their first intercourse. Nor did their hymens (or cherry) pop. It's a myth that hymens are supposed to pop or tear their first time. To understand more about this, please read Chapter 13: *The Hymen.*

During their first intercourse, some women don't feel a thing hymen-wise, others feel a stretching or a sting, and some feel a level of pain that you might when you get your ears pierced, or worse. But if you do the exercises with your fingers ahead of time, the chances are good you won't feel pain. If you do, tell your partner to stop.

If you are getting a gynecological exam before your first intercourse, ask your gynecologist if your hymen has become stretchy enough for intercourse. If not, your gynecologist can give you some estrogen cream that you can rub on it which will help it become more elastic.

Now, for advice for members of both sexes!

Pillows and Lube

Two accessories that might really help with your first time are lube and pillows. You have no idea how much a carefully placed pillow under a woman's rear end can help with the angle of penetration and with her ability to spread her legs. This can allow her to better relax her legs and her vaginal muscles. As for lube, put a few drops on the penis and a few drops in the opening of the vagina and you are good to go. If you don't have lube, spit can help. Just make sure things aren't dry when you try to have intercourse.

Putting It In Your First Time

The finest GPS in the world won't help a guy with this one, and it doesn't matter how much porn he's watched. Guiding a penis into a vagina can be a challenge whether it's your first time or fiftieth. In Chapter 26 on intercourse, some really experienced men admit to still needing their girlfriend or wife to guide it in.

Asking for a hand (or fingers) isn't a sign of being dumb or a dork. It means a man is smart enough to know when to seek help. Otherwise, he can cause his partner unnecessary pain and himself unnecessary embarrassment. On the other hand, not all women are able to be helpful in guiding a penis into a vaginal opening. Perhaps some playful fingering ahead of time will help both of you figure this one out.

Go Slow, Do Not Ram a Penis In, and Don't Start Thrusting

After you've made out for a long time and are ready for intercourse, start with the head of the penis gently pushing against the bottom of the woman's labia or lips. (It can be very helpful if she separates her labia and guides his penis to her vaginal opening.) If she's okay with the head of his penis pushing against the opening of her vagina, he should ease it in a bit more.

Once the penis is all the way inside of her vagina, just keep it there—don't start thrusting. This is the first time the woman has ever had a penis in her vagina. She should spend as much time as she needs adjusting to it being inside before there's any thrusting. This can be the most important moment of your first intercourse. It will be the only "first stroke" that either of you will have in your entire lives. Stop and savor it. Once you start thrusting, go slow unless she says otherwise.

Also, a nice sensation can result if the guy pushes his pelvic bone against her clitoris when his penis is all the way in. He might try doing a slow up and down or circular motion with his hips. Hopefully she can guide him with her words or hands on the sides of his butt.

The Best Position for Your First Time

Your first time is no time to get fancy. Go with the old-fashion missionary position where she is on her back and you are on top. There's plenty of time later for her to be on top. Missionary is better for the first couple of times. For many couples, it's their go-to position.

Where to Do It

"Our favorite place was on the floor in the room over my parent's garage when they were out somewhere. When the garage-door motor clicked on and started vibrating the floor we had just enough time to finish, clean up, button up, and act natural before my parents walked in." *male age 26*

For your first time, a quiet, familiar and comfortable setting is best. But finding a private unhassled location can be a challenge any time you have sex. Ideally, find a time and place when roommates, friends or parents won't be barging in. And please don't do it your first time in a spare room at a party. You might not care now, but maybe you will in a few years. Thinking back over that could be a big regret.

Once you have lots of experience under your belt, exotic locations are fine places to have sex. But for now, safe and familiar is best. If you try it in a bathtub or hot tub, chances are good the water will wash away your natural lubricant. If you do it on a beach, the sand will find its way inside the woman's vagina.

Make Time for Afterward

The time you spend together after your first intercourse can be as important as the time during and before. So don't try to do the deed minutes before your team bus is leaving for the state finals or when your parents have made a quick trip to the store. Spend time together afterward and be aware of each other's emotions. Maybe you'll want to hold each other, or maybe you'll want to run downstairs and raid the refrigerator. Hopefully you won't feel the need to text your friends before the condom is barely off.

You can't predict how you will feel afterward. Perhaps you will be relieved, maybe happy, disappointed or sad. Perhaps you'll feel extra close to your partner, or maybe you'll feel alone and isolated. That probably depends more on the quality of your relationship than anything else. Allow for a full range of possibilities and the time to experience them in the hours and days that follow.

No Time for Sex Toys

If you are so inclined, there's plenty of time in the future to bring out your private stock of dildos, cuffs, and strap-ons. But when it's your first time, it's best to stick to the lovemaking basics.

The one exception might be a vibrator, assuming the woman already uses one and enjoys it. It could be helpful for her to get herself off right before you try intercourse. This can help her relax and it might help her first intercourse feel really nice. Perhaps her partner can hold her as she's using the vibrator, but not even experienced couples are able to pull that off particularly well, let alone first-time couples.

If He Comes Really Fast

Some of us guys can come pretty quickly the first couple of times. Some of us don't even get a penis inside before blowing a wad. Anxiety can do that, and there's nothing wrong with being anxious.

Coming quickly might not be such a bad thing at the start. When a woman hasn't had a penis in her vagina before, there will be some rearranging and familiarizing that needs to go on inside of her pelvis. So less thrusting might be better than more. It might even be that nature intended for first-time males to launch early—to spare first-time women from getting more of a workout than their vaginas are ready for.

Advice for Guys

Look over the following advice that our female readers have for women who are doing it for the first time:

"Make him go slowly and be sure that you are aroused sufficiently before you let him enter you because it will probably be a little uncomfortable the first time. If he rushes, it will hurt and you won't enjoy it at all." *female age 35*

"Make sure you really want it and it's not about being pressured. Masturbate together first. Be comfortable together. My first time was painful and humiliating; there's got to be a better way. *female age 38*

"Have him read the *Guide To Getting It On* first!" *female age 30*

Men who are virgins can be at a disadvantage their first time if they don't have the courage to admit they haven't done it before. Instead of being honest, guys have a tendency to fake like they know what they're doing. Hopefully, readers of this book won't be so silly.

Your first time can be special and sweet, but not if you need to pretend that you know what you are doing when you don't. Here are a few tips for males who are about to make their maiden voyage, or voyage in their maiden:

During Intercourse: If you are on top, she'll want to feel some of your weight on her, but not the full nine yards. So use your arms, elbows and knees to support yourself and thrust with your hips. Not to worry, you'll eventually get the hang of it. Even your dad did!

Your Lips: You will be hard-pressed to find a single woman who wouldn't enjoy it if her lover planted some tender, gentle kisses on her neck or lips before his penis gets to know her vagina as well as during.

Porn: What makes sex work in a relationship and what makes it work in porn are two very different things. In porn, the camera abhors a tender and loving touch. It comes across as being boring. In real life, tenderness rules. The two of you have plenty of time to explore having rougher sex if that's what both of you want. But not your first couple of times.

Oral Anyone? In some situations, it makes perfect sense to go down on your partner before intercourse. In other situations, this would be too overwhelming for her. The two of you need to decide together.

Erections #1: Not to worry if your erection is flaky. Chances are it's never been under this kind of stress. Keep kissing, laughing or feeling each other up. If you do what's described in the other chapters of this book, she'll be having so much fun she might forget all about your penis.

Erections #2: Guys sometimes rush because are worried they will lose their hard-on. If it goes flat, it goes flat. It's far more important that you take your time and offer lots of kissing, touching, and more kissing. The goal of sex is to share pleasure, fun and intimacy. You don't need an erection or intercourse to do that.

If You Can't Come: It's not unusual to come quickly your first time. However, some guys aren't able to come at all. If it seems like you can't come, ask her to tell you when she feels like she's had enough thrusting. Either way, if you come too soon or not at all, don't stress it. This is about the two of you enjoying each other, not about coming.

Practicing with Condoms—Preparing For Your First Time

Unless you've really got it together and have been to Planned Parenthood, condoms will probably be your default method of birth control. If you are a guy, try to get a stash of condoms and water-based lube ahead of time. Condoms come in different sizes and shapes. It's a really good idea to get a sampler pack of different condoms to find which brands fit your penis best.

Practice putting on a condom and jerking off with it on for at least a couple of days before your first time. Here are some goals:

Learn how to manipulate the condom by feel alone, as you'll often be putting it on in the dark. One of the biggest time-killers in putting on a condom is determining which way the material rolls out. Pull the tip of the condom from the center of the ring in a way that allows the ring of material to easily roll down your penis. (There are about a hundred videos on YouTubes of men putting on condoms. For some reason, guys who are really well hung love doing YouTube videos that show the world how to put on a condom.)

After you've got the condom on, run warm water over your hand so it will feel warmer, like your partner's body will be. Then lube your hand up and start thrusting your penis into your hand. See what it's like to thrust with your hips into your lubed hand. This will give you a better sense of the condom's road-handling abilities.

Keep thrusting until you've blown a wad. Then pay close attention to what happens to your penis. If you are like most men, it will start to shrink. This is why you need to crimp the bottom of the condom around the base of your penis as soon as you come. Otherwise, the condom will slip off. If you keep thrusting you will push the condom inside your partner's vagina.

Semen will soon start running out the end of a condom after you take it off. This is why men who know what they are doing will tie off the end of a condom soon after they take it off. Just make a knot in the lower half of the condom.

If you are a woman, get extra condoms and try putting one on something penis-shaped. Learn how to open the package in the dark and how to roll it on, leaving a bit at the end with no air in it if that's what the instructions tell you to do. Also, try to get the morning-after emergency birth control pill in advance. That way, if a condom breaks or comes off before it's supposed to or you forget to bring condoms, you'll have a better chance of preventing an unwanted pregnancy.

If you find yourself having intercourse without birth control or condoms, the guy needs to pull out before he comes. This is called withdrawal. It's where a man pulls his penis out of a woman's vagina before he ejaculates and strokes himself until he comes. This will hopefully keep his sperm outside of his partner's vagina. While withdrawal is not the best method of birth control, it's way better than doing nothing.

Why It's Okay for Guys to Be Nervous Besides the Obvious

If you're a first-time guy, your orgasms during intercourse might not feel as intense as when you are jerking off. After all, how many times has your penis been in your hand versus the number of times it's been in a vagina? When you masturbate, your fingers are focused on the part of your penis that helps get you off. Vaginas don't have fingers. Also, when you are masturbating, the sole point of contact is your hand gripping your penis. It's way different with partner-sex, because your whole body is feeling her whole body.

You've probably never had an orgasm while supporting your body's weight on your arms or elbows. You will become very used to this, but your body will need a few times to figure it out. And if you wank to porn like most guys do, this is the first time you'll be staring into a partner's eyes when you are getting off instead of up a porn actress's crotch. So it takes time and experience to put lovemaking together in a way that beats beating off.

Even if it doesn't end up being your best orgasm, more than 80% of males still come their first time, where it's less than 15% for girls. This is why it's important to become the best lover you can possibly be. You want your partners to enjoy sex and to value having sex with you.

If The Sex Wasn't Mind-Blowing...

"Relax and don't expect it to be like the romance novels."

female age 32

"Be choosy. Take your time. Touch and explore everything."

female age 36

Who knows what makes for mind-blowing sex, but don't be disappointed if it doesn't happen your first time. If you are thinking that finally having sex will change your life or transform your relationship, it probably won't unless the two of you get pregnant or end up with a sexually transmitted infection. If having sex ends up being special or helps the two of you become closer, it will be because of the things you bring to it as a couple, and what you do with it going forward.

If You've Waited until Marriage

The average reader of *The Guide* is not necessarily the kind who waits until the first night of marriage for sex, so it's not like we have a huge data-base of advice to pass on. But if you think about how stressful a wedding and reception can be, the night of your wedding might not be the best time to make it your first time. Maybe if you cuddle together and get some sleep, and make the next day all about your first time. Then again, all that adrenaline might be just the ticket! Talk it over ahead of time.

16 vs 26

Plenty of people don't lose their virginity until they are in their twenties. The nice thing about waiting is that you tend to be more sensible about it and you will often have a better experience. Many of the late-bloomers we have heard from say it's a much better experience. The following is from a reader who didn't lose her virginity until she was well into her twenties:

> "I was surprised at how tricky losing my virginity proved to be. The first couple of times my boyfriend and I tried, my vaginal muscles were very tight and penetration was painful. So we slowed down and tried other ways of loosening the muscles (fingers, a vibrator, etc.), I visited the ob-gyn to make sure nothing was wrong (there wasn't), and we waited for a night when I was nice and relaxed. The first couple of times we successfully had intercourse were amazing—I felt a bit of pain with initial penetration, but once my body got accustomed to him the physical sensation was wonderful, and we had a lot of fun trying different positions and experimenting with what felt good!"

No matter how old you are, hopefully you can plan ahead and make your first time a good time.

A **Very Special Thanks** to Angela Hoffman for advice and help; to Carrie Veronica Smith, University of Mississippi, to Chris, a contented average dude from Canada; to Figleaf; and to Dayna Henry and her students at Indiana.

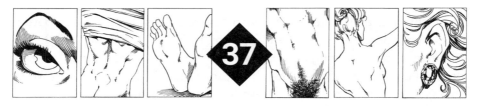

Sex When You Move Back Home

Dear Paul,

I just graduated from college and had to move back home with my parents. Everyone says I need to get on with the next phase of my life, but I have no clue what that should be. I'm so depressed I don't even want to have sex. But if I did, I still wouldn't feel comfortable bringing a woman home to have sex here. I feel like I'm eleven instead of twenty two. Do you have any advice?

Mike from Manitoba

Dear Mike,

Like you, I moved back home with my parents after five years as an undergrad. I was depressed, dejected and had no clue what the future would bring. During my years at college, I had not been lacking in initiative. I had ducked tear gas canisters from antiwar riots on my way to class and I'd worked long shifts in a mental hospital at night. I'd coached a winning woman's football team and had been on the staff in the dorms.

Yet when I moved back home with my parents, I had no idea how to be an adult in their household. I quickly returned to being the same son that I was when I was in high school. It wasn't until years later, after my dad became old and started to get dementia, that I could be the same adult in his presence that I was in the rest of my life. And it wasn't until my mom could no longer manage on her own that I learned to be an adult in her presence.

I don't envy the task you have in changing your family dynamics. I totally sucked at it myself, and I understand how challenging it can be when the structure and safety net of college disappears. So I wrote this chapter for you, to help while you are ending one stage of your life and trying to begin another.

From Rusty Parent-Child Dynamics to Squeaky Bed Springs

If you want to have a normal sex life when living in your parent's home, you'll need to act like an adult. That's how parents begin to accept their children as sexual beings with sexual needs. Even if your parent-child dynamics get rearranged in all the right ways, you still might not feel comfortable having sex in your old room. And your parents might not feel comfortable when the child they used to read *Goodnight Moon* to is having sex with a lover whose name they hardly know.

Boomer-What?

The media has invented the term "boomerang generation" to describe former college students who move back home. This is misleading, because when you toss a boomerang it comes back the same as when it left. That's not true for someone who left home at eighteen and comes back after years of answering to no one. Worse yet, before you left, it was as much your house as your parents. And when you had friends over, it was usually just friends and not someone you were going to have sex with, or not someone your parents knew you were having sex with. Expectations are different and adjustments must be made.

You're Not the Only One Who Likes to Walk Around Naked

If you were an only child or the last of your siblings to leave home, your parents have now had a couple of years to walk around naked, get stoned or drunk, have sex in the kitchen and learn to cherish their privacy. (Where do you think your "walk-around-naked" and "I'm horny, let's fuck now!" genes came from?)

Returning home might force your parents to give up some hard-earned freedom. Be sensitive to this and try to appreciate that they didn't have to let you move back home.

Making Yourself a Grown-Up in Your Parents' Eyes

One way to be a responsible adult is to help pay your share of the expenses. But you probably wouldn't be moving back home if you could do that. So the next best thing is to ask your parents what you can do around the house to help. It may be that your parents will never agree to you having sex with a partner in their home. But the way to give yourself the best chance is to be responsible and helpful:

- Help do the shopping.
- Cook and do the dishes or clean the house and do the wash.
- Be a work-out partner for unmotivated parents.
- Garden, paint, run errands, and chauffeur siblings.

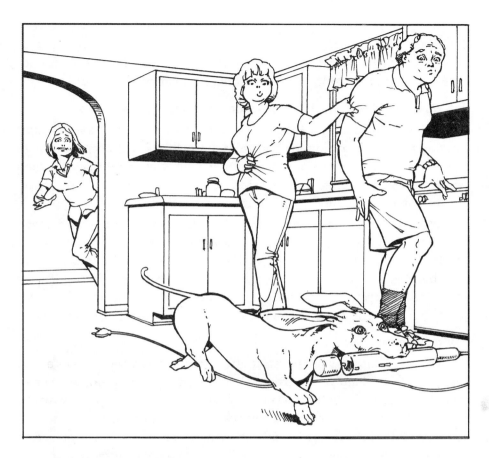

☻ Do the bookkeeping for your parent's business, fix their website, or program their electronics and remotes.

☻ Detail the car or help tutor a younger sibling.

☻ Help with your grandparents.

Doing Yourself No Harm

The moment your parents have to start nagging you, you suddenly return to middle-school in their eyes. Middle school—wasn't that when sex meant your hand in your pants?

Statements like "Oh crap, I forgot to take out the garbage" or "Sorry, mom, I forgot to pick up Davy from baseball practice" will not cut it if you are trying to earn grown-up privileges. Being reliable will probably increase your standing in the eyes of your sex partners as well.

Keep your parents updated about your plans and goals. Even if your chances of winning the lottery are better than landing a job, keep your family in the loop. It can be easy to lose hope. Just making the effort to fake it can be important in making progress or moving forward.

Hot Water and Bandwidth – Two Things You Should Never Hog

Even if you've always taken a shower the first thing in the morning, you don't want your mom or dad taking a cold shower because you've moved back home. Nor does it matter if your younger brother drains every drop of hot water while jerking off in the shower. It's unlikely he gets to have a lover spend the night.

What's true for hot water is also true for Internet bandwidth. Don't be downloading porn when your mom wants to watch a show on Hulu or your sister is streaming a movie. And as much as it might annoy you to cede bandwidth to younger siblings, it will not help your cause if they go whining to your mom or dad about how you are hogging the DSL. (They will tell your parents you are watching porn, even if you aren't.)

Having Friends Over Now vs. Then

It's one thing if your parents offer your friends beer or wine, but your friends offering your parents alcohol or drugs might not go over so well. If your friends walk into your parents' home flashing twelve-packs of beer, it's no different than a terrorist walking into an airport with a bomb. Double that if your friends bring acid, 'shrooms, hash, pills, anything leafy, white, powdery or cause for surveillance by the feds.

Even if it's totally fine with your parents that you are having friends over, it's wise to ask ahead of time. It's different now than when you were in high school and your friends would crash at your place.

Social Before Sexual

When you were living on your own and you met someone new, you might have ended up at their place or yours for a night of sex. This doesn't work so well when you're living with your mom and dad. Meet a potential new lover for coffee, lunch, oat a movie, sporting event, or museum. You won't believe how much you'll find out about a person when you are both sober and your clothes are on.

If you decide sex is a good next move, try making your first time at their place or at a hotel. Some hotels have a special day rate for this exact thing. They are known as hot-sheet hotels. Then, if you decide it's not going anywhere, you won't have to cash in one of your "here's-the-latest-person-I'm-sleeping-with" chips with your mom and dad. And if your new lover is a keeper but screams with wild abandon while having orgasms, you can discuss this before making love in your parents' home.

If your parents pester you mercilessly about meeting your new hookup, tell them you haven't decided if he or she is family worthy. Plus, if your family is a bit odd, delaying a bit avoids scaring away a perfectly good lover before he or she is more invested in you and is more likely to weather your family's unique habits.

Sharing Date Drama With Your Mama

It's one thing to be living hundreds of miles away from your mom and phone her in tears about how terrible your partner has been to you. That's what moms are for. It's quite another thing to have these kinds of conversations when you are living at home. How's your mom going to handle it when you invite the loser over the next day for make-up sex?

This sort of thing makes parents insane, especially dads with a Second Amendment hard on. So if you are experiencing less than domestic tranquility with a lover, consider not discussing it with your mom unless you need moral support.

Explaining Friends with Benefits

What if you have a relationship that consists of really good sex but nothing more? Unless you have the most sexually evolved parents on the planet, finding the right words to explain a casual-sex relationship to your mom and dad is beyond the scope of this book.

Or what if your lover isn't someone you would want to admit to your family that you are spending naked time with? This may not have been so bad when all you had to deal with was disgusted looks from your roommates. But now that you've moved home, maybe it will force you to set the bar higher when it comes to the people you sleep with.

Facebook, Texting, Email and Sexting

It was one thing to be Facebook friends with your parents or have them as Twitter followers when you were twelve. But now? Even if you aren't FB friends with your family, the Internet is an open book. Once you move back home, don't put anything on it that you wouldn't want your mom or dad to see. Or be smart and use Snapchat, Periscope or something your parents aren't likely to use.

Also beware that nothing will piss off parents more than when your little brother hacks into your Twitter or email accounts and shows them your posts dissing them. If you don't want your family to know exactly what you are thinking, don't text it, email it or write it down.

It is unwise to keep a lover's sexts for posterity or masturbation on any device your parents' can access. Assume your mom, dad, or siblings will find them. An upskirt photo from a lover is unlikely to increase your mom's opinion of her. And imagine having to face a partner's father after he found your dick pic to his daughter along with an explanation of what you're going to do to her with it—while under his roof.

Younger Siblings

If the stork made a tragically late visit and you have siblings in elementary school or younger, be sensitive to what an important figure you are in their eyes, either as a friend and mentor or as someone to torment. Also, when it comes to younger siblings, you are in the sometimes strange zone of being more of a parent than their brother or sister. And under no conditions should you ever give siblings drugs or alcohol. Not only is this dumb, but you risk being charged with the criminal act of furnishing a minor with whatever you furnished.

Siblings can form strong attachments to your boyfriend or girlfriend, especially if your BF or GF is being extra nice to them.

> "One of the first big influences I had was when I turned 14 and my older sister became involved with a man who treated me like a brother. He had a huge influence in my life." *male age 26*

This is usually a good thing unless you decide to break up. It's also something to consider when it comes to bringing casual hookups home. Just like a single parent who is dating, you need to be sensitive about the impact that a revolving door of lovers will have on your siblings.

Kids tend to be curious, especially about anything having to do with sex. So it might be wise to put a lock on your door for when a lover is over. You don't want to risk having your third-grade sister asking your mom, "Why does Amy have Trevor's penis in her mouth?"

Arriving Home with Pets and/or Kids

The difference between the family pets you grew up with and the one you are moving back home with is that you and your pets are now guests. In time, your family might grow to like your pet as much as they like you. Maybe more. But if your pet is so obnoxious that your former roommates tried to donate it for medical experimentation, you'll need to become super responsible. Pick up the poop before it hits the ground, or make sure its litter box looks like the sand traps at the Pebble Beach Golf Course. If it's a dog, be sure it gets enough exercise and slap a no-bark collar on if it won't stop barking.

Good luck if you've got a large dog that likes to occupy your dad's favorite chair or bares its teeth at your mom's yappy Poodle.

Strategic Room Choice for Better Sex

If sex in your parents' home is a possibility and you have a choice of rooms, place acoustic considerations at the top of your list. While you might love the room in the attic, think twice if it's directly above your parents' bed. A room at the opposite end of the hall from your mom and dad's bedroom might make for a better sex cave, even if it's smaller.

Another plus is having a separate entrance. This means you won't need to introduce hookups to your parents, which can save all kinds of embarrassment if you can't remember the hookup's name.

Loud Music Is Not the Answer

Your mom to your younger sister: "What's Kyle doing?"

Your younger sister to your mom: "He just turned up the volume on Pandora, so he's probably having sex with Amy."

Do you think that cranking up the volume is going to fool anyone? Turning up the music announces your fuck fest to the world. Try pushing a towel against the bottom of the door if it leaks sound. It won't keep the smell of pot smoke from escaping, but it can shave a few decibels off cries of "Oh God, I'm coming!" and "Harder, Kyle, Harder!"

Vibrators

If you use a vibrator, find a model that doesn't shake the house off its foundation. Try using a famous-brand pulsating toothbrush that's battery powered and sells for around $8 for a twin pack. It vibrates at a perfect frequency and will get more off than the plaque on your teeth.

Barging In, "I'm an Adult Who Has Sex" and "How To Tell a Lover"

If your parents and siblings are barging into your room at all hours of the day and night, you might try reminding your parents that you don't barge into their bedroom without knocking. Don't mention the reason you knock is that you'd rather not see your parents doing something that could result in your needing years of therapy. Use a respectful tone when asking that they not enter your room without knocking unless the house is on fire or your dad is having a heart attack. Keep in mind that your parents are on solid ground to enter when necessary, especially if your housekeeping habits are causing the rodent population in the neighborhood to triple.

At some point, you may need to have the *I'm-not-a-child-anymore,-I-like-sex! talk* with your mom and dad, but it's usually best to save it for a few months down the line after you've demonstrated how helpful, responsible and adult-like you are. One possible approach is to say "You did your job and did it well. You raised a responsible, caring young adult who, like other responsible caring young adults, has friends he or she spends the night with. It's a normal, natural, biologically okay thing when you reach my age." Then see where it lands.

If you are embarrassed and are sheepish or apologetic when you tell a partner that you live at home, then that's what the take-home message will be. But if you confidently explain that your parents are good people and you moved back home for good reasons, then that's probably how it will be received.

Having Fights with Your Lover and Breaking Up

Even the most perfect lover has habits that will get under your skin. That's why fights are necessary. But how do you have a good fight when your parents are in the next room? Finding a private place to have a fight can be as important as finding a private place to have sex.

When you break up with a partner who your family has gotten to know, they might react in one of two ways: with grief or sorrow, or with quiet cheers and high fives. If they genuinely liked your former partner, be sensitive to the impact that your break-up will have on your family.

Common Sense Considerations

😎 Don't ever flush spent condoms or period gear down the toilet. Condoms, tampons and sanitary napkins will cost your parents $300 or more in plumbing bills. You don't want to be around when the plumber tells your mom or dad what caused the backup in the line

😎 Parents like to meet a partner who is respectful, helpful, and doesn't try to sneak off into the bedroom without saying hello.

😎 When possible, schedule sex during parental time away. Never

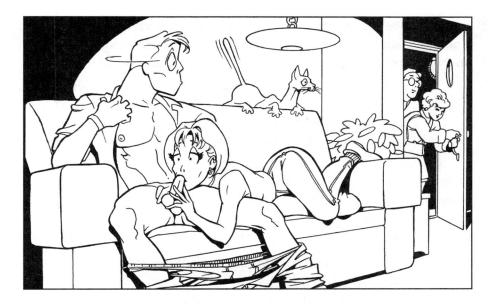

bring a last-minute hookup home for sex. Only bring home sexual partners who you know and can trust.

😎 Unless you have a private bathroom, don't allow a partner to
sneak out of your room naked or in underwear. Sweats, pajamas, a flan-
nel nightgown or a longer robe is essential, especially if your partner is
a woman and your dad tends to leer. This will make some moms insane.

😎 Give your partners tips for having conversations with your family members, eg "My mom had an affair with the tennis pro, so tennis is
a sore subject with my dad," or "When my little brother isn't beating off
to porn, he plays soccer" or "He's had some epic kills in Call of Duty," or
"The sewing stuff belongs to my dad, and the guns are my mom's."

😎 If you use the family car for sex, pack out what you packed in.
Never leave used condoms, wrappers, roaches, or underwear. Semen
stains and wet spots on the upholstery are especially uncool.

😎 Your family dog will ALWAYS find used condoms in the trash.
This can cause an awkward family moment. Also, some parents and siblings will check your trash. So find a safe place to dump used condoms.

😎 Never ever have sex in your parents' bed.

😎 Parents tend to hate it if you text at the dinner table or while
having conversations with them. Texting should be like masturbation,
mostly done behind closed doors. This will make you seem more adult.

😎 If you are the athletic type when making love, try toning it down when your parents are home. Everyone in the house knows what's going on, but there's no point in making the picture frames shake on the walls.

😎 It's never good to leave wet spots on the mattress. Buy a mattress-pad cover and a big, soft, dark-colored beach towel to put down on the bed before having period sex. Be sure to wash the sheets yourself. Lubes that contain silicone can leave wicked stains on your sheets.

😎 Parents tend to worry about their children no matter how old they are. Let your parents know if you are coming home later than planned. Calling or texting are the usual standbys. Turning off a light that they can see from their bedroom will let them know you are home, although there's not much point if the family dog starts howling.

Noisy Beds—Sign of Studliness at College, Not So at Home

Intercourse can turn a bed into a battering ram. The entire bed will sway toward the foot with each outward-thrust and toward the head with each inward-thrust. If it is hitting the wall, try moving the bed away from the wall. If that doesn't work, stabilize it by cramming pillows or gasket-like material between the headboard and the wall.

A frequent culprit is the bedframe. If it's an issue, visit www.Guide-2Getting.com and put "bedframe" in the search box.

When You Have Your Own Kids & Living In a Multigenerational Home

Living in your parents' home with your own children can be complex. Be sure to do research on the kind of issues that can come up. Talk to your parents about what they expect of you, and what you should or shouldn't expect of them. Unless there are good reasons why you should no longer parent your kids, don't dump them on your parents.

If you have casual sex, do it away from home. Otherwise it will just confuse your children. And if your child is living with the other parent, no one will be impressed if you aren't involved in his or her life. Moving home with your parents is not a free pass to be a deadbeat parent. One of the most important jobs in life is to be there for your children.

The chances are good it won't be long before your grandparents need extra care. In some situations, this means they, too, will be moving in with your parents. It's not difficult to see how this can be overwhelming for your parents. Find ways to help your parents.

Sex with a Co-Worker

When you date someone you meet through work, you know what they look like, how they behave under stress and how they treat others. You'll know if they have a good sense of humor and if they have a solid work ethic. If they have personality problems, their fellow workers will usually rat them out. These can be luxuries in the age of digital dating when what you see is not necessarily what you get.

People you meet through work will often be geographically desirable, unless they're in the Omaha office and you're in Maine. You won't have to explain your company's quirks and culture to them, and there's a good chance you'll have each other's backs.

There can also be problems. So think of this chapter as the missing section from your employee handbook, on negotiating the workplace environment when you and a fellow employee are having sex when you are off the clock.

The Downside of Having Sex with a Co-Worker

If you are dating a co-worker, you're not just dating that person. When they are part of a close-knit group, you might as well be dating their entire department. There can also be social discomfort if one of you wants to take it further and the other doesn't.

Another problem is when an employee uses work as a source of casual sex partners. This almost always leads to workplace drama. Casual sex is one of the things employers dislike the most about co-worker dating. So it's your job to keep the drama under control.

Most companies don't have a dating policy, but some do. If your company has a policy, it will probably be in your employee handbook. Some companies have a policy that says it's not okay for a boss or supervisor to date a subordinate, or they can't work together in the same department. At some companies it's okay for co-workers to date, but if they get married, one of them has to transfer or get another job.

Work-related relationships can extend beyond your immediate co-workers. It might include dating a client, vendor, sales rep, consultant, or a patient. Does your company have a policy about this?

In case you are wondering why a company would be concerned about sexual relationships among co-workers, consider the following:

Relationship-related workplace insanity: Companies don't want their employees groping in front of the copy machine or hurling nasty barbs when a relationship starts to sour. They don't want things going on that will make other employees feel uncomfortable or angry.

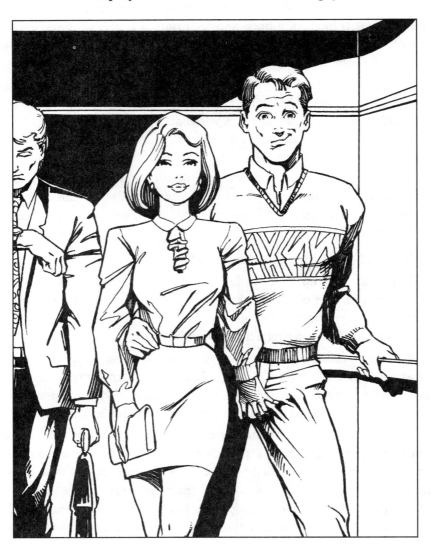

Sexual harassment lawsuits: Lawyers tend to come unglued when an boss or supervisor is dating an underling. What if the couple breaks up and the worker is denied a promotion? This can look like retaliation. There can also be a serious power differential. A worker might feel he or she has to accept advances from higher-ups or else. This is why it can be wise for one of the parties to transfer into a different department when a supervisor is dating someone he or she supervises.

Preferential Treatment: Let's say Austin, who is a middle manager, is dating Brandi, who is an executive vice president. Stormy is another middle manager who is aware that Brandi and Austin are dating. So what happens when Austin, who is incredibly hard working and deserving of a promotion, gets a promotion that Stormy felt she should have had? Stormy can make a big stink about how Austin received preferential treatment due to Austin's relationship with Brandi. Even if nothing was underhanded, appearances can make a difference in the workplace.

Serious Dating vs. Casual Sex

It won't help your career if you're known as the mailroom manwhore or the player from personnel. So if you are hot for a co-worker and value your job, keep it in your pants until you've dated a few times and it has long-term potential. While marriage needn't be the goal, you'll want to aspire to a stable relationship. Otherwise, look elsewhere for a dating pool.

Boundaries and Public Displays of Affection

Talk to your lover about the importance of maintaining healthy boundaries between the two of you at work. Create strategies to achieve this early in your relationship.

Besides bringing relationship issues to work, the quickest way to get fired is to annoy co-workers with public displays of affection. Even if you are in the safety of a locked supply room or have taken refuge in the furthest recesses of a warehouse, do not kiss, grope each other, or have sex at work. Never sext a co-worker when either of you is at work.

While at work, treat your lover the same as you would treat any other co-worker. You have no idea how much better it will work out for both of you if the two of you are discreet at work.

When to Go Public

When people get bored at work, there's no better way to pass time than with vicious gossip. This means that stealth is your friend. So the longer you keep your relationship under wraps, the better. When you are first dating, try not to post photos of yourselves together on your Facebook page. Do not announce, "Ben from underwriting asked me out!" Give your relationship time to develop before telling your co-workers.

This might sound like overkill, but try making "an organizational chart" of co-workers who will be most affected when they learn you have become orgasm-bonded. This will help you evolve a more effective strategy of how to handle matters when your relationship status becomes known. Once you are ready to let the cat out of the bag, plan

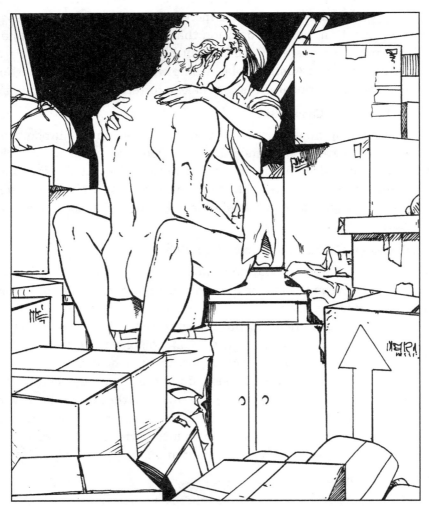

Keep all aspects of your relationship away from work, including quickies.

who you are going to tell. Should you inform your supervisors first? If you have different supervisors, you should probably tell them on the same day. If you have the same supervisor, should you both be there?

If a co-worker pitches a fit because you've been dating another worker and haven't told him or her, explain that you wanted to make sure things would work out first, and that he or she is the first one you are telling. Don't be surprised if everyone is aware of your secret. Still, most will appreciate how you've attempted to be professional about it. At the very least, being discreet will give your co-workers less ammo to say nasty things about you the moment your back is turned.

Extramarital Affairs at Work

One of the most damaging things you can do to your career is have an extramarital affair with a co-worker. You will be shocked to learn how many people will be affected if you are cheating on a partner with someone from work. Even if they don't like your spouse, cheating makes people squirm.

If you and your spouse have an open relationship, it's not cheating. But good luck explaining that to your co-workers!

Breaking Up

If you split up, hopefully you'll be able to remain friends or at least cordial. But even the most amicable of partings can be a challenge.

Just as getting together may have impacted your fellow workers, your splitting up may impact them as well. You never want to pressure them into taking sides or make them feel uncomfortable when they are around either or both of you. As much as it might be tempting, do not diss your ex at work or with a co-worker. In addition to making you look petty, this will not help your career. If you are too hurt to act rationally, don't hesitate to see a therapist to help you keep it together.

A Human Resources Executive Weighs In

Here are the observations of a human resources professional with more than twenty years of experience. He believes that co-worker relationships are inevitable, given how much time workers spend together. However, the relationships don't always work out well.

"Co-worker relationships are probably the most reoccurring cause of employee issues I have experienced. Typically the problems are worse when the relationship is in the end stages. However, I have seen a situation where the partners involved held senior positions and virtually destroyed a division when they were at the height of their relationship."

"It's not unusual for workers to refuse to talk to or interact with anyone if it involves their ex. Essential information will stop flowing. Their friends become involved when things heat up and both sides jockey for position. Absenteeism will rise and one of the former partners will often quit or will be fired, especially if one continues to goad the other."

Comments from Readers Who Have Had Sex with a Co-Worker

"I have seen a lot of horrible office relationships! I have also seen a few great marriages stem from inner-office relationships. It's more common than I thought. I promised myself I would never date a co-worker. However, I have met some of my best friends here at work. And well, I broke my own rule and started dating one of my best friends who is a co-worker!"

"My partner and I have been co-workers for almost six years. We met working on the same project. We continue to work together. We have been lovers for almost four years and have lived together for two. Both our colleagues and our senior management are totally supportive. I totally enjoy working with someone I love and respect and it is a blessing to have a partner who is completely aware of and understands your work environment, stresses, etc."

"I had sex with one of my co-workers and it was fine. He was nice and the sex was good. Even when we stopped seeing each other we stayed friends and work was good for a long time. But I also had sex with my boss one summer and it went so badly that I lied and told him I had an STD when I eventually quit. He was mostly a jackass about it. I think that the sex basically made bad situations worse, and possibly made good situations better."

"I've had sex with co-workers on a couple of occasions, some have ended well and others haven't. Oddly, I've found its been the men in these scenarios that tended to get weird."

Casual Sex

"Some of the best sex I ever had was with an unexpectedly talented stranger, and some of the most awkward sex I've ever had was with a boy I'd known for years and loved. Go figure."

female age 21

"I had a friends with benefits relationship when I was in high school with a good friend. We never really had 'those' kind of feelings, but the sex was just great. I still consider it some of the best I've ever had. Sometimes when I am home visiting my folks he and I just get together for the sex." *female age 24*

People often think of casual sex as being just one thing. But there are at least three very different kinds of casual sex: Sex with No Strings Attached, Friends with Benefits, and Sex with an Ex.

Sex with No Strings Attached is as casual as casual sex gets. It often involves sex with a total stranger who you might have only met in the last hour. Or you may have been on each other's radar for weeks or months before opportunity knocked. It might be a one-night stand, or it may have its own jagged lifeline. The triggers can be many, but alcohol is often involved. Early-morning thoughts such as "Who is this woman I'm sleeping with?" "What bed am I in?" and "Where are my panties?" are par for the course.

As for *Friends with Benefits*, there's a reason why it starts with the word "friends." It's usually with someone you know and it often happens more than once. There's plenty of wiggle room when it comes to defining friends with benefits (aka "booty call" or "fuck buddy"). *Friends with Benefits* can just be for sex or it can include hanging out. It can be with an acquaintance who is maybe a Facebook friend but not someone you'd call when you need a real friend. It can also be with a good friend, which doesn't always end up as bad as you might think. There are times when friends have sex and then stay friends after they stop having sex.

There's no way to know how it's going to turn out ahead of time.

> "When I was involved in my hook-up relationship I would never call him up for a sober booty call. It was always when I was drunk and wanted sex. That is also how I knew there was no emotional attachment because I wasn't even interested in hanging out with the guy unless I had been drinking. He wasn't really my type. We didn't have much in common other than the sex." *female age 23*

> "He was a football player and wasn't someone I wanted to be in a relationship with. We didn't have a lot in common besides the sex. Most people didn't even know we were hooking up."
> *female age 22*

One problem with *Friends with Benefits* is that people who are in them seldom talk about their expectations or feelings. They don't talk with each other about their relationship, which is still a relationship of sorts even if it's not filled with "I love you's." This kind of relationship more or less happens without much discussion.

Another form of casual sex is *Sex with an Ex*. If you are super horny or drowning in loneliness you might call an ex for sex. Or maybe you're both at a place where you realize the best thing about your relationship was the sex, so why not go for it. This might work, but the potential pitfalls in having sex with an ex are endless.

Are there other kinds of casual sex? Of course. Consider this woman's situation, where *Sex with No Strings Attached* turned into something more like *Friends with Benefits*:

> "I hooked up with a guy two years ago. I didn't know him, and I didn't expect to see him again. It's been over two years, and we've become very good friends. We often have sex even if we're not involved in each other's lives by mutual agreement."

Casual sex can take on as many different forms as there are people who want to have it. Is it something you should try? Some people are comfortable with casual sex, others aren't. What works for your friends might not work for you. If you decide to try casual sex, go slowly. The luck of the draw can be a big factor, both good and bad.

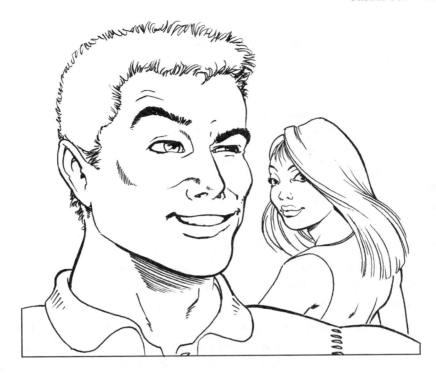

Motivations? Regret?

Casual sex is more about excitement than emotional depth. Men and women often have the same reasons for doing it, but not always. A man might desperately need the touch of a woman. Casual sex is a way for this to happen without having to admit the real reason for the sex.

Casual sex can forestall a woman's worries about being trapped in a relationship. It can provide validation that she is desirable and give her something to talk about with other women. It's healthy and normal to want to know what different guys are like in bed—a curiosity that few women have been allowed to explore until now. There might also be the occasional cross purposes, like having sex with a rival's boyfriend or rubbing it in an ex's face.

Researchers have asked people if they regret casual sex. It turns out that if the sex was good or the person had fun, there are few regrets. Otherwise, it's not unusual to have regrets, especially if a person's expectations were high. Men can have regret as well as women, and there is frequently regret over not using condoms. However, regret about a one-night stand might be miniscule when compared to the regret over years spent in an unhappy relationship or an unfortunate marriage.

Women's Satisfaction in Casual Sex

> "If you go into it knowing that it is just going to be a one-night stand then it is satisfying. If there was supposed to be more and you don't get much, then it is disappointing." *female age 22*

Men have way more orgasms during casual sex than women. Yet almost as many women report being satisfied with casual sex as men. How can this be?

The newness, excitement and risk of casual sex might be factors. Not having to invest as much effort and not worrying about what a partner thinks are big pluses. Alcohol can also make us remember a situation in a better light, and the vapor of alcohol is no stranger to casual sex.

Maybe all Cinderella wanted from the Prince was a good fuck. Or maybe she wanted him as a friend and lover, minus the castle, crown and demand to squeeze out a royal heir. Whatever the case, women today are just as likely to dive into a man's pants as he is into theirs. If a relationship happens, it happens, but the fact that a relationship is not part of the mix can make casual sex appealing to a lot of women as well as men. If anyone ends up being jealous or hurt, it's just as likely to be the guy.

The Double Standard

The double standard still exists, but it's not as bad as it was generations ago when virginity was still a commodity. The new question is *how many men a woman can sleep with before she's slept with too many.*

> "How many partners are too many? How much is too much? How assertive is too assertive? What is experimental vs. promiscuous? These are questions that are always in the back of women's heads, and I don't think a lot of men realize that, or maybe they do and just don't care." *female age 22*

> "The double standard still exists. If a guy sleeps with a lot of girls then all his friends think he's a player, but if a girl sleeps with too many guys she's a whore and no one wants to be her friend. I think girls have a lot more freedom sexually, but that

doesn't mean the times have changed enough to have the girl start making every first move. I would never sleep with a guy who's had an outrageous number of women, but I also would not sleep with a guy who hasn't ever been with someone, not because of how they would be in bed but I just don't want to be someone's first because then they have to remember me forever." *female age 23*

"When a guy asks me how many people I have slept with, I am ashamed to say eight. I feel like it is so high. However, then when you ask a guy he will proudly say twenty." *female age 21*

One thing that hasn't changed is that it's women who are often the biggest enforcers of the double standard:

"Women who sleep around are very much put down by other women and men, but mostly put down by women. Men, on the other hand, are pressured and encouraged to sleep around."

female age 21

"Girls are also calling girls sluts. We don't like to be called it ourselves, but we use it to put down other women. It's a vicious cycle." *female age 22*

Older Feminists Shake Their Heads in Disbelief

Some women assume that having casual sex is a sign of liberation, but older feminists might have misgivings. It's not the lack of commitment that would bother them or needing to drink before having sex. They would have sympathized and perhaps offered some weed or suggested you ditch the dick and try some pussy.

What would have made them crazy was the idea of hooking up with an anonymous guy when you didn't know how he voted in the last election. What if he is filling you up with his baby-making sperm but voted for politicians who want to end your freedom of choice and force you to have his child? What if he voted for politicians who are trying to shut down the Planned Parenthood clinic where you get your birth control?

When it comes to sexual freedom, being liberated means being able to make choices you are pleased with when you are sober, not ones you had to get drunk to make.

Alcohol & Awkward, Horny & Excited

Dating is seldom as formal as it used to be, nor is it the major social event it once was. But dating can still feel as stressful as ever. Not only do you have to make eye contact and use your tongues instead of your thumbs, but once you've said something, there is no option to edit.

Given that casual sex is way more about changes in the traditional roles of women than men, a number of women were interviewed for this chapter. The two words they used most often in describing casual sex were *alcohol* and *awkward,* but *horny* and *excited* were up there as well. In more than 25 pages of women's comments, *love* was used only twice. *Comfort, comforting* and *uncomfortable* were used often. *Abusive, unhappy,* and *pain* were not used at all. When it comes to casual sex, the kind of emotions the women value in a long-term relationship are not a big part of it, nor are the emotions they dread.

While the media coverage of casual sex often has poignant accounts of how empty it can be and how hurt one of the partners ends up, that's not what the women who took our survey focused on.

"When you are not in a relationship and you want sex, you have casual sex. At times it can be satisfying sexually, but not emotionally. To have just casual sex you need to be able to separate the emotions. When I was involved in casual sex it was with the same guy, but there were no attachments. If one of us hooked up with someone else then the arrangement would be over. Now that I am in a committed relationship, I think that the sex with someone you know and are emotionally invested in is so much better. Knowing the person cares about you makes sex a lot more worthwhile." *female age 22*

"The hook-up guy never, ever asked me how it was for me. He always quit after he finished and there was rarely foreplay. You could tell it was strictly sex. My boyfriend always asks how it was for me; he is always worried that he is not doing it good enough." *female age 21*

Almost all of the women said that alcohol was their gasoline for hook-up sex, but they didn't seem particularly concerned about it.

"I definitely think random hook-ups have more to do with alcohol than what is believed in the media." *female age 22*

"Alcohol plays a big role in hooking up. Many (including myself) have used the excuse 'I was drunk.' It's almost like a free pass."
female age 22

"Alcohol is a huge influence on casual sex, especially for girls! I don't think I would ever hook up with a guy I didn't know unless I have the comfort of saying I was drunk at the time so I had an excuse in the morning." *female age 21*

"When I drink I want sex, so I knew I could get it from him. Drinking just makes sex more interesting to me because I am more open to trying things, and I am not worried about what I look like or how I am doing. I am more worried about my receiving sexual pleasure than anything else." *female age 22*

"You may think this person was attractive when drunk, but when you wake up the next morning and see him, you are like 'Whoa... I'm out of here.'" *female age 23*

"I see casual sex more when alcohol or substances are being used, especially in college. People don't think about what they are doing until the next morning when guilt settles in. I know this because, unfortunately it has happened to me and a lot of my friends." *female age 23*

"Alcohol is more of an excuse than a reason sex happens. When I drink I act on my sexual needs more than when I am sober."
female age 22

"Alcohol has a huge impact on my sexual activities. If I drink enough I have no moral rules with myself anymore. The next day I can wake up and make it okay by just saying, 'I was drunk.'" *female age 21*

"Alcohol is a big part of my life as a college student. I know it sounds like a crutch, but on the weekends, everyone I know is drinking." *female age 21*

When it comes to casual sex, getting drunk allows some women to have the same kind of sexual freedom as men. It's a testosterone patch in a bottle or can. But when we asked the women if they needed to hammer down a few Stolis before having sex with a boyfriend as opposed to a hook up, you could hear the "Hell no!" loud and clear.

Technology's Impact on Relationships Today

Here's what college students who use this book in their sex ed class had to say about casual sex. The students are no strangers to casual sex:

"We're impatient. We don't want to miss anything, so we don't take the time to really get to know anyone. We are always in 'go mode.' Maybe that's why we hook up. There's no energy left to do anything more complex."

"There are no rules anymore, at least not that anyone agrees on. There is no social code, everything is open to interpretation and it's all a gray haze."

"There is no more formal 'asking someone out.' Rather, they group text a bunch of people about possible plans for that night and see who shows up. That way, the guys don't have to ask one person out and face rejection. Plus, they don't want to limit their options. OPTIONS MUST STAY OPEN UNTIL THE LAST MINUTE!"

"Guys will google pick-up lines to text rather than trying to think on the spot. They also wonder, how soon do I text? If I call first am I coming on too strong? One male called a girl and she did not answer. He texted and she responded. You meet, text and then see what happens."

"We are so used to communicating via text or social media that we are socially stunted when it comes to one-on-one."

"Texting is the easy way out. Plus, if you text, you can get help from friends on what to say, and how long to wait before you text back."

"This girl essentially asked me what I was doing this weekend. So I sent her a message. She accepted, but during this process I never once considered calling her. An abundance of secure choices have protected me from vulnerability: technology is the brick wall."

"I can't imagine calling seven girls and having insightful conversations with them all; however, I can imagine texting seven girls the same thing at once. This form of impersonal communication has replaced the art of conversation and serves as a way to avoid potentially stressful interaction."

"We have a hard time committing. All of these strange, unclear relationships exist that have no formal rules. It seems we are just using each other to have sex. At the same time we do share mutual feelings of romance and passion, yet we do not call ourselves boyfriend/girlfriend in any aspect of the word. There might be someone better out there, which is constantly suggested by our friend count. It scares us out of committing to someone who could be inferior to the next bidder."

"It's better to keep it simple and casual so it's easier to detach when the inevitable moving on occurs."

"I've had the stereotypical 'who is this girl next to me?' mornings. Although those have not been my best decisions, I've learned from each one. But some people get very confused. My most recent 'friends with benefits' relationship went spiraling into disaster when she got too clingy and tried acting like a long-term girlfriend. At the same time, I've found that girls are as likely to want sex-only relationships as guys."

"I've been with easier girls for random nights of sex, but there's nothing better than a girl who does not mind spending a Saturday night in the library studying. They tend to be more responsible, trustworthy, and able to have an intelligent conversation that does not include alcohol, drugs, blackout, and vomiting."

"Relationships are complicated and the rules are puzzling. I have a hard time figuring them out. Most of our communicating is done through a screen. There are hardly any face-to-face interactions, unless you are wasted at a party, and in most of those situations, you're looking for someone to hook up with that night."

"We're making up the rules as we go along, pretending we don't have feelings. We're sex-fueled young adults trying to figure out who we are by sleeping with as many people as we can."

"When trying to ask a girl out, I need to Facebook friend her. Once she accepts, I write her a comment about something that happened when we first met. If she responds in a positive way, I send her another comment saying we should meet up the next time both of us go out. If she responds with a yes, then I ask for her number and give her mine. After the numbers have been exchanged, I will text her during the evening of the day I plan on going out. She can then take this wherever she wants to: sex, kissing, just a hug at the door. If things go well, I ask her via text when I can see her again, because calling comes off too strong and can be seen as creepy. When I have tried calling or skipping one of these steps, I have failed. I believe this routine is somewhat messed up. The structure is flawed."

Between Dating and Casual Sex

There is an in between kind of dating or "dating adjacent" that's a hazy area between dating and casual sex. It's where two people are checking each other out as possible relationship material. It's like an interview with your clothes off. It's how a lot of relationships do or don't begin. There's also the matter of sex roles:

"Girls want to be on the same playing field as the boys, but when it comes to paying, asking out, approaching, calling and everything like that, a lot of girls still want the boys to be the initiator." *female age 22*

With dating, there are still well defined male-female roles, although they don't scream at you like they used to. One defined role is that it's usually the guy who does the asking out, although that is often massaged and manipulated through interventions ranging from friends encouraging him to text her, to strategies where you "casually" run into each other

Casual Sex and Birth Control

A college instructor from a rural area who uses *The Guide* in her sex-ed course sent in the following regarding her students:

"I'm concerned about some of our students using morning-after pills and abortions for birth control. They often hook up with guys and have unprotected sex. Their doctors prescribe them three months' worth of morning-after pills. Some of the young women use the pills as many as three times in a month. I am not certain what impact this type of use may have on their bodies. Additionally, some of the girls admitted to psychological challenges following abortions."

Anyone who is having sex, casual or otherwise, needs to have a sound birth-control strategy. While emergency contraception is not meant to be used as regular birth control, it can be taken several times a month without causing worrisome side effects for most women.

Two of the last things you want from casual sex are unwanted pregnancies and sexual infections. Using condoms not only helps prevent pregnancy and decreases your chances of getting most sexually transmitted infections, but it helps decrease morning-after regret.

Random Facts about Casual Sex

Oral Sex: Guys seldom go down on women during one-night stands. A woman is more likely to receive oral sex in a friends-with-benefits arrangement where her sexual pleasure is one of the motivators.

Was it consensual or forced? This is a very real concern for women in casual sex situations, especially those with less experience who go to parties where there's a punch bowl of "jungle juice" or "panty dropping punch." This should concern young men as well as women, given how life-changing a charge of rape can be, whether well-founded or not.

Orgasms: The estimate is 80% of men have orgasms during casual sex, while 20% of women might have orgasms. However, the women's orgasms count can go way up in a friends-with-benefits situation.

Cuddling: Plenty of men and women want physical tenderness in casual sex that's more than just intercourse or oral sex. So men and women aren't always running out the door as soon as the media wants you to think.

More Responses From Our Female Survey Takers

"Hook-up sex cannot be with a guy you are wanting a relationship with. It has to be just for the sex."

"I think relationships are still the goal. It's just more relaxed on how we get to that point."

"To me hooking up/one nighters are just that. Generally there are no feelings towards the person. If you're horny you call them up and have sex and that's about it. Alcohol is a huge factor. More than likely we will both be drinking with the same people at the same bar and then one thing leads to another."

"I know people that were friends with their significant other and then started having sex. I also know people who have sex and then a relationship happens. I have tried both. I can't tell you which one is better. They both worked for me."

"I still see relationships as a goal, but if you aren't near to finding someone to meet your goal, why not have fun until then?"

"For me casual sex can be uncomfortable or awkward. You don't know what to expect or what they expect. There is some excitement, but there is excitement in a relationship. You know what the person likes, what they are willing to try, and their comfort level."

"I think that guys look at girls who sleep with them early in the relationship as slutty. If you sleep with a guy before you really know him he assumes that you do this with everyone. He is not considered unfit because of the double standard. It doesn't matter how many girls he has slept with, but it does matter how many guys a girl has slept with."

"If I am at a party and meet a guy and I really like him and we start fooling around and he calls the next day well then great, let's hang out. Not because we fucked, but because I liked hanging out with him. It's always scary when you don't have sex in the beginning and you get into a relationship and your lover is horrible, then you're stuck in a bad-sex relationship and if we're being honest, sex is a huge part. I like to meet the guy first, enjoy being with him and then sleep together, as scary as that is. Then I'll invest time and a relationship in him."

A Very Special Thanks to Dr. Dennis Waskul and his students at Minnesota State University, Mankato, to Janet Minehan and Marian Shapiro at Santa Barbara Community College, to Elaine Hatfield at the University of Hawai'i, to Justin Garcia at the Kinsey Institute, to Heather Flores at Madera and Clovis Community College Centers, California, and to Abigail Nitzel and Dr. Joan Chrisler of Connecticut College for some very thoughtful research done on Hooking-Up ("Hooking-Up versus Dating").

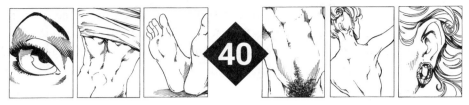

Threesomes

One of the first couples I ever interviewed about sex were in their early 70s and had been married for more than 35 years. They were church-going pillars of the community. The most important thing in their lives were their kids and grandkids. When I sat down in their tastefully-decorated living room, the woman said, "Why don't you look through the photo album of our last vacation that we took with some good friends?"

Within minutes, my grad-student mouth nearly fell off its hinges. Not a single person in the pictures had a stitch of clothes on. Their vacation had been on a cruise for swingers. They said that just last weekend six couples had been going at it in this very living room. And then the man looked lovingly at his wife and said to me from the depth of his heart, "Mama here is the best little cocksucker of any woman in the group!" His wife beamed with pride and gratitude.

The second couple I interviewed had never had a single threesome, let alone done any swinging. They were soon to be married. They were madly in love and very pleased with each other sexually. They even invited me to their wedding. They had a traditional relationship in every sense of the word. We stayed in touch for the next two years, when their marriage suddenly ended in divorce. I never heard from either again.

A few years later, I was having a conversation with a young woman about computer software. She asked me what I did. After I told her I'm the author of a book on sex, she said she lived with two men and had sex with both of them. One was her husband, and the other was their roommate. This had been going on for a couple of years, and she said they were all very happy together.

So I gave up long ago on trying to predict what makes a relationship work or fail, and whether having a threesome was a good idea or bad. I figured it is a good idea for some couples, and a bad idea for others. I do know that of the thousands of women who have taken our sex survey, having a threesome is one of the two most common sex fantasies. So if you are considering a threesome, this chapter was created to help you sort out the possible pluses, minuses, and what you'll need to consider if you want it to be a good experience.

A War on Tradition

Threesomes can evolve in many different ways. They can be a once-in-a-lifetime event when your husband's old college roommate visited for the weekend, or something you do a couple of times a month.

Adding a third person in sex isn't like adding another cherry to your banana split. Threesomes are a declaration of war on two-thousand years of marital tradition—namely, that if you want to include another person in your sexual mix, you are supposed to lie to your partner and cheat on the side. So caution is in order. A threesome revolves around the emotions of three people instead of the usual two. The potential for everything goes up—from the level of sexual excitement to the degree of hurt and anguish.

The Definitions

There are many ways that people have sex in numbers, with a threesome being just one of them. It used to be that there were more set boundaries between the following groups, but not any more:

Threesome: This usually means two males and a female, or two females and a male. One of the Ms and one of the Fs are frequently in a committed relationship, with the third M or F being a free agent.

Open Marriage: This is when a primary couple agrees that each person can hook up with outsiders for sex. The past few decades have seen an increase in couples who agree on the open-marriage option from the start. However, they usually don't announce this at their wedding.

Swinging: This is when an established couple gets together with a larger group for sex. It has many variations, from when two couples get it on in tandem, to sex in large party rooms where almost anything goes. While the swinging couples often form friendships or microcommunities or tribes, it is the recreational part of sex that initially draws them together. (The original term for *swinging* was *wife swapping*.)

Polyamory: This is when a relationship involves more than two people with the consent of everyone involved. It can include group relationships, or it can be a single person who chooses to have multiple relationships without an agreement of monogamy. It used to be that poly-people prided themselves on not being the type to have sex with anything that moves. There was often romance, friendship and intimacy, but with more than just a husband or wife. But now, a date for coffee or lunch can be relationship enough to have sex. People who describe themselves as polyamorous tend to be more liberal and younger than those who describe themselves as swingers and they tend to welcome diversity in sex roles more than swingers, but there is now an increasing amount of line-blurring between *swinging* and *polyamory*.

Let There Be Three

Why do people have threesomes? For starters—alcohol. Plenty of threesomes occur when three friends have been drinking enough to lose their inhibitions, but not enough to lose their erections. Threesomes created on the vapors of ethanol are seldom planned or repeated. Threesomes that endure usually take forethought and planning.

Threesomes are often structured like a triangle or pyramid. At the base of the pyramid is a male-female couple involved in an ongoing love relationship. The third person is the extra at the top. There's no reason why a threesome can't include three males or three females, but for most people who are straight or bisexual, threesomes are MMF or FFM. The decision to have two males and one female, or two females and one male is often based on the preference of the primary couple.

While some successful threesomes just fall out of the sky, most take a great deal of planning and thought. Here are some things to consider:

In MMF threesomes, the chemistry between the men can range from "I'm fine with you doing her, but touch me with your dick and you're dead!" to "Oops, your dick kinda slipped into my mouth!" Regardless of whether the MM contact is casual or planned, when two guys are having sex with one woman, there's going to be body contact between the two men. This is important to consider if one of the men is homophobic.

In FFM threesomes, the over-riding dynamic is often the desire of the women to experience more than the usual girl-hugs and kisses. This kind of threesome is often about letting the women explore, with the man providing a safe, solid, masculine backstop.

There are many ways the male in an FFM can help the FF exploration

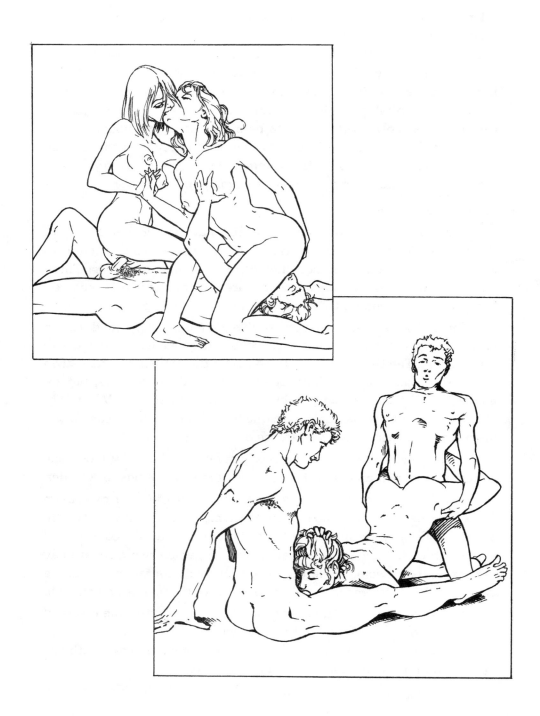

feel safer. The women might want him to be lying on his back, with one of them sitting on his penis while the other is sitting on his face. Both women are facing each other and they can kiss and caress while being connected to a man sexually. (This combination might be more comfortable when all three are on their sides.) Or maybe the women will be happier if he just watches and strokes himself, or if he joins one in doing the other.

Unless both women are totally into the guy, it's usually not a good idea for an FFM to focus around pleasing the man. FFM threesomes tend to work better if the man takes a background role and allows the women to lead. He should never try to script the threesome or attempt to set the tempo, unless it's a BDSM scene with a master and his two naughty slaves.

In a threesome, the women's orgasms are seldom the end of anything. They're more like the "fasten your safety belt" sign. However, the men's orgasms in a threesome can put a dent in the sexual build up. This may be one of the reasons why FFM threesomes often spend the night together, nestled in each other's arms, while in MMF threesomes the third-wheel guy often goes home after the men have come a couple of times.

Planing and Logistics

Spontaneous sex is a gift of the gods that is bestowed upon couples who have undemanding jobs with predictable hours, no children, and friends and relatives who live in other states. For everyone else, planning and compromise are essential to a good sex life. Triple that for sex with three. So the next part of this chapter is divided into four sections:

1.) Things to consider when considering a threesome; 2.) *From* how to find a third wheel to pre-penetration negotiations; 3.) Possible positions and positions on what's possible; and 4.) Don't let the dawn get you down.

More Than a Fantasy, But Not Yet a Plan

This chapter assumes that your threesome is made up of an established couple and a third wheel. That's how it usually is, but it doesn't need to be that way. There are debates about whether threesomes are best when they are made up of three individuals versus a primary couple and a third wheel. There are also debates about whether the third wheel should be a friend, an acquaintance, or a stranger. There are no absolutes. But since it usually happens with a couple and a third wheel, this part is for the couple, and a separate section for "the third wheel" follows. (A number of these suggestions are from Suzy Bauer's e-book, *Step By Step Threesomes*, *Nina Hartley's How-To Threesome* series of videotapes, and Violet Blue's chapter on threesomes in *The Ultimate Guide To Sexual Fantasy—How to Turn Your Fantasies into Reality*.)

👓 When you are first discussing the possibility of a threesome with your partner, avoid blurting out a list of potential lovers, such as "Your friend Ally would be sensational!" or "I'm sure Jason would add a lot!" What your partner will hear is that you can't wait to screw someone else. If your partner is receptive to having a threesome, you might ask who he or she thinks would make a good third.

👓 Anticipate that the threesome could sour your relationship. What if one of you fell for the third wheel or the third wheel fell for one of you? Discuss these possibilities and strategies to deal with them ahead of time.

👓 Try to imagine the sight of someone attractive having sex with your partner. Your partner is laughing, flirting, sighing, and enjoying being with this person. Talk about ways you can signal to your partner if jealousy is getting the better of you.

👓 In a threesome, an erotic connection can sometimes build between two of the participants, with the third person being left out. This is fine as long as the third person enjoys watching, but if not,. discuss how you would deal with this.

👓 What if the third-wheel MMF guy drops his drawers and you and your partner drop your jaws? What if nature blessed him with a package of penile perfection? Ditto if you are a woman and the second women in your FFM has the kind of body that someone only gets when she's cut a deal with the devil? Are you prepared for a bit of envy?

👓 Before trying a threesome, watch some threesome porn together that shows the different positions and possibilities. Talk about what you'd like to try and what you'd like to avoid.

👓 You can get a better sense of an FFM threesome by going to a strip club where you can pay one of the women to do a lap dance for each of you. However, it's not necessarily a good idea to take nude dancer or prostitute home for a threesome. She might be so experienced that it gets strange. It's better to stick with someone whose sexual perspective and experience level is closer to your own.

😎 If you are considering an MMF, both of you might see what it's like to be in a strip bar where male dancers are the ones who get naked. Since they usually don't allow males in the audience during male stripper shows for women, you might need to visit a bar or club where there are gay dancers who get naked. It will give both of you a sense of what it might be like to have another naked male in your presence. And it could be worth a chuckle to see other guys trying to pick up your husband.

Creating a Pre-Penetration Plan

😎 To prepare for your first MMF, the woman might get a dildo and butt plug for practice. She can simulate different penetration scenarios with her partner by using the toys, which can help the eventual threesome to be more manageable rather than overwhelming. (Most MMFs don't do double penetration, but even having a penis in your mouth at the same time that you've got one between your legs will provide more stimulation than most women are used to.)

😎 Having a threesome with a friend can deepen your friendship or it can mess it up. While it might be good to have a threesome with someone you know and trust, it's not such a good idea if he or she has a secret crush on you or your partner. Likewise, an ex boyfriend or girlfriend could make a good third or a horrible third. This is why you should talk it over ahead of time.

😎 To find a third wheel who is not a friend or an acquaintance, you might attend the clothes-on social gatherings that swingers groups have. Other possibilities include ads on websites and apps. The ads need to be carefully worded and carefully placed.

😎 Don't overlook single moms for an FFM threesome. Suzy Bauer and her husband were thinking back over the numerous women who had joined them for threesomes over the years, and it suddenly hit them that the majority were single moms.

😎 If the prospective third wheel is an unknown entity, protect your identity. Do not tell them where you live. Set up a face-to-face meeting at a neutral location where you can meet with your clothes on. Discuss things like setting up personal boundaries, safe-sex precautions, and what you hope to get from your threesome. If the pre-penetration meeting doesn't increase your desire or the chemistry doesn't feel right, consider that you don't have the right combination. If you go through with it, try having your threesome in a hotel room instead of your home until you get to know the person better.

😎 Before your pre-sex meeting, decide what is and isn't off-limits. For instance, one woman might be fine with a third wheel giving her husband a blowjob, but will melt into a psychotic puddle if the third wheel and her spouse French kiss. So make a list of the things that you'd like to encourage and discourage. Discuss them during your pre-sex meeting.

😎 If a man is being invited into a threesome with an established couple, he needs to have a thumbs-up from the primary-couple's male partner, as in "Don't worry, I won't kill you if you fuck my wife." One way to do this is for the male of the primary couple to be the one who brings up the subject of a possible MMF threesome to possible candidates. Likewise, for an FFM, the alpha female needs to invite the other woman to join. There are exceptions to these rules, but respecting them will serve you well.

😎 As with any situation where a new partner is involved, you need to protect yourself against sexually transmitted infections. Do not take a stranger's word that he or she is disease-free. Be sure to use condoms and lube, and protect against unwanted pregnancy. If you are having an FFM, the M will need to change condoms when going from one woman to the next. So have a bunch of condoms and lube handy.

Let the Party Begin

First and foremost, consider the following advice by Nina Hartley from *Nina Hartley's Guide to Threesomes* videos:

"Start slow, with lots of teasing and foreplay, kissing, petting, massage. It's likely two of you will be part of an existing couple where you know each other's sexuality better than the newcomer, so don't rush. Take your time bringing the newcomer into the situation. Unlike us [porn stars], you aren't making a movie. You don't have to be so goal-oriented. Let things unfold naturally instead of pushing for the kind of acrobatics you see in porn. It may take more than one get-together to make it all work, so don't be discouraged if the first threesome ends up with a double blowjob or handjob. It may take time for the three of you to get comfortable enough for actual intercourse. It is not necessary for all three partners to be equally engaged at the same times. Kicking back and watching can be exciting, too. Don't assume that dicks in every hole at all times is a measure of a successful threesome. Do the easiest things first, and see what develops. Don't forget to talk about your feelings afterward. You'll want to learn as much as possible from each experience."

👓 Be sensitive that you are inviting a stranger into your love-making lair. Don't assume that he or she has a clue of what to do or how to be. This is the moment when what used to be a total fantasy becomes reality, which is not always the prettiest of transitions. Be gracious, kind, and offer lots of reassurances. The third wheel is not a fuck-bot who is there at your convenience, unless you are paying them by the hour.

👓 Just being naked together, feeling relaxed, and opening up sexually is a major accomplishment. Pay attention to the chemistry of the threesome rather than to your own need to get off. Don't try to script your threesome. It may take a couple of times together before the three of you find your groove.

👓 Your primary concern should be that your partner feels loved and valued by you. This may mean paying more attention to your partner than to the third wheel—unless you agree that one of you mostly wants to watch.

👓 Be sober enough to legally drive. If you are too anxious to proceed without getting stoned or plowed, consider it a sign that this isn't something you should be doing.

👓 Don't be afraid to stop half way through the lovemaking to talk about what's going well and what could be going better. With three, you need to huddle often.

👓 There could be a time during an MMF when the woman is on all fours and is doing oral on the guy who's in front of her while the other guy is behind her and thrusting, aka "spit roasting." The male who is thrusting into her vagina or rectum needs to check in with her about rhythm and depth, since his thrusting might be causing her to gag on the penis of the guy who's in front. Likewise, the guy in the front needs to establish a comfortable pelvis-to-face distance. Both males need to be aware that the woman is between a rock and a hard place. You will probably need to work out a nonverbal signaling system, given what's in her mouth and all. In an FFM, if the man has his penis inside one of the women who is giving the other woman oral sex, he needs to check in with her about the best speed and depth for thrusting. Otherwise, his thrusting might be making it difficult for her to perform oral sex.

😎 Make sure your phones are turned off and the kids are safely away at their grandparents'. Use a hotel or another location if there's any chance that teenagers might show up, and don't even think about doing this when you are on-call.

The Morning After

No matter how enjoyable your threesome may have been, it's possible you will wake up the next morning with worries and bad feelings. Some people in this day and age still feel shame after they masturbate, and that's nothing compared to having two penises in them at the same time or their first same-sex experience while their spouse was watching.

Try to make sure no one leaves with self-doubt. Take the time to express your thanks and gratitude to one another—to both your primary partner and to the third wheel. If you enjoyed the experience, it's important to send the third wheel something like flowers if she's a woman, or perhaps something manly if he's a guy. Be sure the card has both of your names on it, and maybe a separate line from each of you if you are an established couple.

An established couple has each other to talk over any morning-after doubts with; the third wheel has only him- or herself. The flowers or gift will help with that process. Do not slip up on this one. Doing something nice for the third wheel and talking over your post-threesome feelings with your partner are as important as all the planning that went into making the threesome click, especially if you had a good time.

When You Are the Third Wheel

There is a certain freedom in being the third wheel in a threesome. If things don't go well, you can avoid seeing the other two again. They probably live together and won't have the option of avoiding each other, although they can also comfort each other.

👓 Always meet with the couple ahead of time to get a sense of your chemistry together. Talk about the things the three of you might like to try. Whether you are male or female, it's an important time to discuss the kinds of things you will and won't do. Come up with safe words that will either slow or stop the action if you find yourself feeling overwhelmed. Discuss everything from STIs to birth control. Don't assume that because they are a couple they have their act together.

👓 You will most likely be joining an established couple with lots of history together. As a third wheel, you will need to deal with the reality that you are the third wheel.

👓 If you are a woman, it's likely that a big part of an FFM threesome is for you to explore sexually with the other woman. If it ends up being all about pleasing the man, consider bailing early unless he's the chair of your dissertation committee.

👓 You will be having an intimate experience with three separate entities as opposed to two. You will be dealing with each of the others as individuals, as well as with them as a couple. The couple may have its own dynamics that are different from those of the individuals who make it up. In some threesomes, being mind fucked can outpace the body-fucking. You didn't sign on to do couples therapy. If you find yourself being placed into that role, BAIL!

👓 Things might go spinningly well, or they could get very weird. If the threesome starts to get weird, don't hesitate to suddenly remember an important meeting or a sprinkler you are sure you left on. Don't be afraid to call it a day, no matter what stage the threesome is in. Do not for a moment be intimidated because it's them against you. If you start feeling this is the wrong situation, grab your pants or purse and make tracks for the door. Be sure to drive to the location separately, or have an escape route that doesn't depend on them.

👓 The three of you will have a much better time if you don't feel the need to prove what sexual all-stars you are. This is a time to blend, rather than stand out, unless they have specifically asked you to have your way with one member of the couple while the other watches.

👓 If you are a third-wheel guy in an MMF, seek the other M's approval before trying things with his partner, even if she's inviting you to do it. It's not like you need to check with his attorney, a simple moment of eye contact and a confirming nod are all that's needed. Like-wise, if you are a woman in an FFM, you're not there to upstage the other woman. Be respectful, and the chances are good you will receive pleasure in spades.

👓 Ah, the single-dude dilemma. It is going to be significantly more difficult for a single man to find a willing couple for a threesome than it is for a single woman. It's the same problem with almost every species on the planet, be it a single male elk, sea lion or homo sapien.

👓 This is probably just psychobabble nonsense, but try to think about any less-than-conscious reasons that might be propelling you, as a single person, to have sex with an established couple. Freud might wonder if it has something to do with unconsciously wanting to outdo one of your parents. Some of Freud's followers might wonder if it has to do with wanting to be loved and taken care of by an idealized mommy and daddy. Again, we all do sexual things with motives. That's no reason not to enjoy the experience. But being more aware of it can sometimes help us from getting stuck in situations that aren't always the best.

👓 Make sure that someone knows where you are going, including the address and phone number. You don't have to tell them what you are doing, but leaving a trail and an expected return time is never a bad idea. This is just as true for males as for females. The only exception would be if you already know the people. While joining an unknown couple for sex is probably no more dangerous than joining an unknown single for sex, taking precautions is in order.

👓 Just because they are married and say they are disease free, don't believe it. Be sure to bring your own condoms and lube.

Threesome Resources:

For a list of the resources mentioned in this chapter, as well as others, visit www.Guide2Getting.com and put "threesomes" in the search box.

Double Penetration

Some women will tell you one penis is trouble enough. But if you've got two in your crosshairs or shorthairs, this might be the chapter for you. Double penetration is for the woman who wants a pelvis full of penises. It requires two male partners or a male partner and a dildo. One penis is in her top bunk (vaginal intercourse) while the second is in her bottom (anal intercourse), although double penetration can also refer to two penises in a woman's vagina. We'll discuss that as well.

Is Double Penetration (DP) Safe?

There have been no studies done on DP and there is little in the medical literature about the safety or danger of it. Since the tissue between the vagina and rectum isn't exactly made of Kevlar; it could possibly tear. It's thin enough that if you put a finger in a vagina when you are having anal sex, you can easily feel the penis. So appreciate that there may be risks.

If you enjoy anal and vaginal insertion, remember to scrupulously clean anything that's been in the bum before it touches a vagina. These are two different environments with two different sets of microbes. Brown should never see pink.

Nina Nails It

In porn star Nina Hartley's *Guide to Double Penetration* video, Ms. Hartley is very vocal about guiding the other actors. She tells them what feels good and what doesn't in no uncertain terms Think about that. Here's a very intelligent experienced porn pro who has hand-picked her double penetration partners. You would think Ms. Hartley wouldn't need to say a word to them about what feels good. Shouldn't these veteran porn stars automatically know? But the opposite is true. Nina Hartley doesn't expect anyone else to know what's going on inside of her body. She uses humor and respect, but she lets her partners know what is and isn't working for her. If you are going to try DP, consider doing the same as Nina Hartley.

Also keep in mind that even Nina Hartley avoided doing double penetration until she was more than forty years old and her financial backers "encouraged" her to do a *Nina Hartley Guide to DP.* If DP is something you are interested in, it is important for a woman to know her body and to be able to communicate what is going on inside of her. If she can't do that effectively, there's no way she should be hosting a double penetration. The same is true for having partners who value feedback. Perhaps Nina Hartley hand-picks her porn partners not so much for their physical skills, but for their ability to listen and learn.

One Woman's Experience with Two Different Sets of Dudes

Consider the experience of a reader who has tried double penetration with two different sets of guys. She hated it with the first set, but liked it so much with the other two that they've repeated it a couple of times.

The first pair of men were homophobic, so their need to avoid touching each became more important than her pleasure. She said they also had a macho "slam-her-hard" thing going on. She thinks they had watched too much porn.

The second set of men weren't gay or bisexual, but they weren't afraid to make physical contact with each other. They could work as a team instead of as two men who were trying to out-straight each other. This allowed them to focus on what was and wasn't working for her, and they quickly became three partners in sync.

If you are a man who would have a meltdown if another guy's arms, legs and testicles were touching your own, DP is not for you. If you would be uncomfortable feeling another guy's penis through the thin wall between a woman's vagina and rectum, forget the Robin-Batman thing, not that Robin and Batman wouldn't have been overjoyed.

The position this woman liked best was for the man who was doing the anal insertion to be lying on his back. She would sit on top of him facing his feet (reverse cowgirl) while sliding his penis into her butt. She would then lay all the way back, resting her entire body on top of him. That way, she didn't have to worry about him getting too aggressive with his butt thrusting. The other man stood at the edge of the bed or knelt in front of them and entered her vagina from above.

Or perhaps the position that will work best for you is when all three of you are on your sides, or maybe with the woman on all fours above the guy who's in her vagina while the buttman kneels or stands at her rear. You'll need to try different positions and rhythms to see what works best for the three of you. Also keep in mind that most porn actresses have rectums that can handle big rigs. Your bum might not be nearly as well practiced.

Thrusting and More

Like every other aspect of DP, who thrusts and how hard should be the woman's call. She may want one partner to be thrusting while the other is still. Or maybe she'll want one to thrust slowly and stay shallow while the other thrusts hard and deep. There can be dozens of possibilities. You won't know what works until the show has begun.

Also be aware that a woman might become so overwhelmed by getting twice the bang from her bucks that her ability to speak can become less than optimal. So before zippers get unzipped, work out a nonverbal signaling system. If she doesn't know her body's cues for when it is getting overwhelmed, she shouldn't be trying double penetration. This is no time for passivity when so much male energy is coming at her from both sides. *If there is any pain or discomfort as opposed to feelings of fullness, you need to immediately stop.*

People who are attempting double penetration should not be drinking, getting stoned or doing drugs. These will keep you from being aware of important body signals and sensations. And do not use lube that causes numbing or reduces sensation.

All three of you need to agree that your goal is having fun together as opposed to achieving double penetration. If the chemistry is right but DP feels like a stretch, you can try to make it work during your second or third time together. If the chemistry or timing isn't right, why force it?

A woman who is having DP needs to be comfortable receiving anal sex. To practice, she should try popping a butt plug into her rear while having vaginal sex with her regular partner. However, doing this the other way around (dildo in vagina, penis up butt) can result in the dildo turning into a missile and shooting across the room once her vaginal muscles start to contract.

Things to assemble ahead of time include towels, condoms and lube. Banish your phones and arrange plenty of uninterrupted time. Since a double penetration involves three people, the previous chapter on threesomes should be helpful. It has info on everything from hooking up with a third to the dynamics of three people having sex together.

Double Vaginal Penetration

In spite of this being a chapter on double penetration, it's not something every woman wants to try. And that's double penetration done the "old fashioned" way, with one of the penises in her vagina while the other is up her bum. There are even fewer women who want to try double vaginal penetration (DVP) which is when two penises are in a woman's vagina at the same time. However, some women do have DVP and enjoy it immensely.

If you are considering DVP, a way to simulate it or practice is for a woman to have a dildo in her vagina at the same time as her partner's penis. As for the different positions for DVP, you can do a search for "double vaginal" on porn sites such as Pornhub or Xhampster. However, it's important to remember that porn actors and amateurs who upload porn are way more experienced at doing this than just about anyone else on the planet. They will be doing it far more vigorously than is advisable, and they will magically know what to do as opposed to going slowly and finding what works best. Unlike Nina Hartley, porn actors rarely give each other feedback and they almost never stop if there is pain or discomfort.

So if you are going to try double penetration, it is essential that you give each other an abundance of feedback and that there be collaboration among all three partners. Talk about it beforehand. Discuss how you will signal each other if you are experiencing pain or discomfort, as well as how you will inform your partners when it's feeling just right.

You will need to experiment with different positions and ways of thrusting to find what works best for the three of you. If the woman feels any pain as opposed to fullness, you need to immediately stop.

If you have doubts our questions about double penetration, be sure to discuss them with your healthcare provider beforehand :-)

Resources:

Nina Hartley's Guide To Double Penetration from Adam & Eve (thanks to Sinclair Intimacy Institute for sending it) and Michael Ninn's *Double Penetration*, *Double Penetration 2*, and *Double Penetration 3*; not yet available at Target.

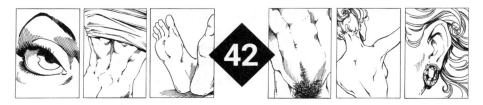

Between Vanilla & Kink

"Why is it that some men just can't deal with the idea that a smart, together, professional woman like me can actually deserve their respect and still want to be thrown down on the couch and pounded like a cheap steak now and then?"

—Hanne Blank in *Clean Sheets Erotica Magazine*

In the world of sexual pleasure, "vanilla" is usually defined as masturbation, hand jobs, finger fucking, oral sex and vaginal intercourse. Then there's kink. Kink is harder to define. It can be anything from spanking and biting to what goes on in your local BDSM dungeon.

So what happens when someone who is usually in the vanilla camp wants to borrow from the kinky side to spice up his or her sex life? That's what this chapter is about that. It's made up of your answers to this question about kink our sex survey:

Are there types of non-vanilla sex that you enjoy having? ("Non-vanilla sex" includes being spanked or spanking a partner, having rough sex, biting, restraining or being restrained, acting out a rape fantasy, fisting, peeing on a partner or being peed on, having her put fingers or anything else up your rear, etc.)

Only about 50% of the people who took the survey answered the question. So if half of you have no desire to do anything that's mentioned in this chapter, you're in good company. But if you are interested in the occasional walk on the wild side, you are in good company as well. And if you have fantasies about doing things that are kinky but are afraid to tell your partner, you are in very good company!

Your Answers

"Yes or yes, yes, yes, yes or yes, no, no, no or no, no or no."

male age 18

"Love some hand spanking and rough sex. Love it when he holds my wrists tight." *female age 22*

"Biting is fun. Also giving orders or being fucked hard." *fem 18*

"I don't do vanilla sex, haven't in years. It's one of the reasons I divorced my ex... he wasn't interested in anything but vanilla. I'm eager to try anything short of urine/fecal involvement."
female age 25

"I like rough sex occasionally (being held down and penetrated hard) and some light biting. I have done some role-playing which can be fun." *female age 28*

"We're pretty wild. We're up for everything besides pain, peeing, or scat." *male age 27*

"I drool thinking about rough sex. I scratch very nicely. I love biting. I love being restraining and being spanked. I love it when he gets ready to come and gently grasps the back of my head while I blow him. I love being controlled." *female age 19*

"Anal play and fantasize about eating cum out of her pussy or off her body." *male age 42*

"My partner and I are in a relatively new relationship, and discussing what we might be interested in trying - I've never had anything non-vanilla before (neither has he), but we have experimented with very light restraints, biting (but more like nipping – nothing hurtful), and I am interested in forceful sex. I'm not yet sure about a full-on rape fantasy." *female age 29*

"I would really like to try out some bondage, but we haven't yet. Maybe tonight." *female age 26*

"Well, I like it when my partner spanks me during sex... I think I would enjoy being tied up. I would also like to add a vibrator into the mix." *female age 20*

"When I was having sex with my best friend, she loved it rough. I slammed her up against a door and she got so horny. She loved getting her hair pulled, and wanted me to tie her up. It was a lot of fun, but definitely needs to be with the right person and talked about beforehand." *male age 22*

"I enjoy biting. While I've never been completely restrained, it's a huge turn-on to be held down." *female age 19*

"Everything, but fisting and peeing. No poop, blood, or fire. I'm OK with everything else. Not into lots of pain but a little is rather fun sometimes. I love getting bit. Being marked means I was claimed." *female age 35*

"We do anal play and both enjoy it." *female age 27*

"I love getting bit. I love restraining her, spanking her and being scratched." *male age 22*

"I like being restrained and blindfolded because it makes everything more intense. My boyfriend feels uncomfortable about it so there goes that..." *female age 25*

"I really enjoy anal play. She is happy to do it, although she would prefer to use anything other than her fingers. We are looking into toys right now." *male age 25*

"I like light bondage, being tied up and blindfolded, pinned, and having the control taken away from me. Unfortunately, it hardly ever happens." *female age 35*

"Being spanked, being restrained (tied down, blindfolded, etc.), rough sex, dominance play and a rape type scenario here and there. We're a rather kinky couple." *female age 19*

"I like to be bitten, controlled and restrained. I love the tease. The enjoyment is the wanting to be touched somewhere and not getting it. Oh, and being marked by bites, bruises, and hickeys." *female age 21*

"My boyfriend and I really like rough sex and sometimes he bites me. We also will sometimes have one partner give directions to the other or have one partner be 'frozen' while the other does whatever the other wants to the frozen partner."
female age 21

"Being spanked, nipples bitten and rough sex. I do like it when he holds me down, but I wouldn't want it to last the entire time and I don't want to pretend that I'm feeling raped. I do really like it when I feel like he knows exactly what he wants and will take it; I guess I like it when he's very dominant, but I also like being dominant on occasion, too." *female age 23*

"I love having rough sex. When my boyfriend and I are role-playing a robbery or kidnapping, rough sex adds to the 'appeal' of the role play. It also like spanking, biting, restraining and acting out of a rape fantasy. We also have sex on every surface we can get to when we're acting out a fantasy." *female age 24*

"I would enjoy being anally penetrated with toys and fingers, but my significant other isn't into that idea." *male age 38*

"I love everything minus rape fantasies and being peed on. I would be fine with all of that every time we had sex." *female 21*

"I like playful, gentle biting, giving and receiving hickeys, back-scratching (but not necessarily to the point of bleeding), mild bondage and leather play. I have a love for piercings and tattoos and find getting them a bit of a sexual rush." *male age 31*

"I enjoy being spanked while having sex with my partner, but only if we're having sex doggy style and I'm already very turned on. I enjoy rough sex some times, but not regularly or when I'm tired. I like being restrained occasionally, although my husband rarely does that to me. He has also pretended to rape me a couple times, which I enjoy, but he doesn't do it very often because of the aggression of the act." *female age 20*

"I enjoy anal play occasionally. I wish we could be more open about what we like." *male age 36*

"I love being 'taken.' I love rough sex, biting, being restrained or restraining him, and spanking. I also really like using sex toys, like dildos and vibrators. They enhance our experiences a lot." *female age 20*

"I love fingers and toys up the rear. Piss play intrigues me but I haven't tried it." *male age 28*

"Does anal and sex in public count? I enjoy anal for most sexual encounters. Sex in public took some convincing from my ex."
female age 32

"Rough sex, spanking or being spanked." *female age 32*

"I think biting can be enjoyable and a quick smack on the ass during doggie style is nice. I like it when my husband pulls me toward his body aggressively and restrains my hands. If you saw the size of my husband's hand you would understand why I would never want to be fisted by him. Fisting seems more like a girl/girl thing with small dainty hands." *female age 30*

"Having rough sex. I love that a lot." *female age 26*

"Sometimes I like getting spanked lightly. I also prefer to be the aggressive one and not the other way around. I would rather I bite him instead of him biting me. I would rather I pin him down instead of him pinning me down. My fiance enjoys fish nets, and I swear he could almost get off just by looking at them on me or touching them." *female age 20*

"Rough sex can be really amazing if we're both in the mood. I also enjoy women wearing plaid skirts." *male age 30*

"I have tried rape sex.... don't really enjoy it. It felt pretty weird. I do enjoy light spanking. I like being restrained as long as I know I can say 'get off' and he will right away. No peeing or fisting though." *female age 20*

"I love being spanked, handcuffed to chairs and blindfolded. I also love schoolgirl role playing, biting, and occasionally being thrown around like a rag doll. I am a very submissive partner."
female age 19

"Rough sex, biting, clawing, fighting a little, being restrained and hair pulling (mine and my partner's)." *female age 20*

"I love everything plus the piss. For some reason I am turned on by urine. It's not something I advertise for or roll out early in a relationship. I love light BDSM, especially getting tied up. My interest wanes as soon as the actual pain ramps up." *female 28*

"I enjoy performing anal sex on myself and being fingered while being jacked off. I like to watch women pee, I like to be peed on and pee on my partner. We enjoy public flashing and public sex and nudism. I enjoy watching others naked and having sex, and I also enjoy being watched while I have sex."

male age 25

"I guess if anal sex qualifies as "non-vanilla," that's something I enjoy, but only if I'm particularly aroused, which happens less and less often these days." *female age 27*

"(Blush) I like peeing (both giving and receiving) although it's been very rare that I find a partner who is like-minded. I enjoy anal play, both giving and receiving. Frankly, if my partner enjoys it, I'm not really above doing anything. Her pleasure is the greatest aphrodisiac there is." *male age 40*

"Being on the giving or receiving end of spanking, biting, scratching, wax play and bondage. There's of at least one of these every time I have sex (about once a week)." *female age 29*

"I love biting, but I hate being bitten. I really want to have sex with someone who won't stop every time I say "ouch." I want it rough." *female age 19*

I'm intrigued by hard fingering and fisting, but I have never done it. I don't think she is physically able and I don't want her to get hurt. *male age 35*

"I enjoy strapping on a dildo and having anal sex with a man. My current boyfriend does not want to try this, but I enjoyed it immensely with a previous boyfriend. I also like the idea of restraining my partner, but I have never tried it." *female age 38*

"I like being spanked, and occasionally doing the spanking; having my hair pulled, pulling my partners' hair; being bitten (gently), doing the biting; I keep my nails long and it turns me on to scratch or dig my nails into my partners during sex—and most of my partners are very turned on by it. I also like group sex." *female age 25*

"Light bondage! Both sides, please. I love rough sex, although not to the point of pain. And anywhere that's not a bedroom is sexy, even though beds are comfortable." *male age 25*

"I like being spanked, biting, being restrained and eating desserts off each other. I am open to most things. Just not peeing, pooping, screwing animals or eating flesh. Oh, or fucking dead people. That's a no-no." *female age 23*

"Love being spanked and caressed and receiving love bites. I love holding my feet in the upside down straddle stretch and being pounded and adored. Being restrained by strong arms is nice." *female age 23*

"My partner and I are rather kinky. We enjoy spanking, rough sex, rape fantasy, fisting, biting, restraint sex, role-playing, and on occasion, we've even yiffed. That was a bonding experience." *female age 21*

"I like to spank, and dominate my partner. I'm always switching between slow caressing and dominance. I would like to restrain her and try role playing." *male age 21*

"I really enjoy being bitten and restrained." *male age 41*

"I love rough sex when I'm in the mood for it. I love being restrained and restraining others! I can get a little kinky at times. I still don't think my current partner knows how to take me sometimes." *female age 23*

"Whoa! Yeah, I like to spank. If I like the girl I want to be spanked. The more involved I am with a girl, the more I want from her. If she likes to bite - awesome. But if she's doing it because she saw it in a video and is trying to impress me – lame." *male 19*

"I like being spanked and spanking my partner, having rough sex, biting, restraining or being restrained, being dominated, acting out a rape fantasy, fisting, peeing on a partner or being peed on, taking dumps together and having a finger in my rear - especially hers. I love non-vanilla sex." *male age 18*

"Nearly every time I have sex, there's some sort of rough element, whether it's spanking, scratching or biting. I definitely enjoy being restrained or restraining my partner. But if I don't want my hands held down I'll move or try to move them. I love the idea of being dominated or overpowered. On the other hand, I hate the idea of a being a "submissive bitch", but there's something about being controlled and dominated that is erotic. Don't get me wrong, it's a give and take. I'll be restrained, but I'm going to want to give it back." *female age 21*

"Yeah, I enjoy being tied up and I tie her up. I love blindfolds and anal play. We'd like to find a way to wrestle and have sex at the same time, but keeping the penis in the vagina while wrestling doesn't work very well. At least, we haven't found a way to do it." *male age 24*

"With some girls it feels appropriate to be gentle. With other girls it gets rough. I guess I'm a sexual chameleon or something."
male age 25

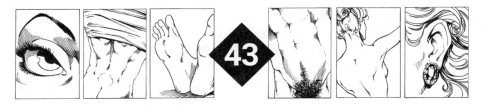

Kinky Corner-Spanking and More

If serious kink is what you are into, then you should probably find a credible group of people in your community who are into the kind of kink you like. This chapter is more for couples who occasionally want to spice things up with a bit of kink. It also gives an overview of fetishes, fisting, and crossdressing,

Spanking

After asking more than a thousand women on our sex survey about their most favorite sex fantasies, the two that were at the top of the list were threesomes and being spanked. Nothing else came even close. Since Chapter 40: Threesomes and Chapter 41: *Double Penetration* have that subject covered, let's take a page or two to focus on spanking. Janet Hardy, who is the author of *Spanking for Lovers,* was kind enough to list some of the basics:

1. Talk beforehand about the "flavor" of the spanking. If one person wants something strict and punitive, and the other wants something playful and erotic, you're headed for trouble. If you find that one of you wants one thing and the other wants something else, perhaps you can find a compromise, or make an agreement to take turns. However, you'll need a way that either of you can signal "this is more than I want to do right now," an agreement that "no means no," or a codeword or "safe-word" that allows you to joyously scream "No please no stop!" while still having a way to end the spanking if something goes haywire.

2. Do some warmup first, starting with not much more than pats, and gradually build up the intensity from there. A warmup gives both players a chance to fall into the mood, as well as giving endorphins an opportunity to flow. I strongly recommend that you start with hand-spanking. A hand has a built-in feedback device (it may not "hurt you more than it hurts them," but it does hurt you at least a bit), and almost all spankees love and appreciate the intimacy of a handspanking.

3. For most people who are being spanked, the lower inner quadrant of the buttock is the sexiest part, and the lower buttock in general is better padded and more likely to respond well. Very few spankees can eroticize strokes to the upper part of the butt. Opinions vary about being spanked on the upper thighs, and for almost everyone it's harder to take than strokes to the lower buttock. Also, have the spankee show you where her or his tailbone is, or feel for it yourself. Many people think that the tailbone is at the top of the buttcrack, but it's usually a couple of inches lower. Strokes to the tailbone, which has almost no muscular or fatty protection, hurt in a very non-erotic way, and can sometimes land someone in the hospital.

4. If you've done a few sessions with handspanking and feel like you want to move onward to implements, I recommend a small leather paddle. (I like the ones that have fur or fleece on the B-side so that you can soothe between spanks). For now, avoid hairbrushes, wooden spoons, wooden paddles, etc., which are *much* more intense than many people realize - I've met very few people who actually like them. If you're using any kind of flexible implement, like a switch, cane, strap or flogger, practice for at least an hour or two on an inanimate object like a throw pillow (look for one that has a "target" like a central button

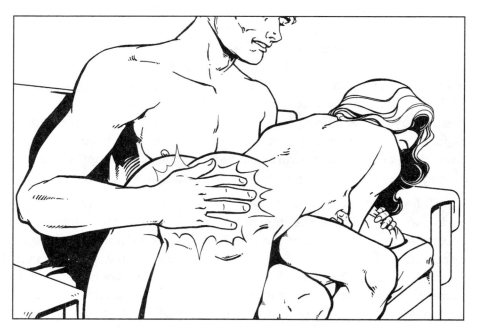

or a visible pattern) or quilt, to make sure you can land the end of your implement on the place you want it to go.

5. Many spanking fans are turned on to over-the-knee positions, but if you're not young and thin, they can be so uncomfortable for both parties, and they can detract from what you're trying to achieve. A compromise is for the giver to sit on a couch or on a bed with their back supported by the headboard, and have the receiver lie across their lap so that their chest and legs are supported by the surface.

With a very special thanks to Janet Hardy, author of *Spanking for Lovers, The Ethical Slut,* and many other fine books.

BDSM

BDSM often involves fantasy, role playing and an exchange of power. It can include the application of pain, humiliation or restraint. If it's what turns you on,it can be an endorphin rush that's like a runner's high. BDSM frequently includes one person taking power and the other giving it up. It can involve physical or psychological surrender, helplessness and trust.

An out-of-date perception about BDSM is that the person who takes the dominant role makes all of the decisions. Deciding on the scenarios and what's being done should be shared equally between all partners. Before anyone surrenders to anything, BDSM requires full consent.

People who are drawn to BDSM often enjoy being rendered passive. They don't have to worry about being a "good" partner who provides pleasure in return. Performance anxiety is eliminated. This can be especially appealing to individuals whose jobs require them to be in charge and in control.

Bondage by Choice — A Feminist Contradiction?

Feminists or social progressives (whatever that means) sometimes feel they are deserting their cause if they enjoy being submissive. Consider a feminist lawyer whose favorite fantasy is being tied up and sexually violated. She acts out this masochistic fantasy with her male lover. The reason this doesn't contradict her political beliefs is because she's the one with the freedom to choose what to do with her own body and who to do it with. In the criminal-rape cases that she handles in court, the rape victim had no choice. The act was forced upon her, rather than being part of a shared fantasy between two consenting adults.

Serious and Heavy Bondage

"Maddie's path to discovery was a gradual process. She'd been kinky for pretty much as long as she could remember. She remembered the teacher finding her tied up to the swing set at the end of recess. She didn't just play 'doctor' as a young child, she played mad scientist. Her vision was pretty dark, involving elaborate punishment scenes in a neighbor's basement. Not surprisingly, she was usually the one who got punished. She has a half-formed memory of having a bucket of coal poured over her crotch while she moaned and writhed in semi-protest. She can still remember the absolute feeling of erotic surrender, the feeling of loss of control. That memory has a sexual charge for her even today. These dirty little games continued until the inevitable discovery by a parent, at which point they abruptly ceased. She doesn't remember seeing those kids much after that. During the teenage years, her sexual awakening seemed to always involve some sort of power exchange dynamic. She chose older boys, the dangerous ones, who would use her. And she submitted to this, sometimes with great drama, but some weird little part of her loved it. The pain of losing her virginity was one of the hottest moments of her life. Unhealthy? Hell, yeah. Self-destructive? Absolutely."

—From *The Kinky Girl's Guide to Dating* by Luna Grey.

BDSM can be a world of whips, chains, ropes, melting candle wax and devices that might put a chill up the spine of just about anyone. In BDSM, the following acronyms apply: B&D = bondage and discipline; S&M = sado masochism; D&S = dominance and submission; BDSM is a blanket term for pretty much all of it.

In BDSM, having an orgasm isn't nearly as important as the scene itself, with its undercurrent of domination, submission and sometimes humiliation. People who are into bondage seem to process pain differently than people who aren't. They find doses of sexual pain to be invigorating and intimate, assuming it's done in a context they find arousing.

If you'd like to get into BDSM, don't pick up a stranger who enjoys beating the crap out of people and confuse that with bondage. In BDSM, there are established rules and etiquette that keep the participants

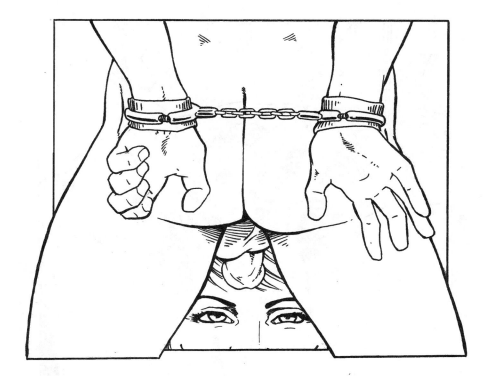

from getting seriously hurt. Mind you, the definition of seriously hurt is a personal matter. If bondage is what turns you on, learn the rules and make sure that your partners know and respect them.

In almost every large city, you will be able to find an established bondage club. These clubs often have extensive calendars of events, including talks, demonstrations and social gatherings. You will often be safer in joining one of these established clubs than by experimenting on your own. You might also be amazed at how many educated, kind and helpful people you will meet at the established clubs. You might even meet some PTA parents from your kids' school!

Also, don't get roped into thinking that mild-mannered people prefer being bottoms (slave or submissive role) and that aggressive types prefer being tops (master/dominator/dominatrix). There are plenty of business executives, lawyers, doctors, politicians and policemen who prefer being on the bottom. In fact, it's well known in the bondage community that a good top is hard to find. It's also true that a number of people into BDSM enjoy alternating roles between top and bottom.

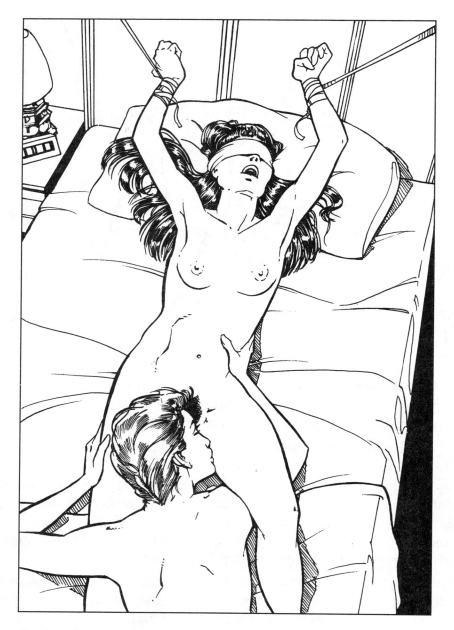

Look at how her wrists are bound! This can cause wrist damage and is NOT the way you want to do it. Splurge and get some fake sheepskin cuffs or look online for the latest in restraints and bedroom bondage accessories.

BDSM — Safety Considerations

Whether you only use bondage once a year or are a dungeon regular, Jay Wiseman, author of the highly regarded book on BDSM titled *SM-101*, makes the following suggestions:

😎 Anytime a body part that is tied up feels numb or goes to sleep, untie it immediately. Never tie anything around a partner's neck.

😎 In anticipation of catastrophes like fires, earthquakes or an unexpected visit from your mom and dad, be sure to have a flashlight and a pair of heavy scissors handy. *SM-101* recommends paramedic scissors, which can be found at medical-supply stores. They cut through almost anything except handcuffs. Keep the scissors and flashlights in a place you can readily find in the dark. Ditto for the handcuff key if that's what you are using. Better yet, tie the key to the handcuffs with a string.

😎 Never leave the person for long, and check them often. If any injuries were to occur, you would be legally and morally responsible.

😎 Always establish a safe word or gesture which means to stop. Some people use "red" for stop and "yellow" for easing up a little. No one who is seriously into dominance and submission uses "stop," "don't," or "no more" for safe words, since any good bottom says them often and seldom means it.

Breath Play or Erotic Asphyxiation—DO NOT DO THIS

A reader reported that he puts his hands around his partner's neck and squeezes tightly when they are having sex—at her request. She says it makes the experience feel more intense. He is concerned. This is called *breath play* or *erotic asphyxiation*. It's also referred to as *scarfing* or *terminal sex*. The side effects can include death and brain damage. There are two groups of people who enjoy *breath play*: males who partially suffocate themselves while masturbating, and couples where one partner likes to be choked.

Boys and young men who are known as *baggers* or *gaspers* put plastic bags over their heads or tight ropes around their necks while they masturbate. *Baggers* are often white, straight and middle-class.

They fit in well socially and they keep their sexual secrets well hidden. Up to a quarter of them wear women's underwear while they are masturbating on death's doorstep.

Several boy baggers die each year in this country. Their deaths are often reported as suicides. But people who are trying to kill themselves don't hang from door knobs and they don't design safety releases into their death devices. Boy baggers fully intend to free themselves after squeezing out their blurry-eyed orgasms.

Horrified parents will often spruce up the death scene before the ambulance arrives. Instead of being reported as masturbation gone awry, the coroner thinks it's a suicide. None of the kid's friends can understand why someone who seemed so well-adjusted would want to off himself.

The other group who are into breath play are normal-appearing couples. They have no fear of the boy-bagger's fate. They assume the person who is applying the pressure is like a designated driver who can put the brakes on before it's too late. "Not so!" says BDSM expert Jay Wiseman:

> "As a person with years of medical education and experience, I know of no way whatsoever that either suffocation or strangulation can be done in a way that does not put the recipient at risk of cardiac arrest. If the recipient does arrest, the probability of resuscitating them, even with optimal CPR, is distinctly small."

You could be hooked up to state-of-the-art heart monitors and have a board-certified cardiologist for a sex partner, breath play would still be like playing Russian roulette. Another thing that has healthcare providers concerned is the risk of brain damage. Charles Moser, a physician who is highly respected in the world of kink, worries about the long-term consequences of breath play. Yet choking and breath play continues to be prominently featured in a popular genre of porn known as *rough sex*.

Fetishes: An Overview

There once was a popular song where a man was imploring his lover to take off all her clothes, except for her hat. If a man can't enjoy sex unless his partner has a hat on, we might say he has a hat fetish:

FETISH—1. Reliance on a prop, body part, scene or scenario in order to get off sexually. 2. The prop can either be fantasized or exist in actuality. 3. A philosopher has described "fetish" as being similar to when a hungry person sits down at a dinner table and feels full from fondling the napkin.

If both people in a relationship enjoy the same fetish, then its presence is a welcome event. But if only one partner is into the fetish, the other person might feel that she or he is not nearly as important as the fetish itself. For instance, the woman in the *Leave-Your-Hat-On* song might start to feel like a human hat rack.

Fetishes come in many different forms; some include objects, others include actions that need to be repeated over and over.

Normal Sexual Turn-on vs. a Fetish

Let's say your boyfriend loves to feel your legs when you have pantyhose on. You enjoy the extra attention, but your sister says it's a fetish. As long as it feels like your partner is more turned-on by you than the pantyhose, they are probably just a fun prop for him. He won't go into sexual mourning if you swear off pantyhose for no-show socks. But what if he can't become aroused unless you are wearing pantyhose, or he gets off more and more by your pantyhose and you feel like a mannequin? That's when you're probably dealing with a fetish.

Some people have fetishes for objects or materials like leather, rubber, latex, underwear, shoes, socks, boots, smelly feet, hair, breasts and even adults who wear diapers as a sexual turn on. Other people with fetishes have scenarios or fantasies that they get off to, for example, the guy who likes his partner to urinate or defecate on him. Or the fetish might be as hidden and subtle as the kind of haircut his partner has. He suddenly goes bonkers if she changes it. (Ever notice how some guys date or marry only women who are the spitting image of each other? Is it the woman he loves, or a certain look she has?)

People with fetishes sometimes get comfort from the fetish that they can't get from human beings. The fetish becomes the missing piece that completes their sexual circuit. It isn't demanding or humiliating like a real-life partner can be. (It's far easier to control a pair of pantyhose than to control the woman who is wearing them!).

One problem with having a serious fetish (aka paraphilia) is the loneliness that can sometimes be a part of it. No matter how many

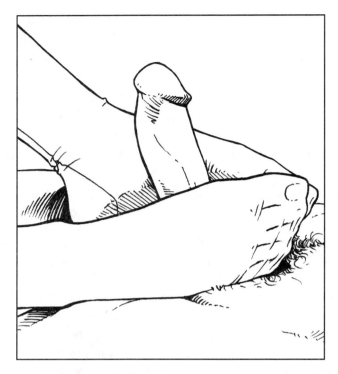

This wouldn't be considered a foot fetish if it is something you enjoy doing but can also do without. Psychologists would call it a fetish if the man couldn't become aroused without seeing or touching a woman's feet, or if her feet were so important that he needed them to become sexually excited. How do psychologists know? Because they are as kinky as anyone else.

times you fondle them, a pair of rubber panties or a woman's feet can go only so far in providing the closeness that many of us value in a sexual partner. This is why fetishes are sometimes referred to as a compromise between the fear of human closeness and the need for it.

Crossdressing

Some women occasionally dress up like men, to the point of wearing a fake penis. This is a form of accessorizing known as "packing." But most crossdressers are men, where a penis just gets in the way. Crossdressing is the way that men who have an inner woman or an inner vagina allow her out to play.

The only reason crosdressing was placed in this chapter is because none of the other chapters of this book felt it belonged, which is the dilemma that most crossdressers face. The following is Amy Bloom in her book, *Normal–Transsexual CEOs, Crossdressing Cops, and Hermaphrodites with Attitude:*

> "Heterosexual crossdressers bother almost everyone. Gay people regard them with disdain or affectionate incomprehension, something warmer than tolerance, but not much. Transsexuals regard them as men 'settling' for crossdressing because they don't have the courage to act on their transsexual longing, or else as closeted gay men so homophobic that they prefer wearing a dress to facing their desire for another man. Other straight men tend to find them funny or sad, and some find them enraging..."

There are hundreds of thousands of male crossdressers in the United States alone. Many are quite masculine when they aren't wearing a bra and panties, and many appear quite masculine when they are wearing a bra and panties. These men are often married to women and enjoy having sex with them. A lot of crossdressers value their sports-page loving side as much as their inner girlfriend, but struggle with finding ways to enjoy both at the same time.

Contrary to what you might imagine, male crossdressers aren't necessarily drawn to professions that welcome a guy's feminine side. The average crossdresser is as likely to be a baseball player, fireman, policeman, auto mechanic or business executive as a hairdresser or florist.

Crossdressers have a crush on their female persona. She often calls to them, imploring them to give her life by dressing as a woman. The bra becomes her breasts, the panties her vagina that crossdressers so often love. Standing in front of a mirror, admiring his "breasts and vagina," will allow some crossdressers to have the erection they need in order to masturbate. Other crossdressers don't want to be reminded of the male genitals that are tucked beneath their frilly lingerie.

Therapy will not change a crossdresser's need to crossdress. However, if a man is compulsive about crossdressing, therapy can help him with that. Many crossdressers hope that marriage will cure them of their desire to dress like a woman. But the envy and allure of a wife's underwear drawer will soon rear its head and so much for good intentions.

Men who are reading this book while wearing their favorite DKNY dress might be concerned about being found out. This is a fear shared by many crossdressers who are not out of the closet.

If you are a wife or girlfriend who suddenly discovers your man has a secret cache of frilly garb, try to give yourself a three-month chilling-off period. Talk to your partner about what he does and why. He must love you a great deal if he's worked so hard to hide something that's so darned big. If you can, check out the site of the Society for the Second Self or Tri-Ess at www.tri-ess.org. This national organization is for crossdressers, their wives and their families. Search out anything written by Francis Fairfax, particularly the *Wives' Bill of Rights*. Some women also find the books by Helen Boyd to be helpful.

Given how this is not the sort of thing you can necessarily call your mom or sister to talk about, see if there is a support group in your area for wives of crossdressers. The folks at Tri-Ess can help you find them. Ask these wives about what they will and won't put up with. There are plenty of things you don't need to agree to, like meeting your man for lunch when he's dressed like Britney Spears. And if for some reason he thinks he can dress up in front of the kids or gets so deep into the crossdressing scene that he stops being a good husband or dad, crossdressers' wives will offer all the support you need to confront him. In other words, you don't have to condone what he's doing but you don't need to divorce him either.

For a lot of women, it would be easier to accept their husband if he said he were gay. But to see him dressed up like Little Bo Peep and hear him say he's straight? Wives tend to fear they will lose the manly part of their crossdressing man. Hopefully, he'll be the same man he was in bed before you found out about the heels and gown. Part of a wife's fear may have to do with humiliation that someone else will find out.

After chilling out, a wife or girlfriend might appreciate there are worse things a man could do than wear women's clothes, fashion crime that it might be. She might also realize that he has the same good characteristics that he had before she found out about his hidden side.

There's no shortage of publications on crossdressing. Some people value the books by Peggy Rudd, a therapist and the wife of a crossdresser. Others aren't so comfortable with her crossdresser-as-visionary point of view.

Highly Recommended: The book "Alice in Genderland" should be at the top of any crossdresser's reading list. It's by Alice Novic, a cross-dressing psychiatrist. And don't ignore www.wayout-publishing.com if you need a gift for a man who crossdresses.

Phone Sex—When 911 Won't Put Out Your Fire

Ever wonder what goes on in phone sex, when a man pays several dollars a minute to get a good talking to? A woman who worked as a phone-sex operator after graduating from an expensive private college was kind enough to offer the following description:

> "The fantasies ranged from men who wanted me to physically beat myself on the phone with a hairbrush, to those who wanted me to force them to have oral sex with other men and those who just wanted to hear me have an orgasm. What struck me is that men have more gay fantasies than I would have expected. There seems to be a correlation between men who have powerful jobs and their sexual fantasies. One client, who I later found out was a senior partner in a financial firm always wanted me to 'force' him to do things, mostly to other men and sometimes to me. Others wanted to escape from their life, shed their responsibility and their male-ness—they explored their imagination with me and pretended I was their dominatrix, their she-male, their whore. I gave them permission and encouraged them to be who they wanted to be and that's what they needed."

> "I always wondered about clients. I was madly curious. I wanted to know who they were, how much money they made, if they were married, if they were straight and if they were the kinds of guys I knew. And often, I'd 'interview' them and I'll admit that I looked up what I wanted to know why they were calling me, how it played into their real sex life and what I was to them. In some instances, I was the woman on the phone who was their mistress, but in the most controlled way. Some got attached to me and I was fired and then rehired and in my absence, I was missed (as I learned later)."

Vaginal and Anal Fisting (Handballing)

Vaginal fisting is finger fucking times five, with a fist thrown in for good measure. Some women enjoy having a partner's fist inside their vagina. But keep in mind the sex of the partner. Most women have significantly smaller fists than men. A fist the size of a man's could take a potentially pleasurable fisting experience and turn it into something akin to childbirth. Or not.

If vaginal fisting is something you want to try, read everything you can on the subject. Stop immediately if you experience anything but the slightest amount of discomfort. You should never attempt fisting if either of you has been drinking or doing drugs, and you certainly shouldn't try it before reading the advice of women who do it.

Some couples, straight as well as gay, are into anal fisting. Don't even think about trying this unless you really, really, really know what you are doing. The classic book on anal fisting is Bert Herrman's *Trust— The Hand Book* as well as Tristan Taormino's *The Ultimate Guide to Anal Sex for Women, 2nd edition*. Also, there may be organized groups of fisters in your area who give talks and demonstrations.

Dear Paul,

Do you have any advice about going to a dominatrix?

Policeman by Day, Schoolboy by Night

Dear Officer,

To help answer your question, I called my friend Lorrett, who runs a house devoted to BDSM and fantasy play. Here's her advice:

1. BDSM is about creating a fantasy scene, and then acting it out. In creating the scene, you need to talk to the person you are hiring about things like boundaries, safe words, and how you want the scene to play out. You should feel comfortable with the person, and feel that they are comfortable with you in negotiating the scene. If they come off as being abrupt or domineering when setting up the scene, then what follows isn't going to be play. Instead, you are going to be acting out their agenda, and what follows will be anything but consensual.

2. Trust your instincts. It's fine to be nervous or anxious, but if you feel frightened or uncomfortable, go elsewhere.

In domination and fantasy games, the dominatrix doesn't actually get you off. You are free to get yourself off in her presence, but she won't actually give you an orgasm the way a prostitute will. That's why it's not illegal for you to hire a dominatrix.

A Special Thanks to Lorrett at Fantasy Makers in Berkeley and Janet at Greenery Press—two of the nicest people around.

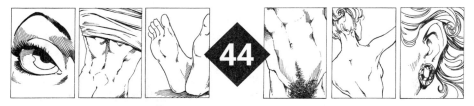

Sexual Orientation

Sexual orientation refers to the gender that turns you on. If are a male who is turned on by women, then you considered to be straight or heterosexual. If you are turned on by both men and women, you are bisexual. And if you are turned on by other men, you are gay. There are also the "mostly" categories, as in mostly straight and mostly gay.

People used to think of "straight male" and "straight female" as being opposite sides of the same coin. Not any more. Some of the top researchers in sexual orientation were kind enough to offer readers of *The Guide* their current thinking about sexual orientation. Consider what Richard Lippa from Cal State University at Fullerton has to say:

> "Recent research suggests that the nature of sexual orientation may be quite different for men and women. (I've conducted some of this research.) Women's sexual orientation seems to be more fluid and flexible than men's, whereas men's sexual orientation seems to be more fixed, 'black-and-white,' and perhaps biologically wired in. For example, recent studies of people's physiological arousal to sexy male and sexy female stimuli show that heterosexual men are turned on by sexy women but not by men, and gay men are turned on by sexy men but not by women (as you would probably expect). However, women—both heterosexual and lesbian—get turned on by both sexy men and women (which is perhaps not so expected)."

> "Western society has become more open about variations in sexual orientation and more tolerant of non-heterosexual orientations and relationships. So it will be really interesting to see how the expression of sexual orientations develops in coming years."

Here's what Michael Bailey from Northwestern has to say:

> "Increasingly, people are understanding that men and women do sexual orientation differently. Men are straightforward. A man's sexual orientation results from what causes him the greatest

sexual arousal, what kind of person (or animal or thing) gives him the most intense sexual excitement and the most dependable erections.

"Women are different. Increasingly, it appears that women's sexual orientation is not closely linked to their sexual arousal patterns the way it is in men. I even question whether women have something called a sexual orientation, although they clearly have sexual preferences. Women's sexuality seems more fluid than men's, in that it can vacillate between different types of people, and women are known to fall in love with each other and then to revert to a heterosexual identity and life."

What Do We Mean By "Women's Orientation is More Fluid?"

When sex researchers ask women to put tampon-like probes in their vaginas that measure their blood flow, they find that just about any kind of sexual stimulus can result in an increase of blood flowing around their vagina. A picture of two hippos humping would probably do the trick. But before you take a woman to the zoo hoping she'll want to have sex with you, what flows between a woman's legs and what she's experiencing in her mind can be very different. As the researchers say: there can be a huge disconnect between vagina and cranium. This makes figuring out women's sexual orientation much more difficult than figuring out mens'.

There is also the assumption that a lot of women are turned on by other women. This is certainly true for a number of women in certain situations. But if you look at who most non-lesbian women have sex with, a large majority of the time it is with men.

So just because researchers are saying that female sexuality is fluid doesn't mean that waves of women are going down on each other. Perhaps a better way to put it is to say that when it comes to sex, the theater of the female mind has more potential for variety than the male mind. If the stars are lined up right and the chemistry with another woman is exceptionally hot, all bets are off. But most of the time, most women want to have sex with men.

Beware How the Research Is Interpreted

Just because sensitive probes in women's genitals can detect an increase in blood flow when women are presented with a certain stimulus doesn't mean a woman is feeling sexually aroused. This is something people don't take into account when they hear about studies that show "women are turned on by videos of bonobos fucking" or "women are turned on to videos of rape." There may be an increase in blood flow in the tissues around the vagina and increased activity in certain parts of the brain, but we still have no clue if and how this is related to sexual arousal. So if you are reading studies about women's sexual arousal, pay close attention to what the women actually report in addition to what the MRIs and sensors in their vaginas find.

Mostly Straight" vs "Totally Straight"

If women's orientations are more fluid than men's, it might explain the results of our own totally unscientific sex survey. Over the past years, we have received approximately 10,000 sex surveys from visitors to our website. One of the first questions has been, "Please state your orientation as *totally straight, mostly straight, depends on the time and day, mostly gay or totally gay.*" Here are the approximate results:

	"totally straight"	"mostly straight"	other categories
males	80%	15%	5%
females	45%	45%	10%

We've also tried to design a nonthreatening question about same-sex interest. We have tried to make the question as safe to answer as possible, since even a hint of same-sex interest can make male survey takers come unglued. Here's the question in one of its many incarnations:

> "If our society did not care or notice, and if your girlfriend and best friends thought it was perfectly normal and OK, do you think you might ever consider experimenting sexually with another guy to see what it was like?" (For the women's version, we changed *girlfriend* to *boyfriend* and *guy* to *woman.*)

The vast majority of the women replied, "Sure!" or "I have already thought about it and am wondering how to make it happen," or "It's nothing I would seek out, but if it happened, I might go with it."

It was a very different story for the male survey takers. A number of them flamed in all caps, "NO FUCKING WAY" or "I'M NOT GAY!" Around 30% did say "Maybe" or "You never know." Most said, "It's nothing that interests me." (We are pleased to report that the amount of angry flaming has gone down in the last few years. Maybe society is changing, or maybe it's because there are more gay males in hit TV shows. Unfortunately, given the rhetoric of the last presidential election, there still seems to be a strong undercurrent of homophobia in America.)

As for why most males describe themselves as being either totally straight or totally gay, it could be that most males come out of the womb with an orientation that says "either straight or gay" with no wiggle room. But what about males who are sitting on the fence? Perhaps they are part of a smaller group of men whose orientation isn't set in stone. It could be that culture and their family environment can have a significant influence on the sexual orientation of some men.

Wet Panties Have Their Advantages

If a woman becomes aroused at the sight, smell, or touch of another woman, she doesn't have to worry about being found out. If she's undressing with another woman and finds the situation to be arousing, she can smile inwardly and enjoy her feelings without having to camouflage an emerging erection. She doesn't even need to think of her feelings as sexual or as homosexual.

But if a guy gets an erection when he's around other guys, it's not something he can ignore. He knows who is turning him on, which is not always the kind of feedback that women get from their genitals.

Given how the penis is one of nature's more obvious feedback devices, it might give men more of an all-or-nothing or black and white interpretation of sexual feelings.

Do Social Factors Influence Women More Than Men?

Psychologist Roy Baumeister believes women are more sexually flexible than men, and not just in terms of intercourse positions. He says the reason is because women's sexuality is more influenced by social factors such as religion, education and parental pressures. Women with college educations are more likely to masturbate than women without, while a guy who is a high-school drop out is just as likely to masturbate as one with a Ph.D.

Women may be more flexible, but they often see themselves as guardians of the family and champions of the status quo. If a woman in a woman's church group is romantically kissing another woman during their annual anti-pornography potluck, she'll have hell to pay. Women are also the first to call other women "sluts" or "whores." Perhaps women are more flexible about some things and more rigid about others.

Women's Genitals vs. Men's Genitals When Watching Porn

Since men watch more porn than women and women read more romance novels than men, you'd think that male genital arousal would be more visually driven and women's less so. However, women's genitals are just as responsive to porn as men's. The blood around women's vaginas flows more to hardcore porn than to erotic stories or sex fantasies. But there are major differences in the kinds of porn that make women wet.

Straight men often get more of a penis response when porn shows female-female sex. For gay men, the boner raiser is male-male sex. So if you show men either male-male or female-female sex, the chances are good you can determine whether they are straight or gay based on what their penis reacts the most to. (It's different if you show them heterosexual porn. The penises of gay and straight males often have similar responses to heterosexual porn, but probably for different reasons.)

With women, there is an increase in the blood flow to their vaginas no matter what kind of porn they watch: male-male, female-female or male-female porn. It's difficult to tell what this means, because it is not consistent with what the women are consciously feeling.

When It Comes to Sexual Orientation, Men Are Judged More Harshly

When it comes to same-sex experimentation, we tend to be far more judgmental about boys than girls. If you doubt this, consider the following:

If a therapist is consulted about two teenage boys giving each other hand jobs or oral sex, she'll assume they are probably gay. You can't talk a child out of one orientation and into another, and as long as they are well-adjusted and happy, she wouldn't be concerned. (This would not be a case of parallel sex-play; it's highly unlikely the boys were thinking about girls when they were given each other blowjobs!)

But if two college sorority sisters had been drinking and had sex together at a party, people wouldn't think much about their sexual orientation as long as they were popular or didn't have the kind of

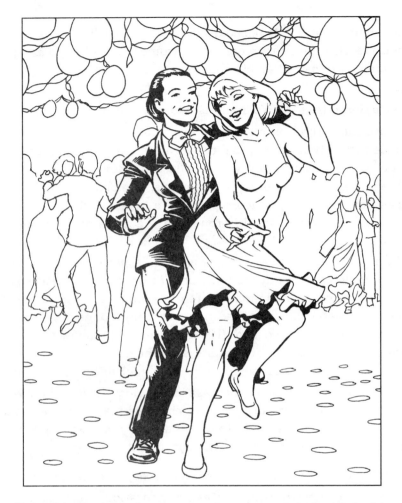

masculinized behaviors that is sometimes associated with lesbians. Or they would dismiss the girls' behavior with terms like "Lesbian until Graduation!" In our culture, we have an understanding that women can be all over the map when it comes to sexual orientation,but not so with males, who we expect to be either straight or gay.

"Mostly Straight" vs "Bisexual"

Few people would be surprised if a woman who identifies as totally straight says that she is attracted to another woman. At least we wouldn't be after reading hundreds of women's sex surveys where they describe themselves as being "totally straight" but ten questions later say they would have sex with another woman if she were really hot.

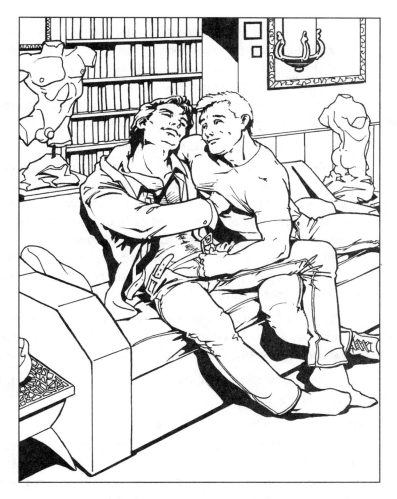

It's different for men. Very different. While close to 50% of women describe themselves as being "mostly straight" rather than "totally straight," fewer than 15% men describe themselves as being "mostly straight." And those who describe themselves as being "mostly straight" are pretty much totally straight when it comes to their sexual behavior and fantasies. While they might find themselves being attracted to other men on occasion, they prefer being with women.

As for men who truly are bisexual and enjoy having sex with women and men, current best estimate is 1% and 2% of all men. If the number of bisexual males were higher than this, there would be dozens if not hundreds of porn sites that feature bisexual males. Yet there are only a handful of sites with bisexual males. Most porn sites go out of their way to exclude male-to-male sexual contact unless they are sites for gay males. Even when there are two men having sex with one woman, they almost never make sexual contact with each other. The world of mainstream porn would come unhinged if two men had sex with each other. It's fine for women to have sex with each other in porn for straight males—it's even a bonus. But male-male sex is forbidden.

Bisexual Men and a Lack of Social Acceptance

While people are at least somewhat accepting of bisexuality in women, this is not the case for bisexuality in men. In most straight circles, it's better to say you are a serial killer than a bisexual male. Among gay men, bisexual males are often accused of being afraid to come out as gay. And while many straight people are accepting of gay males, this would not be the case with how they feel about bisexual males. Recently, a male student who is openly bisexual at a liberal college wrote a letter to his school's newspaper saying:

> "I am out as a bisexual male, but the degree of discrimination is worse than most know. So I don't exactly advise bi-men to be out unless they are ready and able to emotionally endure the abuse."

The abuse he is describing comes from both gay and straight students on his campus.

The Influence of Having a Higher Sex Drive

You would think there would be a tendency for both men and women who have higher sex drives to also be more open to bisexual exploration. Yet the research shows that this is only true for women. Men with a higher sex drive will only want to have sex with partners whose sex they prefer in the first place. Having a higher sex drive does not make it more likely that a man will be bisexual.

While straight women who have a higher sex drive are more likely to want sex with both men and women, gay women who have a higher sex drive follow a pattern that is more similar to men: they only want sex with partners of their preferred sex, which is women.

Sperm-Drinking Males and The Influences of Culture

A number of years ago, an anthropologist discovered people on a remote island who believed that in order to become real men, male adolescents needed to drink the sperm of the adult males in the tribe.

Given how the adult males didn't exactly have sperm spigots that could be turned on and off without sexual arousal, the way the young boys harvested the sperm was by giving the older men blowjobs.

Unfortunately, people in the modern world who read these studies assumed that the sperm-drinking adolescents were sexually aroused by giving the older men blowjobs, and that this was an indication that we all are bisexual in nature and learn to hide that part of ourselves due the influence of culture. But the reality is, the sperm drinking young men probably viewed blowing their elders as an anticipated experience like a teenager today looks at having to take a driving test or or a college entrance exam. Taking and passing the test means you achieve a certain level of independence, not that you want to keep taking the test again and again.

A few decades after the initial research, an anthropologist returned to the island to see what was up with the off-spring of the sperm-drinking tribe. Time had done a number on the people of the island. Many of its members had moved to a more urban part of the island, and Christian missionaries had also helped put the kibosh on any ideas that swallowing sperm confers magical properties. (The women who read this book could have told them that!)

The teenage grandsons of the sperm-drinking granddads were wearing wrap-around sun glasses and listening to iPods in front of the island's equivalent of a 7-11 store. Satellite dishes meant that this was the first generation of the island's natives who had grown up under the influence of Netflix and YouTube.

When the researcher inquired about rites of manhood and what the boys needed to do to be regarded as manly, they wondered if he was talking about doing extreme skateboard tricks. He eventually broached the subject of the sperm-drinking to some of the boys, who became very grossed out and said, "My granddad did what?"

Homophobia in the Homeland

Let's take a look at a study on homophobia that was done at the University of Georgia. The University of Georgia is one of the finer institutions of higher learning, and not simply because they have used the *Guide to Getting It On!* in their sex-education classes, although it does speak well of them.

Psychologists gave a questionnaire about homosexuality to a group of sixty-four men. Based upon their responses, the men were divided into two subgroups: those who were homophobic and those who were not. The testers then showed the subjects hardcore X-rated videos of men having sex with women, and men having sex with men. They did this after placing sensors on the guys' penises to see if they were having a penis response while watching the different videos.

When watching the tapes of gay men, 80% of the homophobic men had penile arousal, while only 34% percent of the non-homophobic men did. Yet almost all of the homophobic men denied feeling aroused while watching gay guys having sex.

Unfortunately, the penis does not always tell the truth, and studies using genital sensors can raise as many questions as they answer. It's possible that anxiety or anger caused the homophobic men's penises to change size enough to be confused with a sexual response. Also, keep in mind that men who are truly homophobic don't care how they got to be that way. If they are viscerally enraged, one needs to assume they are dangerous. They might believe that their very existence is being threatened by the mere presence of a gay guy.

Happy Trails

This might be a good time to return to something that researcher Richard Lippa wanted you to know:

> There is no good or bad when it comes to sexual orientation. You are who you are. Sexual identity and sexual orientation may not be fully fixed in young people, and this may be particularly true for women. Whatever your sexual orientation is and whatever gender (or genders) you're attracted to, learn to accept yourself and enjoy your sexual feelings. Sex is always a process, but not necessarily a fixed process. So learn to go with the flow—in particular, learn to go with your flow—but do so in a safe, sane, and sensible way."

A Special Thanks to Richard Lippa of California State University at Fullerton, to J. Michael Bailey of Northwestern University, to Ralph Bolton of Claremont College, to Ritch Savin-Williams of Cornell, to Meredith Chivers of Queen's University, to Adam Safron of Northwestern University, and to members of the SexNet listserve for their generous help.

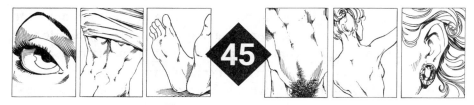

Premature Ejaculation
When Your Penis Has ADHD

It's easy to understand why most men would be too embarrassed to call a healthcare provider about premature ejaculation. The receptionist always asks why you want to see the doctor. "Uh, 'cause I come in about three seconds?" Worse yet, most healthcare providers know more about the rings of Uranus than they do about premature ejaculation. That's why this chapter is kept as up-to-date as possible, and why some of the world's top researchers are consulted. Perhaps you and your doctor can learn together.

Terms like premature ejaculation, PE, early ejaculation, and rapid ejaculation are used interchangeably, but they all mean the same thing. You would think it would be easy to define premature ejaculation, but it was only recently that researchers and clinicians finally agreed on a working definition. Even then, their definition is more limiting than many would have wanted. You'll see why in the pages that follow. You'll also see that there are many myths and misperceptions about PE.

This chapter begins with a look at what PE is and ends with the treatments that are currently being used. One of the biggest problems with premature ejaculation is that a man's partner is seldom part of the conversation or the solution. That's not good. This chapter is for sexual partners as well as for men with PE. Hopefully you'll both read it and discuss the sections that are meaningful for you. There's no reason why PE needs to ruin your enjoyment of sex.

ISSM on Jizzing

According to the International Society for Sexual Medicine (ISSM), premature ejaculation is when a man usually comes in less than a minute and has little if any control over it, and he feels distress as a result.

Depending on whose statistics you use, almost 98% of men are able to last for more than a minute. This leaves between 1.5% and 2.5% of men who qualify as having PE. But if you add another thirty seconds to the ISSM definition by including men who come in less than a minute and a half, up to five times as many men have premature ejaculation, as long as they feel a lack of control and it's causing them distress.

The reason ISSM has taken such a conservative approach is that it wanted to limit its definition to what is truly known and can be validated with research. Otherwise, there is a chance PE would not be accepted as a legitimate diagnosis in the medical world. Treatment would not be reimbursable and drug companies might stop their research. Unfortunately, using only a minute as a definition of PE allows drugs that don't work very well to appear to be more effective than they are.

The Problem with "What's Average"

In a study of nearly 500 couples from five countries who timed their intercourse, the lion's share of the men lasted between two and nine minutes. Few men lasted longer than eighteen minutes and half of the men lasted for less than six minutes. Condom use and circumcision did not have an impact one way or the other.

The men over-estimated the amount of time it took them to come by an average of 31% or almost two minutes. So guys who came in six minutes thought they lasted for close eight. There is also more variation in how long each individual male lasts than was previously thought.

A lot of PE researchers don't think it's relevant to list an average time for intercourse. That's because there are men who last for a minute and who satisfy their lovers with all the things they do rather than just intercourse. And there are plenty of men who can last for ten or more minutes and aren't satisfying lovers.

Researchers would want you to remember there's way more to being a good lover than how long you last. Consider this book: only one chapter is on intercourse. That should tell you there is way more to satisfying sex than when a penis is in a vagina.

Parallel Parking and Premature Ejaculation

Another problem with defining premature ejaculation based on the clock alone is that it doesn't speak to the speed and intensity of the thrusting. Some of the men who were part of a huge study said they are able to last more than a minute but that they ejaculated within ten thrusts or less. That works out to about six seconds per thrust. ("One Mississippi, two Mississippi, Three Mississippi, Four Mississippi, Five Mississippi, Six Mississippi" for each thrust.) This would be like having intercourse in slow motion, which is what some men do in order to last longer. Also, some men think about dead animals or when they dropped the winning touchdown pass in a championship game in order to last longer. This makes sex less fun for themselves and their partners.

Most men who don't have PE are able to get control by stopping for a bit or pulling out and changing positions. They don't have to slap a governor on their sexual excitement from start to finish. Doing so is one of the burdens of having PE. Female partners will often keep their hips still and mute their excitement in an attempt to help a partner with PE to last longer. They throttle down their sexual excitement, which results in their being less satisfied.

The Grim Reaper of Sexual Fun

For most men who come in less than a minute, premature ejaculation feels like a joke their body is playing on itself. Their penis feels like it's had hundreds of thrusts before their partner barely has her panties off. As much as they would love to have intercourse, they start to dread it because they feel like losers who can't please their partners.

Some women feel that premature ejaculation is "his problem" and their partner is the one who needs to fix it. However, a man with PE can no more will himself to delay coming than he can will world peace.

Erections don't fare well in an environment of dread. So a lot of guys with PE not only worry about coming too soon, they also worry about not being able to get it up or keep it up once they do. Their orgasms are not always as enjoyable as for men who have better control. There are plenty of men with PE who fear new relationships or avoid them rather than having to face the embarrassment of PE.

Is Premature Ejaculation Inherited?

According to the latest research, there seems to be a genetic influence that impacts some men who have PE. So it is possible that a man with premature ejaculation may have more in common with his father and brothers than meets the eye. Or maybe not.

While genetics might be a factor in PE, there is not a specific gene for premature ejaculation. To quote one researcher, "PE is influenced by many things, most of which are not understood. The genetic influence on PE is likely to be indirect." This means the genes that effect PE probably influence other things first, such as your mood, appetite, emotions, and temperament. These may or may not have an effect on your ability to control your ejaculation. So it's a long and winding trail from what's happening in your genes to what's happening in your jeans. Saying that genetics can influence whether you have PE simply means the chances are greater that you will come sooner than someone without that particular gene configuration. Beyond that, we do not have enough knowledge about PE to be more specific.

If you are the partner of a man with PE, it's best to leave the genetic research to the geneticists. Do not succumb to the temptation of asking your lover's mother, "Mrs. Snappy, does your husband come as quickly as your son?" But in case you do, be sure to let us know what she says.

El Prematuro Loco

There are a number of men who are sure they have PE when they don't. The majority of the men who describe themselves as having premature ejaculation do not have anything close. When a man assumes he has PE but doesn't, we say he is *El Prematuro Loco.*

Someone with a real case of premature ejaculation can hardly last a minute. But a man with *El Prematuro Loco* can go for several minutes during intercourse while thrusting at a satisfying clip for both he and his partner. He is within the range of average, sometimes at the high end of average. Being able to last that long would make a man who really does have premature ejaculation smile from ear to ear.

Education, reassurance, and sometimes counseling is enough to help a man with *El Prematuro Loco* stop focusing on what he perceives to be his short-comings, and to work instead on finding ways to give his partner extra pleasure besides just thrusting. So if you are a man who feels he has premature ejaculation but doesn't really, why not start talking to your partner about your concerns? It could be she wants something different in bed than for you to last longer.

If she does want you to last longer, some of the retraining techniques mentioned later in this chapter might help. If you can already last for a few minutes, you've got a lot more room to teach yourself to improve your hang time than a guy who lasts for 30 seconds. You might not have to be fighting your body's genetics, neurology or psychology in order to last longer.

Also, a reality check is in order for today's porn-inspired couple who assumes that every guy can thrust like a robot. The vast majority of men in porn take nearly toxic doses of boner drugs, and they wouldn't be in porn if they didn't have excellent control to begin with.

Control Issues

Surveys have shown that 50% of men feel they can control when they ejaculate during intercourse. Being able to control when you come is beyond the comprehension of a man who has premature ejaculation. Unfortunately, research also shows that partners of men with PE often believe that a man can control it if he tries. For most men with PE, this is not possible.

While some women blame themselves when a partner has erection problems, they tend to blame their lover for PE. Couples would have way more fun if they learned to have sex that's based less on what a man can do with his penis. Making it safe for your partner to act out some of her sex fantasies with you would make you a better lover than most.

Lifelong vs. Acquired — How Psychology Can Impact Biology

Most men who have PE have had it in varying degrees from the time of their first intercourse. This is known as lifelong premature ejaculation. However, there are some men who had decent control until the PE Fairy waved a wand of quickness over their penis. So if you were okay to begin with and then start to ejaculate rapidly, you might have "acquired PE."

Consider the case of Bill, who is a construction worker and who scheduled an appointment with a urologist to deal with his premature ejaculation. Bill rarely had trouble with his ejaculation until recently.

If Bill's urologist had been too busy to ask about Bill's relationships, he would have missed that Bill recently started dating Jenni who is a corporate CEO. She is high-powered and white-collar, while Bill carries a hammer and is blue-collar. Bill has felt inadequate from the start with Jenni, given that she's drop-dead gorgeous and makes about ten times as much money as he does. Bill's premature ejaculation started soon after he began dating Jenni.

Bill got his PE along the way as opposed to always having struggled with it. What Bill needed were some sessions with a therapist to help him deal with his conflicted feelings about being in a relationship with Jenni. (Thanks to sex therapist Stan Althof for providing this example.)

Possible Risk Factors

If you have recently started to ejaculate rapidly and no earthshaking life changes have occurred that might explain it, such as finding your wife in bed with the teenager who mows your lawn, then it is a good idea to have a complete physical exam.

Before assuming PE has a physical cause, be aware there has been little evidence to support a medical or psychological cause of premature ejaculation. As of press time, the best that can be said is more and better studies need to be done.

To date, one study found that between 50% and 70% of men with a hyperthyroid have PE. After receiving successful treatment for their thyroid problem, the rate of PE dropped from 50% to 15%. On the other hand, there was not a single case of hyperthyroidism in a study of 620 men who have lifelong PE. So while any man with acquired PE should get his thyroid checked, it's unlikely that thyroid is the cause of PE in a man who's always had premature ejaculation.

There are some indications that prostate infections might be a cause of PE. The trouble with these studies is they aren't particularly sound from a scientific point of view. Prostate infections are something to be aware of regarding PE, especially PE that is acquired, but that's about it.

There is a high association between premature ejaculation and erectile dysfunction in men who have diabetes, and a moderate association between PE and erectile dysfunction in general. In these cases, trying one of the boner drugs like Viagra is something to consider.

Early ejaculation has been reported as a side effect of withdrawal from SSRI antidepressants. Some recreational drugs might also contribute to premature ejaculation.

Aside from genetic influences, one study suggests that a short frenulum could help trigger PE in men who have lifelong premature ejaculation. Theoretically, having a shorter frenulum could cause excessive tension in the area of the glans corona, which is one of the most sensitive and nerve-filled parts of the penis. However, controlled studies need to be done regarding the short-frenulum theory before any credence is given to it.

In time, it's possible that physical causes of PE will be discovered. Currently, the data is limited and sometimes contradictory.

Your First Time vs Youthful Exuberance

In a recent study in Finland, a lot of men who don't have PE reported ejaculating in under a minute the first time they had intercourse. Many of these men ejaculated before their penis got its first feel of their partner's vagina. But they've had normal ejaculation times ever since. So there's a big difference between mastering the anxiety and inexperience of your first couple of times and coming quickly for the rest of your life.

In most men with PE, ejaculation control doesn't improve with age. And in many cases, premature ejaculation gets worse as relationships get longer. That wouldn't be the case if time and experience were the cure for premature ejaculation.

A Reality Check with Your Partner

Women often assume their male partners are not concerned about having PE when the man himself might be an anxious mess. At the same time, there is often a major disconnect between what a man thinks his partner wants and what she really wants.

So if either of you is concerned about PE, the first thing to do is to talk about it together. She might prefer that you spend more time kissing, caressing, or giving her oral sex. Maybe she wants you to be more of a take-charge kind of guy when it comes to sex. Or she might want you to last longer, but hasn't let you know because she's been afraid of hurting your feelings. Either way, talking it over is an important step when one or both of you is concerned about premature ejaculation.

Myths To Fry

In trying to understand more about PE, it is helpful to look at what people used to believe caused it. Some sex educators and therapists still adhere to these myths:

Goat Gonads! Premature ejaculation was first described in medical literature in the late 1800s. That's when PE, impotence, and just about everything that could possibly go wrong with a man was blamed on masturbation or "self-pollution." Even having intercourse more than once a week was a concern among the anti-ejaculation fanatics of the day. To help revitalize and rejuvenate the body, more than a thousand men were given testicular grafts from sheep, monkeys, goats, deer, and other men.

Vasectomies to Prevent the Spilling Seed: In the late 1800s and early 1900s, there was so much concern about losing semen that men would get vasectomies to keep their sperm inside their bodies. That's how vasectomies originally became popular—not for birth control, but as a way of returning a man's "masculine essence" into his own body. Even Freud got a vasectomy when he was 67, clearly not for birth control.

Being Pissed Off: In the 1920s, a psychoanalyst by the name of Karl Abraham suggested that PE resulted from a man's unconscious anger at women. Rapid ejaculation was a man's way of symbolically peeing inside of his partner's vagina. How charming. We have since discovered that men with PE aren't more angry at women than men without PE.

A Headache in Your Penis: In the early 1940s, another German psychiatrist, Bernard Schapiro, speculated that PE was a psychosomatic illness, like anxiety-related headaches. He said that PE was the result of a man's psychological conflict expressing itself bodily. This, too, is false.

PE from Jerking Off Quickly: In the late 1970s, renowned sex therapists Masters and Johnson changed the premature ejaculation landscape by claiming that PE was a learned experience. They believed PE was something males taught themselves when they rushed their way through masturbation or had rushed sex in a car or did it with a prostitute. We now know that popping out quick ones is not the cause of premature ejaculation. However, it is possible that if a man was born with a shorter fuse to begin with, the rushed experiences he had when he was a teenager could have had more of a lasting impact than if he had been born with a penis that was wired like a porn star's. In this situation, the squeeze-technique that Masters and Johnson suggested might be helpful in extending his hang time (explained in the treatment section of this chapter).

From Zero to Sixty in 2.46 Seconds: In the late 1980s, sex researcher Helen Singer Kaplan proposed that men with PE never developed the ability to experience a gradual buildup of sensation in their penis. Kaplan believed most guys have an early warning system in their penis and are able to say to themselves, "It's starting to feel like I'm getting close—I'll slow down my thrusting or change positions so I can delay coming." But for the man with PE, ejaculation arrives like a sneak attack. He gets no warning signals until it's too late to delay. Kaplan also felt that anxiety fueled PE.

Kaplan's theories held sway for many years, and they shouldn't be quickly dismissed. But when men with PE are given medications that allow them to delay their ejaculation, they can have the same range of sensory awareness in their penis as guys who don't have premature ejaculation. It is also interesting that tramadol and SSRIs, which are drugs that help with anxiety, also help decrease PE. However, it's more likely these drugs delay ejaculation by impacting the centers in the nervous system that trigger ejaculation.

Porn Causes PE: This is one of the most recent and more bizarre theories about the causes of premature ejaculation. If porn were a cause of premature ejaculation, we would have seen a huge increase in the number of men with PE during the past two decades. There has been no such increase. However, if this theory were true, it would be interesting to know if men with DSL come faster than men with dial-up used to!

Research Findings on the Man with a Pronto Penis

When researchers placed sensors on men's penises and showed them sexually exciting materials, they expected the men with PE to have a more rapid sexual response. Yet they weren't able to find any differences between men with PE and those who had good control. Time to erection was about the same.

So the researchers made the situation more like real life. They put "pleasure devices" on the men's penises so the men would feel physical stimulation while they were watching dirty movies. And that's when they found that nearly 60% of premature ejaculators would quickly blow a wad as opposed to only 5% of the men who didn't have a problem with coming too soon. This finding helped give credence to the idea that men with premature ejaculation might be wired to come sooner than men who don't have PE. But it doesn't mean they can't retrain themselves.

Semen Samples

Anxiety about sex with a partner does not appear to be the cause of premature ejaculation. Researchers have had premature ejaculators and controls masturbate in the lab to give semen samples. The men with PE came out of the rest room with their semen in a cup faster than the men who were controls. Given that they were masturbating, anxiety about sex with a partner was not the reason why the men with PE produced their semen samples sooner than men without PE.

Research Findings–Neurology and Heart Rate

When men who don't have PE are having intercourse, their heart rate slows down after their penises get hard, even though they are getting aerobic exercise from thrusting during intercourse. When they are about to ejaculate, their heart rate speeds up again.

But when a man with PE becomes sexually aroused, his heart beat is likely to remain rapid from the moment he gets hard until he ejaculates. His nervous system doesn't shift into the intercourse version of cruise-control. He is on the verge of ejaculating from the get-go. It is possible that by doing the retraining techniques listed later in this chapter, a man with PE can learn to drop his heart rate like one who doesn't have PE.

Erection Issues

You would think that men with PE would get erect sooner than controls. However, the opposite is true for some groups of men with PE. A number of men with PE also have varying degrees of erectile dysfunction. This dovetails with why some men with PE respond well to erection drugs such as Viagra, Cialis, and Levitra. Perhaps these are men whose PE is related to erectile dysfunction. Or maybe their erectile dysfunction is due to their distress about having PE, and the erection drugs help alleviate the fear that they won't be able to get it up.

Some men who don't have PE complain that the boner drugs make their penis feel somewhat wooden. This would be a case of one man's poison being another man's cure.

Even if the erection drugs don't help a man last longer the first time he ejaculates, they do help most men to get a subsequent erection sooner. Most men will be able to thrust longer the second time around.

Emotional Reaction

Men with PE often have more negative feelings about sex than men who have control over their ejaculations. Therapists used to assume it was the negative feelings that were causing the premature ejaculation rather than being a result of it. But the men with PE did not look forward to having intercourse because they believed they were going to disappoint their partner. Many of the negative feelings that men with PE have about sex stop once they are able to get more control over their ejaculations.

Lasting Longer Doesn't Make Partners More Satisfied

The results of a recent FDA trial on a treatment for premature ejaculation trumpeted how it added extra minutes to the men's thrusting times. But in spite of the great results, the men's partners didn't report significant increases in their own sexual satisfaction.

So maybe the problem wasn't as bad as the guys with PE assumed. Or maybe sexual satisfaction is more complex than we think. Sexual problems don't exist in a vacuum. When it comes to sexual intimacy, mutual pleasure can't always be measured with a stopwatch. This takes us back to a central theme throughout this chapter: men with PE are often so focused on their failure that they aren't able to enjoy ways of making sex more fun and rewarding. By the time a man with PE tries the retraining techniques or uses drugs for it, sexual excitement in the relationship might need to be rekindled.

Plenty of men learn to compensate for PE by becoming really good at pleasing a woman with oral sex or different kinds of massage. Some couples act out fun scenarios and kinky fantasies together. There's no reason why coming quickly should get in the way of having great sex.

The Other 97% of Your Body and Mind

It can be helpful for a man with PE to become more aware of the sensations in other parts of his body in addition to his penis. Not enough can be said about allowing a partner to touch you from head to toe while you let your body relax. This kind of non-pressured exploration is often the cornerstone of sex therapy. Some couples enjoy using different materials and fabrics to massage each other from head to toe. Good results can be had with feathers or furry mitts, as well as a silk scarf or piece of rayon. Some couples might be into leather, latex, or rubber. Others find the feel of a partner's fingertips to be exquisite.

The Most Important Ingredients

In helping a man to last longer, don't forget to have a sense of humor. Humor is the sexual lubricant for the soul. The chances are, a man with PE is angry and frustrated with himself. Humor and a tolerance for frustration can go a long way.

None of the treatments on the pages that follow are a cure. However, they can help, and sometimes a great deal. But they do require motivation and a long-term commitment by both partners.

The couple must find ways for the man's partner to get off besides having intercourse. That way she won't feel resentful, he won't feel guilty, and they will both get to experience what it is like when she can open up and no longer needs to mute her excitement. This is one of the first things a couple should work on, as opposed to just focusing on the man's penis.

Relationship Fears & Resistances

Helen Singer Kaplan said that the men who were unable to complete her program for rapid ejaculation usually had wives or girlfriends who did not necessarily want them to last longer. The two men mentioned below were rapid ejaculators as well as contributors to *The Guide.* They were kind enough to share their personal stories for you to read.

Zeus suspected his wife didn't want him to improve his sexual function and that she would resist helping him do something about it. He was right. His wife didn't enjoy sex, or not with him anyway. The faster he came, the better. In addition, she didn't want him having sex with anyone else. She assumed he would be less likely to have extramarital affairs if his problems with PE remained.

Heathcliff had a secret and didn't know if Catherine would want to help. While caring greatly for each other, their sex life had never been a central part of their relationship. After several years, he finally asked for her help with his premature ejaculation. He received an unexpected reply. She told him she often masturbated after he went to sleep, keeping her sexual needs to herself because she didn't think he was interested. They began masturbating together and started feeling sexually intimate for the first time in their lives. They found many ways to please each other sexually. By this time, Heathcliff had become such a changed man that not even his neighbors could recognize him.

Rather than bulldozing ahead with the treatments that are mentioned in this chapter, why not start by having talks about it first? You might want to include a discussion about what it would be like if you were able to make changes in your sex life. Even if you both want changes, each of you might have your own fears and concerns.

Treatments for Premature Ejaculation

The rest of this chapter lists drugs, creams, condoms, and behavioral techniques that are being used to treat PE. Since PE isn't a disease and it doesn't have a specific cause, the best treatment will depend on your biology, psychology, and partner situation. In exploring treatment options, you will need to be flexible and adventurous—two qualities that can be in short supply when you are frustrated with yourself.

A logical treatment to try first would be exercise and the retraining techniques. One version is free, and these methods have no side effects.

Can Exercise Help Decrease PE?

Shortly before this book went to press, one of the top researchers of premature ejaculation published the result of a study where he found that men who exercised less were more likely to have PE symptoms. The researches found a slight connection between alcohol use and PE, and no association between PE and BMI (body mass index) which is a measure of body fat based on height and weight. Obviously, more research is needed.

Teaching an Old Dog New Tricks: The Squeeze Technique

The squeeze technique for premature ejaculation has been around for almost as long as the penis itself. It has had different variations, one being called "the start stop technique." It's goal is to take you to the edge of ejaculation, but not over. This will help your body learn how to be in a high state of arousal without ejaculating.

You would think there would have been dozens of studies investigating the efficacy of this technique; not so. Since the squeeze technique is free, drug companies haven't lined up to fund the research. And

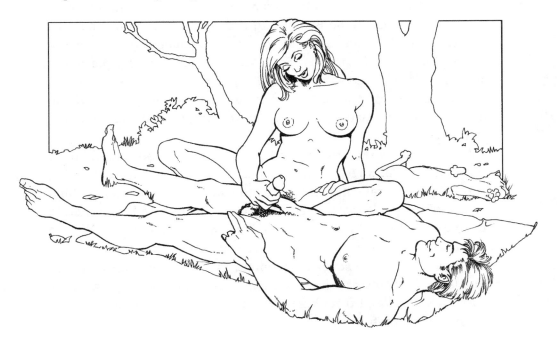

our government rarely chomps at the bit to fund studies on improving sexual pleasure. Two studies that were done on the squeeze technique during the 1980s showed that a number of men had success with it initially, but most of the gains were lost over time. This is not unusual regarding sex. Sex therapists often schedule follow-up appointments for any kind of problem every six months after successful treatment. That's because sexual problems have the tenacity of the cockroach. There can also be a placebo effect with any kind of sexual intervention, which means it works at the start because you believe it will. So don't be surprised if you need to do squeeze-technique refreshers every couple of months. But this should be fun. And think about the benefits if it helps you last longer.

Squeeze-Technique Particulars

You both get naked and kiss and fool around. Then you kiss and fool around some more. At some point, which is totally up to the two of you, the female partner says, "On your back, dude!" She then starts stroking his penis handjob style. While it's usually done without lube, there's nothing that says lube can't be used. See what works best for the two of you.

The man's job is to tell his partner what he's feeling in his penis. As soon as he feels like he is reaching the point of no return, he asks her to stop stroking and that's her cue to start squeezing—right below the head for 10 to 20 seconds. Then, after a minute or so, the man's urge to ejaculate should subside, and his partner can start stroking his penis again. Repeat at least three or four times. When the two of you decide his penis has had a good enough workout, she can stroke him to ejaculation.

After a few weeks of doing it this way, the woman might experiment with switching techniques. Rather than stopping and squeezing when her partner tells her he's about to come, she might try rubbing the head of his penis instead. So she goes from choking his chicken to polishing its helmet. As for erections, don't worry about them. What a man should be focused on is trying to tolerate more sensation.

A variation on the squeeze technique is called *the stop-start technique.* Instead of squeezing when the man is close to coming, his partner removes her hand from his penis. It's totally your call as to which technique you'd prefer to use.

From Squeezing to Intercourse: When the two of you feel you are getting more control over the situation, the woman might try stimulating the penis with her lips instead of her fingers, or by sitting on top of the man and rubbing his penis with her genitals. This is called femoral intercourse. It is where the shaft of the penis glides through the labia like a hot dog in a bun. The penis doesn't go into the vagina. The woman can lift her pelvis up when her partner is close to coming.

After another week or two, she might try putting the man's penis inside of her vagina while she is on top. Try keeping it there for a few minutes without thrusting very much. This helps the man get used to the warm sensations, and there's nothing that says she can't be caressing her clitoris or breasts while his penis is inside her vagina.

The Point of No Return: When doing the squeeze technique, it is helpful to recognize when a man is approaching the Point of No Return. This is when nothing short of stepping on a land mine will keep him from ejaculating. Signs that ejaculation is eminent include: the veins in his penis start to bulge, his penis gives a sudden throb, the color of the head darkens, his testicles suck up into his groin, his muscles start to tighten, his hips thrust, and he starts to groan or invokes the name of various deities. Appreciate how well you are doing if the man can stay close to the point of no return for several minutes without going over the edge.

Also, it helps if the couple can cut themselves plenty of slack. There will be times when a guy reaches the point of no return before his partner can squeeze or pause. It's no big deal. Doing the squeeze technique should be fun, and occasionally funny. It's not a competition.

Before Squeezing, Stop Apologizing and Thinking about Other Things

Some of the most annoying aspects of premature ejaculation that women report are the constant apologies and self-criticism that men express after coming too soon. This puts their partners off. If you decide to work on these exercises together, the man needs to promise he will no longer apologize or berate himself for coming too soon.

Men with PE will also try to delay ejaculation by thinking about something unsexy, which would be like a race-car driver thinking about golf when he's entering a high-speed turn. To think about something besides pleasure is not a good way to last longer. It could lead to erection problems, so you'll then have ED and will still come too soon. As you are doing these exercises, let yourself feel totally turned on.

Pelvic Floor Exercises

Researchers from the University of Rome recently published a study titled *Pelvic floor muscle rehabilitation for patients with lifelong premature ejaculation: A novel therapeutic approach.* You are encouraged to do a browser search and read the study. This study seems to demonstrate that a number of men with serious lifelong PE can be helped without drugs.

Promescent—A Delay Spray

Sprays and creams for PE that help numb a penis have been around for decades. All of these sprays and creams contain similar numbing agents, such as lidocaine, prilocaine and benzocaine. The problem has been with the delivery system. Most of the numbing agent molecules have remained evenly distributed throughout the creams they are mixed in and do not make contact with the skin. As a result, they are not quickly absorbed and the man has to wear a condom to keep the numbing cream from touching his partner's clitoris. The creams also have a tendency to numb out the penis.

Drug companies have spent millions of dollars trying to create a delivery system for the numbing agents that allow just enough of the molecules to get to the skin of the penis where they can be rapidly absorbed without leaving a residue that will numb a partner's genitals. The well-funded company that invented Promescent believes they have succeeded. They also believe that Promescent will not numb out a man's penis if he begins to have intercourse within five minutes of application.

Promescent is a cousin of a product called SD502 that is used for pain relief for burn victims, although not necessarily burn victims with premature ejaculation. Promescent is not a cure for premature ejaculation, but something a man can use five minutes before intercourse. Promescent is anything but cheap, but it doesn't require a prescription and there appear to be no side effects.

NOTE: When this spray was in Phase II clinical trials, it seemed like the researchers were having to move heaven and earth to squeeze significance out of the results. However, Phase III trial results looked more promising. The proof will be in the ejaculating.

A concern with this cream and the company that makes it is the degree of hype and the huge amount of marketing dollars that are being spent. If you are looking for a delaying cream or spray, this is probably the one to try. But you might do just as well with the squeeze technique, or perhaps a combination of the two.

Trojan Extended Pleasure and Durex Performax Condoms

These condoms have benzocaine gel on the inside to desensitize or numb out the penis. It is fascinating to read user reviews. They tend to either be 5 stars or 1 star, with guys and their partners either loving them or hating them. The biggest complaint is that these condoms numb out the penis so much that some men lose all sensation, and their erection as well. The biggest praise is that they numb out the penis enough so a man can last longer than he normally does.

Men who have tried both brands tend to prefer one or the other. So you might try both and see if one works better for you. Do not put these condoms on too soon before intercourse. Otherwise, your penis could feel like your gums after getting novocaine at the dentist's office. Do read the instructions, and be careful not to get the gel from the inside of the condom on a woman's genitals. Also, as a woman with a numb mouth flamed on a user forum: "Do not give a blow job after a man takes one of these bad boys off!"

Treatments –The Drugs

Most of the drugs that are now used for PE were not designed for PE, just like Viagra was not designed for ED. The ejaculation-delaying properties of drugs like tramadol and SSRI antidepressants were first discovered as unwanted side effects. Most of these drugs have not yet been approved for treating PE and may never be approved for it. *They do not necessarily work well and all have side effects.* Also, many of the researchers who are doing studies on these drugs consult for the drug companies that make them and receive compensation for doing so.

The Ugly Side of Progress

More and more research is being done on premature ejaculation, especially since the drug companies realize they would have a pharmaceutical gold mine on their hands if they could come up with a pill that helps men last longer without putting them to sleep, zapping their sex drives, or making their penises feel like lead pipes. The problem will be in how drug companies will market the PE drugs. They'll try to convince young men that their sexual self-esteem will rise exponentially if they take the new intimacy-enhancing pills. Soon enough, men who last "only" six minutes—which is close to the amount of time that half of all men last during intercourse—will assume they have premature ejaculation and will want to take the new drug. So while there will be a definite upside to a medication that works for men who truly have PE, there may also be an ugly underbelly.

Treatments—Pills

As of press time, most pills used as treatments for premature ejaculation are not approved for that purpose. Using them would be off-label and the wisdom of doing so is between you and your healthcare provider. The following summaries are for information only and might not reflect the latest research which you are encouraged to keep up on.

Also, all of the medications mentioned have side effects which could be negligible for some men, but truly bothersome for others. The possible side effects include dry mouth, nausea, headaches, weight gain, insomnia, erectile dysfunction, low sex drive, the occasional suicide attempt, drug addiction, fertility problems and liver damage.

Up to 90% of men who start taking drugs for PE discontinue them because they don't work as well as promised or because of the side effects. If the pills alone don't help you last longer, some physicians suggest combining them with the squeeze technique or layering them, such as using an SSRI with a boner drug, or a boner drug with a delaying spray. There are currently only a few studies to guide us on combining medications for PE, and when studies are paid for by the manufacturers of the drugs, we have no idea if the results are truly valid.

SSRI Antidepressants (brand names include Paxil, Prozac, and Zoloft): A common side effect for SSRI antidepressants is delayed ejaculation. The delay in ejaculation can be so significant for a man who doesn't have PE, that taking SSRI antidepressants can make him feel like he's wearing a dozen condoms. This is why SSRIs could be just what the doctor ordered for men with premature ejaculation if it weren't for the other side effects. There are some SSRIs that delay ejaculation more than others, but the additional side effects can be problematic. The front line SSRI that one sexual medicine expert prescribes is Zoloft (generic name is sertraline). He says there are other SSRIs that might be better for PE, but he finds Zoloft is better tolerated. He also likes the fact that Zoloft has a generic version that doesn't cost his patients as much.

Keep in mind that SSRIs can cause ED and kill your libido. They can cause headaches, nausea, drowsiness, weight gain, and other physical and mental nastiness. They may cause an increased risk of suicide in young men. Also, some men with PE who find early success with SSRIs report their PE returns after several months. Do not even think of taking SSRI antidepressants for premature ejaculation if you are bipolar.

Dapoxetine (Priligy): Some researchers assumed that a fast-acting SSRI with a short half-life would be a good on-demand solution for premature ejaculation. While one SSRI by the name of dapoxetine (Priligy) has been approved in other countries for on-demand treatment for PE, our own FDA was not particularly impressed. Up to 90% of men who are given this drug for PE stop using it before the end of a year. This should say volumes about the side effects vs. the lack of efficacy.

Silodosin: A group of researchers has reported that on demand use of a drug called silodosin 4 mg which is taken three hours before intercourse has fewer side effects than dapoxetine and results in a decent delay in ejaculation. Way more research is needed, but you might keep an eye out for this regimen.

Boner Drugs (brand names are Viagra, Levitra, Cialis, and Stendra): Can erection drugs help men with PE? Yes and no. A number of men with PE have erection-related problems. But are the erection problems causing premature ejaculation, or does PE cause men so much distress that they end up having erectile dysfunction? Research to date has not found that Viagra helps men with PE to last significantly longer, but the men reported increased confidence, a greater perception of control, and more overall sexual satisfaction. There might be two reasons for this: Viagra may have resulted in more reliable erections, which would be a big relief. Viagra also helps men with PE to get it up more quickly after coming the first time. Most man with PE can last longer the second time if they can get it up again. (Research by the Levitra people found Levitra to be helpful for PE as well.)

If you and your healthcare provider decide to give the boner drugs a try, it's best to get samples and try each one. You might find one works better for you than the others. Consider using erection drugs with a delaying spray or in conjunction one of the retraining techniques.

Clomipramine (brand name is Anafranil): This is a tricyclic antidepressant that has been used for a long time to help people with obsessive compulsive disorders. One of the side effects is that it delays ejaculation, which is why they started to use it for men with PE. A 25-mg dose taken 4 to 24 hours before intercourse is sometimes recommended. This can be raised to 50 mg, but with that can come increased side effects. A study was done in which a 10-30 mg dose was given on a long-term basis with satisfactory results.

As with SSRI antidepressants, be sure to understand the side effects, as there could be an increased risk for suicide among young men, although it's not known if that would be the case for young men who are taking it for PE and who are using it on demand as opposed to daily. Do not take this if you are bipolar or have erection problems.

Tramadol (brand name is Ultram): This is a centrally-acting opioid analgesic that appears to have few side effects at the low doses being used to treat PE. The doses of Tramadol used in PE studies are between 25 mg and 89 mg (the drug is approved for 400 mgs a day).

There is conflicting and limited research with an on-demand dose of 50 mg of Tramadol for PE. In one study that may not have had the best methodology, men who could only last for 19 seconds started lasting four minutes. Men who took 25-mg dose and who normally ejaculated in a minute went for more than six minutes. This drug is optimally taken two hours before intercourse.

While some studies have found Tramadol to be effective for premature ejaculation, another study comparing the on-demand use of Tramadol for PE with daily use of the SSRI antidepressant paroxetine (Paxil) found paroxetine shredding Tramadol when it came to delaying ejaculation at 12 weeks. The authors of the Paxil study also say that Tramadol had a negative effect on erections, while Paxil had a positive effect. In responding to the Paxil results, the lead researcher in one of the tramadol studies insists that Tramadol humbles Paxil as a drug for PE and claims his team never saw erection problems with men in their Tramadol studies. Plus, it's hard to find ED listed as a side effect for men taking 400 mg a day of Tramadol, let alone only 50 mgs every couple of days. Also, if you are considering Paxil for PE, keep in mind it can have wicked side effects.

Unfortunately, little is known about the effectiveness of Tramadol on PE after being used for extended periods of time. Tramadol is one of the only opioid drugs that is not a controlled substance in many parts of the world. It has been around since the late 1970s and is even sold over-the-counter in some countries. However, in 2010 the FDA listed new side effect warnings for Tramadol, and it is unlikely Tramadol will ever be approved as a PE drug because it is an opioid. Mind you, it is commonly prescribed for backaches in much higher doses.

WARNING — Tramadol has become a highly abused drug worldwide. Some clinicians do not feel it is worth the risk of giving young men prescriptions for Tramadol due to its potential for abuse as a recreational drug. While the dose used for PE is a fraction of that which is needed to get a pain-killing effect, this is an important warning and should be taken very seriously. Tramadol can be a bear of a drug to get off of if you become addicted. Clearly, more research is needed to guide us on the wisdom of using Tramadol for PE.

Treatments—Penis Injections (Do Not Use These for PE!)

Penis injections can be helpful for men with erectile dysfunction who don't respond to the usual array of boner drugs. However, unscrupulous healthcare providers have been advertising the use of these injections for premature ejaculation. The *Journal of Sexual Medicine* has strongly warned against using penis injections for PE. Long-term penis damage can result.

Drug Precautions

Be sure to look up the side effects of any drug you are taking. As new drugs for PE enter the pipeline, posts will be done on them at www.Guide2Getting.com. Enter the letters "PE" in the search box.

A Special Thanks to: Patrick Jern of the Åbo Akademi University in Finland and the Sahlgrenska Academy in Sweden; New York City psychiatrist and sex therapist Stephen Snyder; Jason Feifer, an editor at Men's Health, Donald Strassberg of the University of Utah; David Rowland of Valparaiso University; Marcel D. Waldinger of University of Utrecht; Joseph Marzucco, urology specialist; Stan Althof of the Center for Marital and Sexual Health in South Florida; and Michael Metz, co-author with Barry McCarthy of *Coping With Premature Ejaculation*. Michael Metz has left us. Michael, may you rest each night in emerald meadows surrounded by smiling naked women.

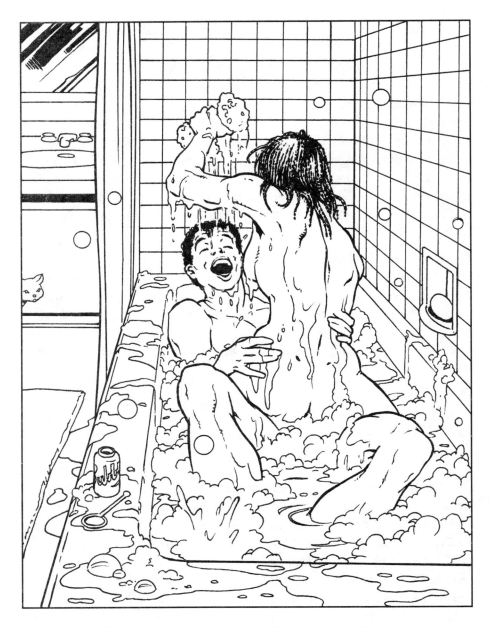

*There's way more to a relationship than if you
ejaculate too soon or too late.*

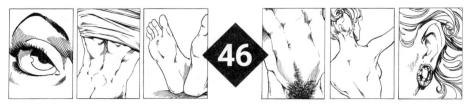

Delayed Ejaculation

Delayed ejaculation is when a guy can get a rock-hard erection and have intercourse for a really long time, but can't ejaculate or he struggles to ejaculate. It doesn't matter if he's having oral, vaginal, or anal sex, or if his partner is giving him a handjob — either he can't ejaculate or it can take him close to forever. Or maybe he can come by masturbating in a certain way, but not with a partner. The problem is not in getting an erection and keeping an erection; rather it's with orgasm and ejaculation.

For those of you who have delayed ejaculation or are dealing with it in your relationship, be aware that very little research has been done on this subject and virtually none of it is the double-blind kind that you can take to the bank. Delayed ejaculation (DE) is poorly understood. No one has come up with a universal set of causes, physical or emotional.

There appear to be two different types of delayed ejaculation: the primary type, where a man has always had it, and the secondary type, where he was okay and then it starts to occur. If you have the secondary type, be sure to rule out physical causes such as diabetes, multiple sclerosis, pelvic surgery, dystonia, spinal cord injuries, or a tumor. Fortunately, these are rare causes of delayed ejaculation. Side effects from medications are more likely to be the culprits behind secondary DE.

Delayed Ejaculation: A Partner Speaks

A sex educator who uses *The Guide* in her college course has been married for more than thirty years to a man who has delayed ejaculation. She offered to write this section for partners of men with DE. What she says is more helpful than much of what's been written on the subject to date. Here goes:

> I've been married to a man for 31 years who has never been able to ejaculate with me in the ordinary way. I married him knowing this was true, but thought we would be able to solve the problem. I didn't know that delayed ejaculation is the most difficult of the

sexual problems to solve, even more difficult than desire discrepancy.

Early in our relationship, I looked this up in a book on sexual problems by Masters and Johnson who were famous sex researchers. I discovered that they had only worked with a handful of men with this problem; mostly couples who were worried about whether the women could become pregnant. They used the technique of the man masturbating to the "point of no return" and then the woman would get on top and the man would ejaculate inside her. If the couple was able to do this, then this was considered a successful outcome.

We were able to do this and have two beautiful daughters who are now grown. However, that did not feel like a success to me and my husband was not really interested in doing this for recreational sex. We have explored a lot of sex therapy and psychotherapy, individually and together trying to come to terms with this.

As Paul describes in this chapter, my husband has a style of masturbation that is very hard to duplicate with my hand, let alone with my vagina. It is very, very fast and very hard. He has had some success changing his masturbation style, but because it is difficult for him to orgasm. Even when masturbating, it is hard for him to want to change his style. Because of this, I have never been able to bring him to orgasm in any way, orally, anally, vaginally or manually.

Overall, I think my husband has come to see this as normal for him; he has never been any different with any other partner. I have had to accept that this sexual style is not something that he really wants to spend a lot more time or energy worrying about. After all these years, we still like to be sexual together, and I count my blessings. He really likes intercourse and has no problem with erections. Unfortunately, I am one of those women who don't come with vaginal stimulation only, so I don't get the benefit of having a partner with this problem that some women do.

Here are some things I've learned that might help the partner married to someone with DE:

👓 DON'T TAKE IT PERSONALLY. IT IS NOT ABOUT YOU! I am a skilled and experienced lover and have never thought that my vagina wasn't tight enough or I wasn't sexy enough to please him. Also, he had this problem with all previous lovers.

👓 Don't decide it is a sickness or a pathology. In one of the articles that Paul mentions, the author talks about a bell curve of sexual responsiveness on which men and women naturally fall. Some men and women orgasm extremely easily and some orgasm with a lot of difficulty. Most are somewhere in between. Rather than thinking there is something wrong with your partner, try to think of DE as something he is born with, like dark hair or intelligence or needing glasses.

👓 Don't marry him if you need him to change. It may be impossible and it's better to go into it knowing that.

👓 Use your sexuality as an opportunity to develop greater intimacy. Talk to each other, use the ideas that are in this book, improve communication, have fun. Focus on loving your partner and feeling emotionally connected and physically close.

👓 Don't fall into the trap of "goal-oriented" sex instead of "pleasure-oriented sex". Goal oriented sex says that all good sex ends with orgasm. Pleasure-oriented sex says that any sexual behaviors that feel good count as sex.

👓 Count your blessings and enjoy the fact that you will never be able to do "cookie cutter sex". Use it as a way to rebel against the Hollywood myth of perfect sex and keep it creative and fun.

👓 Don't tell too many friends about this. They will never have heard of it and will think it is really weird and will make you feel worse, most likely.

Looking Under the Hood of Delayed Ejaculation

Delayed ejaculation used to be known as retarded ejaculation, until we decided that calling a man a "retarded ejaculator" was a bit harsh. Some people refer to it as inhibited ejaculation, and those who are trying to sound medical refer to it as a DED, diminished ejaculatory disorder.

How many men have delayed ejaculation? We aren't really sure. The guesses range from 1% to 4%, but even if it were only 0.5%, that's still a lot of guys whose corks won't pop. This condition can present itself differently in different men. It can be intermittent or it can happen every time. It can be lifelong or something that crept up along the way. It can be mild, moderate, severe, or super severe.

If you are stopwatch obsessed and hellbent on quantifying delayed ejaculation, consider that an average guy lasts somewhere between three and eight minutes during intercourse. One researcher has cooked the various standard deviations of how long an average intercourse lasts and suggests if you can't come after 25 to 30 minutes of thrusting, then you probably qualify as having delayed ejaculation. But here's a problem: for some couples, 25 minutes is just getting warmed up, while for others 25 minutes would be a nightmare of excess. So in order to declare a man has delayed ejaculation, both he and his partner need to consider it a problem. There are also situations when a man is able to come after fifteen minutes, but his partner wishes he were done after five. And forget calling it delayed ejaculation if it only happens when a man is using a condom.

What's particularly fascinating about delayed ejaculation is that the majority of men who have it are able to ejaculate when they masturbate. It's when you put a flesh-and-blood partner between the guy's hand and his penis that he usually has the problem. It can get so bad that his intercourse partner is able to figure out the plot lines to her next three novels before he's even close to coming.

As you'll see, there can be numerous factors that contribute to how fast or slow a man comes, from the biology he was born with to how he processes things like excitement and anxiety. While one man with delayed ejaculation might respond to X, Y, or Z, another man might do better with A, B and C, and a third won't respond no matter what. So we'll take a shotgun approach and mention a number of possibilities. Your job is to decide which, if any, apply to your situation.

Delayed Ejaculation vs. Faster Than a Speeding Bullet

Let's start with biology. A man might be pre-disposed to delayed ejaculation if he has a slow stick for a penis that's not as sensitive as most other guys, or if his body is wired in such a way that he needs to reach a higher level of excitement than others before his ejaculation button gets triggered. He can't do any more to change the way he's wired than you can blink your eyes and your Ford will magically turn into a Maserati or your Suburban into a Prius. So let's focus on some of the possible work-arounds you might consider.

And yes, if you suffer from premature ejaculation and come faster than Han Solo in a Millennium Falcon, you might be thinking, "What's the big deal—I'll trade my premature ejaculation for his delayed ejaculation in a heartbeat." But unless you've been there and done that, it's hard to understand just how cumbersome or what a burden on a relationship DE can be. It can make sex hard work for both partners.

Although premature ejaculation and delayed ejaculation are on opposite sides of the spectrum, they both result in the man's ejaculation taking center stage. Instead of his being able to have fun with his partner and sharing pleasure, sex becomes more about his failure to ejaculate when he wishes he would.

Reverse Misogyny

Here's a caution about delayed ejaculation that you won't read elsewhere. Not many years ago we used to say that a woman who couldn't have an orgasm from intercourse was "frigid." We would give her a medical diagnosis as if she had a disease. While "frigid" is nicer than "retarded" as in retarded ejaculation, we now consider ourselves more enlightened. We tell people today that a lot of women can't have orgasms during intercourse and it's completely normal if they have their orgasms from masturbation. In other words, we've tried to make the female orgasm something a woman is allowed to have by her own hand, rather than it being an experience she needs to put on parade during intercourse.

We are neither as kind nor as generous with men. If a man can only come from masturbation but not intercourse, we call him a retarded ejaculator. He feels horrible about himself, and his partner is sure it's because he doesn't find her sexually appealing. Or she thinks it's because she can't do anything good for him in a sexual way. So sex can become a source of dread and anxiety for both partners.

If you are a man or a couple with this problem, why not at least try to remember that there are plenty of ways you can enjoy intercourse and sexual intimacy without needing an ejaculation to signal that you are crossing the lovemaking finish line. What if you agree on a signal your partner can give during intercourse for when she or he is satisfied and wants to stop? This takes the pressure off of both of you.

Women have used a "Let's stop having intercourse" signal since the beginning of time. It's called faking an orgasm. If men could do that as easily, few people would know there was such a thing as DE.

Beyond the Basic Symptom

Let's look at some of the possible causes and treatments of delayed ejaculation with an emphasis on the word "possible." That's because much of the current information is based on anecdote, which means if it is real science, it's only real science by accident. Please keep in mind that what follows is strictly for informational purposes. This is not meant to take the place of a meeting with your healthcare provider, although few healthcare providers will have a clue on how to deal with delayed ejaculation.

It's important to be sensitive about both sexual partners. A couple's chemistry, ability to talk it over, and willingness to deal with the matter are critical if they hope to make progress. And if a man tends to be the passive partner, helping him deal with his delayed ejaculation will require that he step out of his comfort zone.

Patience, Prudence, Drug Side Effects and More

If you're the kind who's looking for a magic pill, it's unlikely the ejaculation gods will be blowing many sticky kisses your way. If you want it to be like TV talk shows where patients solve massive problems in the span of two commercials, forget it. And good luck if your goal is to be like porn stars—where the male actors are human thrust-and-come machines who have no emotions. (Actually, some sex therapists believe a lot of male porn stars suffer from delayed ejaculation; they've just managed to make a career out of it.)

Speaking of magic pills, you want to rule out the possibility that the ejaculation problem is a side effect of drugs or medications you are taking, anti-depressants are at the top of a list of possible causes that includes antipsychotic medications, methadone, heroin, opiates, other analgesics, tranquilizers, sedatives, medications to lower your blood pressure, muscle relaxers, pregabalin, gapapentin, benzos, GHB, poppers, marijuana, cocaine, alcohol, and possibly cigarette smoking. But don't assume that prescription drugs will include delayed ejaculation as a possible side effect on their warning labels. There are medications that don't list heart attacks as a possible side effect when they probably should, so don't expect them to put "delayed ejaculation" on the side of the box even if they truly do cause problems with ejaculation.

If your problem with DE has not been lifelong, try to think back to when it began. Did you start taking any new medications around that time? Also, delayed ejaculation can be secondary to erection problems, or these conditions can occur in tandem. So if you aren't having good erections, see if your healthcare provider can help you with that.

You want to be sure that delayed ejaculation isn't due to neurological problems, multiple sclerosis, spinal-cord injury, diabetes, thyroid issues, prostate-related problems, certain surgeries, or other pelvic unpleasantries. Low testosterone can be a suspect. Most cases of DE aren't caused by drugs or disease, but it's important to rule out these possibilities.

Religion, Abuse, and Other Possible Semen Stoppers

You might explore whether there were any traumatic psycho-social events that occurred around the time when you started coming slower than a slug in Super Glue. Did you come home unexpectedly to find your wife and best friend going at it with her screaming, "I've never come like this with that loser husband of mine!"?

Religious prohibitions about sex can be a contributing factor for men with delayed ejaculation. One study found that a disproportionate number of men with delayed ejaculation were raised in conservative religious homes or had conservative religious beliefs. Even without a religious upbringing, guilt and shame can be serious issues.

Another possible psychological semen stopper is if a man is having fears about his partner becoming pregnant. Deep-seated anger and having a withholding personality should also be evaluated. However, if anger, conservative religious upbringing and fears of getting your partner pregnant were the sole causes of delayed ejaculation, almost all men would suffer from it at one time or another.

Is Your Penis Lying?

The erect penis of a man with delayed ejaculation sometimes lies. This can be confusing, because when a guy is sporting a seriously hard penis, you assume he's highly aroused. But that might not be the case.

Even though a man is really hard, he might not be allowing himself to experience as much sexual excitement as other guys with hard-ons. To use psychological jargon, his erection might be out of sync with his emotional or internal state. If that's the case, he may need to work on increasing the level of sexual excitement that he allows himself to feel. Focusing on the sensations that make him feel good sexually might be helpful.

Sometimes men with delayed ejaculation are so focused on giving their partner pleasure that they won't let themselves be aware of their own sexual excitement, or they don't take in enough pleasure to orgasm.

Too Much Focus, Too Little Excitement

To help make his partner feel better, some men with DE will try so hard to ejaculate that they focus on their penis at the expense of the rest of their body. This can make a man even more numb to his own sexual excitement. So consider exploring the erogenous zones of a man's body from head to toe—and not just trying to find some magic spot or button that makes him ejaculate. Try to discover some of the subtle things that feel good and work on talking more easily about them. For some men, this might include long lingering kisses up and down the side of the neck or on his chest, nipples, back, or maybe a finger up his bum. Experiment and explore. Or you can get seriously Cosmo and run silk scarves or soft make-up brushes up and down his body. You might try to stimulate his genitals at the same time that you are kissing his neck or nipples.

Again, the goal of this approach is to focus on pleasure rather than on orgasm. You're trying to help him experience more pleasure and excitement. Technically, you're trying to storm the guard that's keeping sensation away from his orgasm trigger. You'll also need to be sensitive to how much he can handle. Some men will enjoy whatever you've got to throw at them. Others will reach a point of overload, after which all you are doing is increasing their resistance.

Note: Some therapists advise that the man not attempt to have intercourse until he can actually feel that he's sexually excited as opposed to just having an erection. Hopefully, you really will focus on pleasure as opposed to ejaculation. Sex is about sharing pleasure. Even if he never ejaculates, he might learn how to feel more pleasure and joy than guys who are able to ejaculate when they want.

Harsh Masturbation Techniques as the Cause? Pros and Cons

One of the few researchers who has actually studied delayed ejaculation feels that super vigorous or unusual masturbation habits can be a contributor in some cases. He thinks that changing masturbation habits is essential in situations where the guy pounds his meat like he's making chicken fried steak. He often tries to get the man to stop masturbating for several weeks or months, with the hope that he will have to rely on his partner to help him come. When the man does masturbate, a goal is to masturbate in a way that is kinder and gentler. She might try using his other hand or perhaps use lube in a way that makes masturbation feel more like intercourse.

On the other hand, it could be that the man's penis is less sensitive to begin with or his threshold to reach ejaculation is higher, so he learned to masturbate the way he did because it's the only way he can have an orgasm. If that's the case, his strange way of masturbating isn't the cause of the problem, but the result of it.

Masturbating face down is also thought by some to contribute to delayed ejaculation. If you have trouble coming and masturbate face down, see if you can teach yourself to start stroking it when you are on your back or while standing up.

However, there are plenty of men who pound their meat mercilessly and have no trouble ejaculating during partner sex. There may also be guys who masturbate face down and whose partners find them to be prolific comers. But still, it's hard to see a downside to easing up on the grip, or to masturbate face up rather than face down, or to turn over the reins to a significant other.

The Role of Fantasies

It's possible that some men with DE have certain fantasies they need in order to get off. But the realities of having sex with a partner might get in the way of being able to call up those fantasies.

Let's say a guy has a secret fantasy where his partner is stroking his penis with her feet, or maybe she's dressed in a corset, or she pees on him, or he or she is being gang raped or someone is forcing him to have sex with another guy. These fantasies might work great for him when he's strokin' it alone, but how does he lose himself in them when he is having intercourse with a real-live partner?

One of the challenges for he and his partner will be to allow enough of the fantasy to safely emerge to help him get off during intercourse. This means that exploring masturbation fantasies might be fruitful in some cases of delayed ejaculation. This might not be a problem if what turns him on is his partner wearing a certain bra or a pair of pantyhose with the crotch cut out. Most women won't be offended by those kind of requests; some will even be turned on by them.

But things can get a little dicey when his fantasies are at the extreme end of good taste and propriety or when he feels guilty about them. It can be particularly difficult to share a fantasy with a partner when he needs the same rigid scenario to get off each and every time.

For That Rare Man Who Doesn't Abuse Himself

There are situations when a man with delayed ejaculation can't or won't masturbate. If that's the case, you might start to explore the reasons and beliefs that are behind that decision. This will require introspection, which is not the hallmark of all men, let alone those with delayed ejaculation. Some men who are too embarrassed to masturbate might try doing it in stages. They can start while they are home alone, and work up to where they can do it when their partner is home but in a different room. Eventually they might try to do it when she's in the same room but with the lights off.

When Porn Might Help

It could be helpful for a man to watch porn just before or while he is making love. I might increase his level of stimulation or excitement. This could theoretically help him learn to ejaculate during intercourse, or at least learn to associate ejaculation with the feelings of intercourse. Think of it as the ejaculatory equivalent of using training wheels. On the other hand, there's absolutely no science to back any of this up.

Streaming your favorite porn while making love might not sit too well with your partner. Or it could be absolutely fine with her. So it's important to talk it over first. Also, porn might help a person with ADHD to focus better while making love.

When Porn Might Hurt

As a result of watching so much porn, a guy may have conditioned himself to need more visual stimulation than most men in order to come.

It's unlikely he'll get the kind of visual hyperstimulation from real-life lovemaking that he gets from porn.

If you watch a lot of porn and have delayed ejaculation, weaning yourself from porn might be a sensible thing to try.

Training Yourself To Feel Less Sensation

A consultant to this book offered his own theory on DE. When most men feel the sensations that tell them they are about to ejaculate, they choose between letting themselves ejaculate or slowing down or changing positions in order to delay coming. However, some men with delayed ejaculation seem to have trained themselves to automatically go the other way once they start to feel an increase in sensation. They mentally decrease what they feel even though they are still thrusting at the same speed.

This specialist advises the men to stop intercourse once they have blocked sensation more than three times in one session of lovemaking. He feels that to keep thrusting simply reinforces the tendency to delay ejaculation, which only teaches men to become even better at delaying ejaculation. This is anecdote rather than science, but it might have meaning for some readers.

Old Advice vs. New

It used to be that the advice for dealing with delayed ejaculation was to try having intercourse in novel situations or in places where there might be additional excitement from the lack of familiarity, like in the kitchen or in the back seat of a car. However, this isn't mentioned as much in the more recent articles on delayed ejaculation.

This novel-situation approach attempts to distract the man from his usual modus operandi where he's thought to be the master of control. The goal is to help him relinquish his need for control, assuming that's one of the things that might be causing the problem.

Another strategy has been to have the man bring himself close to ejaculating with his own hands, and then quickly put his penis in his partner's vagina and begin to thrust away. Hopefully he is able to ejaculate, and he can start to appreciate that he can ejaculate inside of his partner without the world coming to an end. However, this assumes that he and his partner will find this to be of value as opposed to being yet another form of torture and torment.

Imagine What Would Happen If...

Sex therapists sometimes ask couples to imagine what would happen if the problem would suddenly disappear. The point of this is to see if fears or concerns might emerge. Is there something about the problem that's keeping both partners within a certain comfort zone? Would the man's partner worry he'd want sex more often if he didn't have the problem? Would he be tempted to try his newfound skills on other women? Would he be concerned his partner might make new demands on him. Would he sense a loss of control? None of these fears need to be grounded in reality to be impacting sexual response.

ADD, ADHD, Bipolar Issues and Abuse As Contributors

A sex therapist who has treated men with DE believes that some of his patients with attention deficit and bipolar issues could have trouble reaching high enough levels of sexual excitement to ejaculate when having sex with a partner. This is because they are tuning in to everything in the room as opposed to the sex they are having. He wonders whether some of these men watch porn while having intercourse in order to help them focus on the sex so they can eventually ejaculate.

If you have delayed ejaculation and struggle with attention issues, perhaps this therapists observations will be meaningful for you. While no one is encouraging you to have porn blaring on a 60-inch screen during intercourse, perhaps there are things you and your partner can do to help keep you more focused on the sex you are having and on the building excitement in your body.

This therapist has also seen men who were sexually abused as boys who he feels may have trouble ejaculating as a result.

Sex Toys?

Sex toys, including a vibrating cock ring or vibrating butt plug, might provide the extra stimulation that some men need to help them ejaculate. Unfortunately, there's no research to guide on this.

Are There Drugs That Can Help?

In a word, none, as of press time. No drugs have been approved for delayed ejaculation. Dopamine agonists and anti-serotonergic drugs have been tried, but side effects can be significant and there doesn't appear to be anything on the immediate horizon.

Thanks to Stephen Braveman, Joe Marzucco and Michael Perelman.

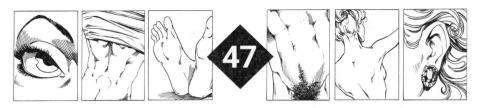

Dead Wood. Boner Down!

Contrary to what the boner drug commercials show, erection problems happen to men of all ages, including teenagers and men in their twenties. They don't just happen to men your dad's age.

Different kinds of erection failure are discussed in the pages that follow, including possible causes and current treatment options. Hopefully you will begin to appreciate that penis problems, regardless of the cause, can be an opportunity to have better sex.

The Bummer in Your Pants

It's not unusual for erection problems to occur at the start of a sexual relationship. Call it performance anxiety, call it fear—a man might need a couple of weeks or months to find a comfortable groove. Insisting that he must have perfect erections is silly and shortsighted. As long as your relationship is solid and you want to have sex with each other, give it time.

The real danger is not with the lack of erection, but with what each of you makes of it. Short-term problems can become long-term problems if the man sees himself as a failure or the woman needs his erection to validate that she's desirable. Consider this from a young man in his early twenties:

> "Last week we attempted to have sex again. Once again I went from an erection to completely unerect in a short amount of time. It happened when she said do you want to have sex. I had a feeling of uneasiness run through my entire body. It's like when you blow past a cop doing 80 and you get that feeling in your chest. There's a penetrating feeling through my body that I won't be able to get an erection and it becomes self-fulfilling and self-defeating. I don't have control over my body and that is what is so frustrating."

A combination of sex therapy and a Viagra-like drug might be the approach of choice for this man. (Only use the boner drug, and he might become psychologically dependent on it; but if he combines the drug with therapy, he'll be getting insight while putting an end to a self-fulfilling prophecy that has become a big part of the problem.)

Soft Hard vs. Hard Hard

A lot of men don't realize that there are at least two separate mechanisms that result in an erection. That's because when they are sexually aroused, their penis goes from the first step to the second step so quickly that it's pretty much a blur.

The first step is when a penis starts to get bigger and becomes just hard enough for intercourse but remains somewhat floppy. It then requires a second step to go from bigger-but-still-floppy to seriously hard. (In urology speak, the first step utilizes the veno-occlusive mechanism while the second requires cavernosal artery perfusion pressure.)

While a lot of men with erectile dysfunction (ED) are able to achieve the first step, failure to complete the second step leaves them with a "soft erection." It's maybe hard enough to stuff into a vagina, but it can result in intercourse that doesn't last very long and isn't as much fun. So there are at least two issues to be aware of if you are having ED problems: first, if your penis can swell up, and then whether it can get hard enough and stay hard. For many men, erection drugs help make the second step more doable. Still, a pill like Viagra isn't going to transform a middle-aged or older penis into that of an 18-year old. It's an assist, not a miracle.

Hard-Ons Don't Solve Everything

Guys who are having erection problems often assume that being able to pitch a tent in their pants will fix everything. Hopefully you will stop thinking that a hard-on can fix all that ails you. Erections are marvelous wonders, but a satisfying relationship they do not make.

Unfortunately, when there are problems with a guy's penis, it begins to suck up all of the energy that a couple could otherwise use in pleasing each other. There are plenty of times when a woman would be perfectly satisfied with her partner if he would focus on her instead of on what his penis is not able to do. Consider the two following situations where having a reliable erection doesn't help:

Some men have a problem called delayed ejaculation. It's when a guy can easily get an erection, but he's not able to come or ejaculate during intercourse. Even though these men often have magnificent

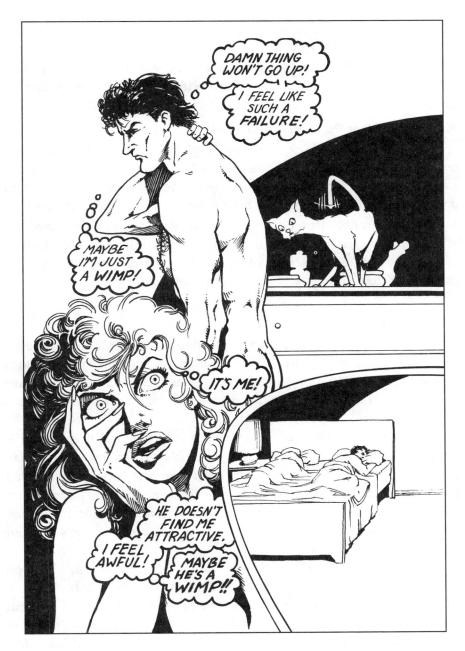

hard-ons, there is little magic and awe when their partner is saying "enough already." Likewise, more than 50% of men who have erection problems stop taking drugs like Viagra even if the drugs totally solve their erection problem. That's because when it comes to making love, relationship issues trump penis issues. When you haven't had sex with a partner in a couple of years, suddenly introducing a hard penis can create as many problems as it solves. As we have learned, it's not always good to give a man an erection without a few sessions of counseling for himself and his partner.

Stop Letting Your Penis Rule Your Sex Life

If your penis stalls out, try not to give it the power to ruin your sexual intimacy. Easier said than done, but what about necking for a long time, finger fucking, learning to give mind-blowing oral sex, using a vibrator or dildo, tying each other up, or acting out sex fantasies?

Success in life often depends on what we are able to make of our shortcomings. The biggest problem with impotence isn't the lack of erection. It's with a lack of playfulness and resourcefulness on the part of the man and woman when they are confronted with a penis that's being contrary.

When Your Posse Won't Ride

People often use terms such as *self-hatred, self-loathing* and *devastating* to describe how a man feels who is boner-challenged. (Guys with premature ejaculation often feel this way as well, and men who have solid erections but suffer from delayed ejaculation usually have less sex than other men.)

Perhaps this book is out of step or insensitive, but *devastating* is what happens when your wife or child dies or when you've just been told that you only have a few months to live. *Self-hatred* is what you feel if your business flops or if you've just blown your life's savings on something dumb. *Self-loathing* is what you experience when you've had a major stroke or accident and can't feed or bathe yourself or wipe your own ass.

There are about a thousand things worse than if a man's hard-on takes a hiatus, even if it's forever. It can certainly be frustrating and humiliating at times, but so are a lot of other things. You still have your fingers and mouth for giving pleasure, and you still have what's in your heart to love your partner with. And if you can't count at least five things in your life to be thankful for, even if your penis never gets hard again, then it's time to change your priorities.

Fortunately, modern medicine has ways to help a recalcitrant penis get hard, but it seems a shame to employ a quick cure without allowing yourself and your relationship to grow in the process. (Boner pills will often result in better erections but not in better sex.)

People who survive heart attacks and cancer learn to approach life differently as a result of the disease. A woman who is overcoming orgasm problems has to welcome a new way of embracing her body and her sexuality. It's a journey and a process. Impotent men, on the other hand, just want their dicks to get hard with no learning and no journey.

The Sufis have a saying that you have to let yourself die before you are truly born. Sometimes a guy has to give up his penis as a symbol of masculinity before he can get on with his life. Sometimes he has to realize that there's more to being a man than getting an erection or lasting for a prescribed number of thrusts. Then he sometimes has to convince his partner.

This is not to say that a man shouldn't inquire about the remedies that modern medicine has for erection problems. He should absolutely have a full physical exam to make sure that the erection problem is not a symptom of something else, because it often can be.

Why It's So Important To Get a Physical Exam

No kidding about getting a physical exam. A gradual onset of impotency can often be the first sign of an impending stroke, heart attack or diabetes. Impotence may be a better predictor of cardiovascular disease than the stress test. That's because the arteries in the penis can start to gum up before those in the rest of the body. There is also a strong correlation between sleep apnea and boner problems. If they discover you have sleep apnea as a result of getting your erection problems checked out, your penis might have just added years to your life.

Also, researchers are now finding a high correlation between obesity and impotence. Who knew that the drive-thru at McDonald's and the Frappuccinos at Starbucks could do your dick in?

A Modern Medical Approach to the Great Groin Grinch

If you aren't able to get it up, it is likely you are muttering under your breath that we can take our Sufi logic and stuff it where the sun don't shine. You want a magic bullet that does not require introspection or lifestyle changes. Good enough.

The advice that follows is a spoof on a modern medical approach to fixing erection problems. While it conveys some wisdom, it still focuses on fixing the penis instead of helping the man behind it and the woman in front of it. It is an approach that attempts to turn the clock back to a time when the penis worked just fine. It's a regressive fix rather than a step forward, one that is oblivious to lessons that might be learned. But it can also be a helpful approach if you are mindful of other issues in your life and relationship that could be going on as well.

> *Dear Paul,*
>
> *My bowling partner recently started having erection problems and is too embarrassed to seek help. Can you offer advice?*
>
> *Bob from Boston*

Dear Bob,

If your bowling partner has stopped throwing strikes for more than a couple of weeks, it's a good idea for him to take his pokey pecker for a checkup. It's important to rule out underlying medical conditions.

Modern medicine has decided that more than 99.999% of erection problems are due to physical causes, and drug companies claim their products can fix almost anything, unless your friend is a cigarette smoker. If that's the case, he might as well call a mortuary and have himself interred.

Is your friend able to get erections at all, like in the morning upon waking or when he jerks off? If so, his urologist might send him home with a device he attaches to his penis when he sleeps. It won't help to get him off, but it does record if he has erections in his sleep and for how long. If a man can get a rigid sustained erection in his sleep or while masturbating, this means the valves and plumbing in his penis probably work.

If all the valves, veins and arteries are okay, some physicians will send your friend home with samples of Viagra, or Levitra or Cialis if they own stock in Glaxo or Lilly.

If the boner pills don't work, a urologist might give your friend's penis an injection that will most likely make it hard. Don't worry, no one's going to pull out a syringe with a hollow nail for a needle and say, "Drop your drawers." It's an itty-bitty wisp of a shot that hurts less than getting a pubic hair stuck in your zipper. If a penis gets hard and is able to stay hard, then the underlying plumbing is intact and the problem can probably be fixed with a prescription.

If the shot does not make the penis hard, or it gets hard but doesn't stay hard, then they will want to rule out a circulation problem. The causes can range from hardening of the arteries (strange term for when it happens in a penis that won't get hard) to leaky valves. More tests will need to be done to peg the exact cause.

It is also possible there is a neurological problem which is disabling the body's ability to trigger hard-ons. This is similar to when you turn the ignition key on your car and nothing happens.

Another thing to check is if your friend is taking medications that might be impacting his penis. Suspicious meds range from alcohol and heroin to prescriptions and over-the-counter drugs. Some say that Tagamet can do a dick in. (Your friend isn't one of those meth-abusing party boys, is he? Recreational drugs can be very bad for a penis.)

If specialists can't find anything medical, they may consider the possibility that your friend's erection problem stems from emotional causes or a combination of something emotional and physical. To explore the emotional possibilities, some questions are in order. What was going on in your friend's life around the time when his soldier stopped marching? Did his ability to get an erection decline gradually, like the fall of Rome, or did it shut down all at once, like Bear Stearns, Wachovia or Lehman Brothers? Was there a change in his job status? Did his team not go to the Superbowl because of a lousy call in the closing seconds? Was there a change in his relationship with his partner? Did his wife leave him for another man? Did she leave him for another woman? Was he pulled from an important project, or did he lose a promotion he had his heart set on? Did he receive an unkind inquiry from the IRS?

Also, it is helpful to inquire about his relationship with his partner. If he instantly says, "Naw, it's fine," ask him to describe some of the things that are fine about it. See if he conveys a sense of love and fondness, or if he sounds like he's reading the instructions on a bottle of Kaopectate. If the relationship has fallen on, dare we say, hard times, then he and his wife need to focus on fixing that in addition to his penis, which might merely be the messenger.

In order to treat erection problems that are caused by relationship problems, your friend and his partner might try to forget all they know about each other and start over again as if they'd just met. This can be difficult, especially if they have had some really terrible times together. They might try taking a month or two doing things like hugging, touching and talking, with no attempt at intercourse. They also might try sharing fun dinners, movies and doing the type of things they enjoyed doing when they first met. How about racking their bowling balls and taking a trip around town or even around the country? They might discover there really is life after bowling. On the other hand, some couples do better when they spend less time with each other. This can be especially true when one or both of them recently retired and they suddenly find themselves in each other's face—uh, company—24 hours a day.

Your friend and his wife should be reminded that the older a man is, the more hands-on play and wooing his penis needs in order to get hard. So a man will need more penis play when he's forty than when he was twenty. And if none of that helps, there's this Sufi saying....

The Best Viagra Quote

One of the finest quotes about Viagra is from the *Boston Globe's* Ellen Goodman:

"I can't help wondering why we got a pill to help men with performance instead of communication. Moreover, how is it possible that we came up with a male impotence pill before we got a male birth control pill? The Vatican, you will note, has approved Viagra while still condemning condoms."

Erection Drugs—Be Sure to Read the Instructions

Viagra should be taken on an empty stomach. This is a major reason why Viagra doesn't work very well for some men: they don't take it on an empty stomach. If you are using erection drugs, carefully read all of the instructions.

There are other boner drugs with names like Levitra, Cialis and Stendra. If side effects aren't a problem, men often prefer Cialis because it lasts for a few days and they don't have to take it just before intercourse. Regardless of what you take, do not buy erection drugs from online sellers unless you know they are a licensed pharmacy. There is a lot of counterfeit Viagra on the Internet.

Viagra in the Cockpit, Cialis in Your Hamstrings

Pilots are not allowed to take Viagra for twelve hours before a flight, and it's not because the FAA is worried the pilot will accidentally grab the co-pilot's erection instead of the landing-gear controls.

Most of the boner drugs in use today are called PDE5 inhibitors. They work by inhibiting an enzyme in the penis which helps the blood vessels dilate. There is a similar enzyme in our eyes that can also be impacted by Viagra which can result in altered color perception. (It's not like the pilots will be seeing flying vaginas. Just a blue haze.)

PDE5 inhibitors like Viagra and Cialis can inhibit other PDE enzymes in the body, and that's where the side effects come into play. The reason Viagra can cause vision issues is because it also inhibits PDE6 which is an enzyme that resides in our eyes.

Cialis leaves PDE6 alone, but it can impact PDE11, which is an enzyme in our skeletal muscles. So a major side effect of Cialis can be back aches, pain in hamstring muscles, and other aches and pains throughout the body. While these side effects don't impact some men, other men find them to be quite severe. (Approximately 7% or more of men who take Cialis have these side effects which can be very painful).

Since each of the boner drugs effects a different PDE enzyme besides just PDE5, the side effect profile is different for each one. This is why it can be a good idea to sample different erection drugs when you are first taking them. See if there's one that helps create a good erection but has few if any side effects. Since each man's body is different, it's impossible to predict which will be best for you.

If you can't find a pill that works without causing side effects, talk to your urologist about the injections that can help make you hard.

Penis Injections and Pellets That Make You Hard

There are compounds that cause an erection when they are injected into the penis, assuming the plumbing is intact and can maintain an erection once the penis gets hard. A compound called Papervine was formerly used for this purpose, but now, different combinations of ingredients are used, such as a combination of papervine, phentolamine, and prostaglandin E1.

There is an erection-inducing pellet or suppository called Muse that a man can place in his urethra (peehole) to help make his penis erect. It can work very well for some men, and not for others. One suggestion, besides carefully reading and following the instructions, is to try intercourse positions where the man is standing or sitting upright.

There are other orally-prescribed drugs that might help some men to get hard. One drug that is sometimes prescribed is called yohimbine.

Yohimbine is native to Africa. It can be found in health food stores, but since the cost of yohimbine isn't much more by prescription, why not get it from a urologist? That way you can be sure you are getting the yohimbine in consistent doses, which is not true for the yohimbine in health food stores. The physician can also rule out possible health related issues.

Levitra as a Thrill Pill for Younger Men Who Don't Need It?

At least the people who make Viagra have had the decency to market their drug toward guys who might actually need it. No such claim can be made by the makers of Levitra, which has run ads that were clearly meant to target younger men who get it up just fine. In one of their ads, they show a young stud trying to throw a football through a tire. It bounces off to the side. After the word Levitra is mentioned, he gets the ball through the tire several times. He is then joined by his smiling wife or girlfriend whose tires he seems to have successfully rotated.

An important thing to know about boner drugs is they don't add much to sex if you're able to get a good erection to begin with. Side effects can also be a problem in addition to the cost. Please read the account of a younger man about his experience with how boner drugs can cause psychological dependence (see page 54).

"Ejaculate Like a Porn Star," "Add an Inch in Two Weeks," "Natural Male Enhancement," "Recharge Your Libido"— Some Seriously Iffy Ideas

There are few living humans who haven't seen ads for herbal pills that promise to get a man horny, big and hard. Some of these products are cleverly marketed to make them look legitimate.

Some of the companies that produce these pills are being shut down for consumer fraud. Also, if you or your in-laws wanted to make herbal supplements in your garage and sell them on TV, you can. Even if there are rodents crawling over the equipment and cats sleeping next to it, there are no regulations on herbal supplements. You could put cow plops in herbal pills and run ads for them; the only way the government will test herbal pills is if about a dozen people suddenly die.

If there really were a pill that could do all of the things the scammers and spammers say their pills can do, don't you think the multibillion dollar drug companies would be selling it?

Pumps & Implants

Some men find vacuum pumps are useful erection aides. Pumps are bulky and cumbersome, but they might be worth a try if you are in search of a lost erection. There are different suppliers for vacuum pumps. Be sure the pump you purchase includes gaskets which keep your scrotum from getting sucked up into the vacuum tube. Some of the penis pumping companies that market to gay males sell excellent units for less than half the cost of pumps that are Medicare approved. Still, expect to pay $100 for a decent rig.

There are different surgical implants, from semi-rigid shanks to implants with little pumps that will give a man an erection. Frequent improvements are being made in the technology. Please research this subject carefully before making a decision.

Bicycle Seats As a Cause of Impotence

Urologists have been saying for years that bicycle seats are causing erection problems in men and clitoral numbness in women. They have been seeing case after case of young male bike riders with numbness in their crotches and erection problems. It's not so much that these young men can't get it up, but that it won't stay up. Instead of wanting to study the matter further, some of the bike magazines apparently tried to discredit the concerned physicians.

But the bicycle industry has underestimated the steadfastness of the crotch docs who have wired bicycle seats in their research laboratories with more sensors than the Sands Casino when it was demolished. They have also done studies on bicycle-riding policemen whose penis heads were connected to oxygen sensors. They found that the typical bicycle saddle robs the penis of 80% of its oxygen and causes a decrease in erections during sleep. Plus, there's a major nerve to the penis that runs between a man's legs. It takes a terrible thrashing when he is using a traditional bike seat or saddle.

If you are a guy, you have probably experienced a tingling sensation in your penis after riding a bike for awhile. It's not normal. It is from crotch compression which can damage the nerves in your penis or in a woman's clitoris.

A good way to explain this is to compare sitting in a chair verses on a bike seat. When you sit in a chair, your weight is distributed across your entire butt and thighs. The circulation in your crotch is not compromised and the nerves aren't damaged. But when you are on a bike, the entire weight of your body is bearing down a very small part of your crotch that provides the oxygen and nerves to your genitals.

Bike saddles with the cut-outs have been advertised to eliminate the problem, but they can actually make it worse. That's because with the cutout, there's even less area to distribute your weight over.

Women are no more immune than guys. Researchers have found a measurable decrease in sexual sensation for women who ride seriously. They've also found a condition on competitive riders called "Bicyclist's Vulva" where one of the labia can grow bigger due to the pounding a woman's crotch takes from the seat.

There are two possible solutions: The first is to raise the handlebars above the level of the seat so you sit up instead of crouching over. This will help somewhat. The other solution is to get a no-nose bike seat or saddle. Innercity cops who ride on bikes swear by them. For a list of no-nose saddles, enter "bike" in the search box at www.Guide2Getting.com.

Pharmaceutical Sex Assassins That Impact Both Men and Women

You wouldn't believe how many over-the-counter or prescription medications can mess with everything from your ability to get hard or wet to your feelings of desire.

One of the most common sources of sexual side effects are antidepressants known as SSRIs. According to the Journal of Sexual Medicine, any person who has been given a prescription for an SSRI antidepressant should be given a warning such as the following:

> "There is a high probability of sexual side effects while on SSRI medications. There are indications that in an unknown number of cases, the side effects may not resolve with cessation of the medication and could be potentially irreversible."

SSRIs are antidepressants that include Prozac, Zoloft, Paxil, Lexapro, Luvox, Celexa, Effexor, Serzone and Remeron. (While not related to erection problems, women who take SSRIs and use hormonal methods of birth control are especially at risk for low desire and other sexual side effects.

Damn That Hurts! When Sex is Painful

Few men understand how painful sex can be for some women. This isn't pain from the kind of rushed and rough sex that's typical in porn. Instead, think of when a Q-tip is pressed against a woman's genitals and it causes her to flinch in pain. Or when intercourse with a gentle lover creates an intense burning sensation in her vagina or makes her feel like she's being stabbed with a knife. Or when the muscles around the opening of her vagina are clamped so tight she can't insert a tampon.

For plenty of women with sexual pain, it's not this severe. But it still makes sex something they endure rather than enjoy.

Many of us assume there are two times in life when sex hurts for women: their first time and after menopause. We don't realize that more than 20% of women in their teens, twenties and thirties can experience pain during sex, and not just once or twice. This is chronic pain for months or years.

What Chronic Pelvic Pain Isn't

A good way to describe chronic sexual pain is to start with what it isn't. While rushed or clumsy lovemaking can make sex painful, this can usually be resolved with effort and education or by finding a new lover. That is not the case when there is chronic pain during sex. Sometimes a woman can have great sex with a man for years, and then suddenly develop pelvic pain. Or she will have pain from the first time she tries to put in a tampon and it doesn't go away, no matter how many different lovers she tries to have sex with.

Chronic sexual pain isn't when a woman is enjoying intercourse and the head of her partner's penis hits her cervix and it feels like she was punched in the stomach. Nor is it the pain a woman feels if she is dry and needs lube. Chronic sexual pain doesn't go away by adding lube. Chronic pelvic pain can't be fixed by changing positions or by wrapping her legs around a partner's waist instead of around his neck. It's not a matter of lube or logistics.

A lover's penis might be three clicks bigger than huge and a woman may need to do exercises like they teach in childbirth classes to fit it in, but that is not usually what causes chronic sexual pain. Chronic sexual pain is pretty much there each and every time a woman has intercourse, assuming she is able to have intercourse. It doesn't suddenly get better if she has sex with someone else like her partner's younger brother.

While menopause may bring its own set of issues that can lead to pain during intercourse, the type of pelvic pain this chapter is about is not brought on by menopause.

The Rest of this Chapter Is Addressed to Women

A problem with defining pelvic pain is that whatever caused it probably occurred long ago. This might have been an infection inside your vagina or it may have started from a dermatological condition in the sensitive area between your lips called the vulvar vestibule. The vulvar vestibule is like a small platform that the urethra (peehole) and the opening of the vagina are mounted on.

The pain might have developed in response to an uncomfortable gynecological exam, or a sudden surge of hormones in your body that went back to normal in a few days, weeks, or months. It could have been caused by taking oral contraceptives, or by an allergic reaction.

As long as there are no current conditions that might be causing the pain, the cause is not what's important. The problem you are probably dealing with now is the reaction (or over-reaction) of your nerves and muscles to something that happened long ago. But as far as your body is concerned, this doesn't make it any less severe or less painful than if it happened yesterday.

Creating a Strategy

There are several books on sexual pain, some of which are recommended in this chapter. Unfortunately, many offer an approach that doesn't take into account the complexity of the problem. Here are some of the steps that may be required to help resolve your sexual pain. Some researchers say it will require all of these steps to fix the problem:

> 😎 Getting a thorough exam to rule out medical conditions that might be causing pain. This can be done by a gynecologist or a physical therapist who specializes in pelvic pain disorders—in a perfect world, you would see both.

👀 Learning all you can about chronic pelvic pain before you try various solutions.

👀 Retraining your central nervous system.

👀 Retraining the muscles in your pelvis.

👀 Involving your partner if you have one.

Eliminate the Obvious

While the original cause of your pelvic pain may be long gone, you will need thorough exam by a competent gynecologist to rule out any causes of pain that still might be ongoing.

Deep-thrusting pain is sometimes caused by constipation or pelvic inflammatory disease. Shallow-thrusting pain has a larger range of possible causes, from adhesions under the clitoral hood or episiotomy scars to yeast infections. There are a number of pain-causing conditions with names that are difficult to pronounce. Some are listed in the preceding chapter. It would seem that most gynecologists would know how to treat chronic pelvic pain, but few specialize in this area. This is why the next step is so very important.

Knowledge—The Key to Any Strategy for Pelvic Pain

Fortunately, pelvic pain is not as hopeless as it used to be—far from it. But to help assure a positive outcome, you need to be well informed from the very beginning. Research is now being done and there are good resources. But it will be up to you and your partner to form a strategy, or just you if you don't have a partner.

Assuming you are in good gynecological health, one of the first things to do is to read the resources that are suggested in this chapter. Please do this before venturing on an odyssey through the healthcare system. Hopefully you will find other resources as well, but a good place to begin is with the *When Sex Hurts* book and at the website of the National Vulvodynia Association. (See *Resources* at the end of the chapter.)

Is the Pain in Your Head? YES!

Whatever caused the pelvic pain in the first place is usually gone by the time you see one of umpteenth healthcare providers who women with pelvic pain often see. So you will soon start to hear that the pain is in your head. And for the most part, this is true! That's because all pain comes from our heads, or our brains, anyway. It doesn't matter if you step on a nail or break your arm. The pain is controlled by your brain, which decides when to turn the pain on and when to turn it off, as well as when to turn it up and down.

What probably happened is your nerves and the muscles between your legs responded to the initial provocation exactly as they should have. Your brain assessed the incoming data from the nerve receptors in your genitals, decided there was a problem, and started setting off pain alarms. And then the muscles in your pelvis probably started clamping down to help protect you from what your brain perceived was a threat.

But after the threat was gone, your brain and the muscles never got the memo. They might still be fighting a in a war that's long been over. They are still on hyper alert, as if the cause of the pain was never resolved. Whatever happened in your genitals created the perfect storm, especially if you have a genetic predisposition to being tense or anxious.

The Pain Is Also on Your Forearm and in Your Feet

Researchers have discovered that women who have chronic pelvic pain are more sensitive to pain throughout their entire body. This is called pain amplification. It's a nice way of saying things are messed up. When researchers put noxious substances on the forearms and feet of women who do and don't have pelvic pain, the women who have pelvic pain notice the pain much more. It's as if whatever went on in their genitals created a hypersensitivity throughout their entire body. The skin all over their body becomes more sensitive to tactile sensation. This is often the case with pain disorders. Pain in one part of the body can make us more sensitive to pain in other non-related parts.

Some women with chronic pelvic pain become so hyper alert that even thinking about sex can cause them pain. Sexual fantasies which may have made them want to masturbate or jump their partner on the spot might now cause them to feel pain in their genitals. This pain is every bit as real as the pain you feel when you hit your finger with a hammer.

The good news is that it's possible to retrain a nervous system that is on hyper alert. To learn more about how, you'll want to read the *Why Pelvic Pain Hurts* book that's listed at the end of the chapter.

Pelvic Floor Muscles — The Pit Bull in Your Panties

The muscles in the pelvis are usually players in chronic pelvic pain conditions. Sometime they are the key players, other times not. But by the time a woman has chronic pain during sex, her muscles are usually doing things they shouldn't.

A pelvic pain specialist who works with elite athletes says that a number of her patients who do repetitive motions on one side of their body have pain during intercourse as a result, eg, tennis players, volleyball players, golfers, shot putters, javelin throwers, etc. The muscles on that side of their pelvis become tense or tight and can make intercourse very painful. So for these women, physical therapy involves biofeedback that helps them learn to relax the muscles on one side of their pelvis.

The sexual pain for these athletes began in their pelvic muscles. In other women with pelvic pain, the muscle problems in their pelvis began after the original cause of the pain. One or more of the pelvic muscles tightened up to help protect the women from the source of the problem. Muscle groups in the pelvis that control the opening of the vagina may have started clamping shut whenever something like a finger or penis touched a woman's genitals, and they continue to do so. The muscles might stay relaxed until there is touch, and then they go ballistic.

For other women, the muscles in their pelvis never relax. They are like a pit bull in your panties. There can also be trigger points along various muscles in the pelvis. Touch or pressure on these trigger points can cause excruciating pain. This is why a strategy to eliminate pelvic pain will most likely need to include teaching the muscles in your pelvis to relax. The *Sex Without Pain: A Self-Treatment Guide* listed at the end of this chapter shows some of the ways it can be done.

Your Partner: Ally for Intimacy or ???

Most approaches to pelvic pain list involvement of the woman's partner as a footnote, if that. Unless your partner is a useless tool, he or she can be your biggest ally.

Women who experience sexual pain often avoid sexual intimacy with their partner. This is a mistake. It almost never turns out well. The job of a couple is to figure out the types of sexual intimacy they can enjoy that don't cause pain. Once a woman can be sure her partner won't reach for her crotch, there are many ways the two of them can enjoy sexual intimacy.

Different partners respond to a woman's sexual pain in different ways. For simplicity' sake, let's assume there are three types of partners:

What a Dick! This is a guy who either doesn't believe your pain is real or doesn't care. He's angry that he's not getting the sex he thinks he deserves. The last thing he tries to be is reasonable, supportive, or helpful. Why you stay with him is beyond the scope of this book and probably has your friends stumped as well. The prognosis for pain-free sex with this type of partner is unlikely.

Mr. "I feel your pain!" This type of partner is so solicitous and afraid of causing you pain that he becomes a pain himself. Rather than being a ray of hope, he ends up reinforcing sexual pain. Pelvic pain has compromised your intimacy. You need an ally who will inspire you in battle, not a wimp who is going to bring you aspirin. You need someone who is strong as well as sensitive.

The Man! This is the guy who is going to help keep sexual intimacy alive in your relationship without creating more sexual pain. This is the partner we all want to be, and on some days, we are! This is a man who wants to learn about your pelvic pain. He wants to backstop your efforts, but doesn't need to take over. He understands the shots are yours to call, but he isn't afraid to offer the point of view of a third party who might understand things about you that you don't.

He's a man who isn't afraid to say, "If that hurts, let's find something we both like to do that doesn't hurt." He's not afraid to be an unflinching advocate for sexual intimacy with you.

Reconnecting with Your Partner

While women who have sexual pain do not have anywhere near the level of sexual satisfaction as other women, their satisfaction with their relationship is often the same as women who don't have chronic sexual pain. It seems that sexual pain can bring some partners closer. However, there are situations where a woman will begin to avoid her partner's touch in order to avoid having sex. Maybe she'll go to bed earlier or later than he does, or when he says sexy things to her she freezes up rather than smiles. He will often assume her distance is because of something he's done, or because she would rather have sex with someone else.

A strategy to treat sexual pain will often involve reconnecting with your partner. Maybe this is something the two of you can do together, or maybe you can use the help of a couples therapist or a sex therapist. At the very least, it would be a good idea to ask him to read this chapter.

Sexual Intimacy With Your Partner When You Have Pelvic Pain

Only one chapter out of all the chapters in this book is on sexual intercourse (penis into vagina). This should speak volumes for how many ways there are to share sexual intimacy without having intercourse. Here are a few suggestions for how a partner can be sexually intimate with you without touching your vagina:

👓 Smother your inner thighs with kisses, avoiding the part of your crotch that hurts when it's touched.

👓 Shower your abdomen with kisses, from your navel to the top of your mons pubis (landing strip area) and from one hip bone to the other.

👓 Did your partner used to be the incredible make-out king? Dust off his make-out skills and give them new life!

👓 Are there fantasy scenarios that turn you on or you used to enjoy acting out together? Have you ever done role playing?

👓 Is it possible the two of you will like reading erotica together?

👓 Perhaps you like breast play. Maybe it's in the form of tender kisses or you like a firm approach and have a favorite pair of nipple clamps. If so, he should be on it.

👓 If you enjoy anal stimulation or anal sex, there shouldn't be anything stopping you.

👓 If you like being restrained or spanked, go for it.

👓 Some women with pelvic pain are able to masturbate. Your partner can hold you or kiss and caress you while you masturbate. Maybe you can masturbate together.

The purpose of this is for the two of you to share sexual intimacy. It is not not a step on the way to having intercourse. This is your safe harbor of sexual intimacy. Making it a milestone on the way to intercourse will only ruin it.

As for the things you can do to satisfy him, stop assuming there are rules that sex isn't sex unless a penis goes inside a vagina! There are dozens of ways you can give a partner sexual pleasure without your vagina being involved. If you are short on ideas, read the chapters in this book on handjobs, blowjobs, the testicles, the prostate, and more.

Just kissing your partner's neck and nipples, or letting him kiss you while he's masturbating might lead to more sexual satisfaction than a lot of couples have.

Dissociation vs. Pleasure

One of the bigger problems in treating sexual pain is when its focus is on eventually having intercourse instead of being about sexual pleasure. If the goal is intercourse, the woman will often dissociate or mentally leave her body to ignore the pain.

While it's easy to understand why she might do this, it is unlikely to work. Besides, is this how you want sexual intimacy to be—where the woman mentally numbs herself so her partner can get his penis inside of her vagina? (Pelvic pain specialist Talli Rosenbaum has written about this. See the references at the end of the chapter.)

A Problem with Hormonal Contraceptives

Contrary to popular belief, women's bodies make testosterone and men make estrogen. The skin on a woman's genitals is sensitive to testosterone and it needs a certain amount of testosterone to be healthy. The problem with hormonal methods of birth control is they decrease the amount of testosterone in a woman's body, often times considerably.

This can cause a thinning of the skin in a woman's genitals. It also could be the reason why women who use hormonal contraceptives are six times more likely to experience pelvic pain than women who don't use hormonal contraceptives. And it's one of the reasons why physicians who specialize in pelvic pain will often suggest you discontinue using hormonal contraceptives that may be decreasing your body's level of testosterone.

Can Bicycle Seats Create or Contribute To Chronic Sexual Pain?

Research has found an association between bicycle seats and clitoral numbness, but there's been no research on bicycle seats and chronic sexual pain. If you have chronic sexual pain and ride a bike, consider switching to a no-nose saddle. *See* www.Guide2Getting.com/bikes for links to manufacturers of no-nose saddles.

Caution about Kegels, Pilates and Yoga for Pelvic Pain

For years, Kegel exercises have been suggested as a nearly universal "cure" for all things going on in the female pelvis. Yet Kegel exercises that are not done properly can contribute to pelvic floor problems. And even when Kegel exercises are done properly, they can make an already painful situation worse. This is particularly true when some of the muscles in your pelvis are already clenching or have too much tone. It's one of the reasons why it is so important to be examined by a physical therapist who specializes in pelvic floor problems if you are experiencing chronic pain during sex. If your personal circumstances prevent this, at the very least, read the books mentioned at the end of this chapter to learn more.

The same cautions apply for Pilates core exercises that are designed to strengthen pelvic floor muscles and certain Yoga regimens. While these exercises can be beneficial when done correctly by women who have no pelvic floor problems, they should not be used as a treatment for pelvic floor pain without an evaluation first.

The Journey Forward

If you have insurance or the financial means and are in proximity of a gynecologist or physical therapist who specializes in female pelvic pain, then a hands-on examination is essential. Women who have pelvic pain tend to dread gynecological exams, but rest assured, if you can find a gynecologist or physical therapist who specializes in sexual pain, it should not be like your past visits to healthcare providers.

BOOKS

Here are two of the most important books you can read at the start of your journey to eliminate sexual pain:

When Sex Hurts: A Woman's Guide to Banishing Sexual Pain by Andrew Goldstein, Caroline Pukall, and Irwin Goldstein, Da Capo Lifelong Books. This book was written by three of the top specialists in the research and treatment of women's sexual pain. You won't find a more competent resource on sexual pain anywhere.

Why Pelvic Pain Hurts—Neuroscience Education for Patients with Pelvic Pain by Adriaan Louw, Sandra Hilton and Caroly Vandyken. This little gem explains what's going on in the nervous system of people with pelvic pain. It is easy to read and incredibly helpful.

Sex Without Pain: A Self-Treatment Guide to the Sex Life You Deserve by Heather Jeffcoat is recommended but with reservations. It does a good job of explaining how to examine your genitals and do the exercises that are often used to help retrain the muscles in the pelvic area. The reservations are because it tends to promise a one-dimensional cure to pelvic pain, when treating pelvic pain can be much more complex than retraining the pelvic floor muscles. Also, the author suggests readers use the resources on her website including her list of specialists, when excellent physical therapists and gynecologists who specialize in pelvic pain are not included. The book does say to not take shortcuts and the advice is sound and up to date.

Other books to consider include Amy Stein's *Heal Pelvic Pain: The Proven Stretching, Strengthening, and Nutrition Program for Relieving Pain, Incontinence,& I.B.S, and Other Symptoms Without Surgery*. This book gets good reviews, but hasn't had a refresh in years. As for "proven," maybe if you are a patient of Ms. Stein's where you and she can tap into her years of experience in evaluating your problem. But this doesn't mean other readers will find a cure by reading this book or any other. —Harold Glazer's book *The Vulvodynia Survival Guide: How to Overcome Painful Vaginal Symptoms and Enjoy an Active Lifestyle*, but it hasn't had a refresh in years. Also, Claudia Amherd's *7 Steps to Pain-Free Sex: A Complete Self-Help Guide to Overcome Vaginismus, Dyspareunia, Vulvodynia & other Penetrations Disorders*.

For organizations, the National Vulvodynia Association is excellent www.nva.org. In Canada, contact the Women's Health section of the Canadian Physiotherapy Association: www.physiotherapy.ca.

For Talli Rosenbaum's article, click on the "publications" section of her website at www.tallirosenbaum.com/en.

A very special thanks to Caroline Pukall, Ph.D., Psychology Department, Queen's University, Canada.

The Pill, Your Sex Drive & Depression

"I have noticed a big decrease in my sex drive since I started taking the pill. I am not randomly horny anymore and I used to be all the time. I used to want sex at least once a day." *fem 20*

"After a not-so-great experience with the first brand, I switched to a low-dose birth-control pill. I like it. I have no side effects at all. My sex drive is back, which is great!" *female age 19*

"I used the pill and saw no effect on my sex drive whatsoever. However, my twin sister took the pill and saw a marked decrease in her sex drive. It just goes to show that everyone reacts differently—even identical twins." *female age 21*

Little research has been done on the impact that birth control pills have on a woman's sex drive and mood. Yet in our sex survey, more than 35% of women have said they experienced unpleasant sexual side effects from using hormonal methods of birth control. However, 65% of women had no complaints about the pill, with some saying their sex drive is even higher now that they are taking it.

As for the pill and depression, a few weeks before this edition of *The Guide* went to press, a study involving thousands of women from Denmark found that using hormonal birth control substantially increases a woman's chances of becoming clinically depressed. This includes the pill, Mirena IUD, the implant, NuvaRing and Depo Provera. The authors believe it could be the progestin that's a major component of hormonal birth control that's the guilty party. That's because women who used progestin-only forms of birth control suffered from significantly more depression than women who took hormonal birth control that also contained estrogen.

Before you begin taking hormonal birth control, write down your answers to questions at the end of this chapter. That way, you'll have a baseline to refer to after you've been using hormonal birth control.

NOTE: It used to be that the only hormonal method of birth control was the pill. Now there are different delivery systems such as the Nuva-Ring, Minera IUD, Implanon implant, the patch, and the Depo shot. For simplicity's sake, this chapter usually refers to all of these as "the pill."

Impact on Your Sex Drive: Less Than 5% or More Than 25%?

"We used to use condoms until six months ago when I started taking the pill. I love the pill! I have noticed no change in my desire for sex since starting it. I was incredibly horny before and am still incredibly horny now!" *female age 19*

"I took the pill for five months but stopped because it gave me horrible side effects (no sex drive although I was a newlywed, depression, paranoia, panic attacks, weight gain, and heart burn). Now that I'm off hormones my sex drive is a whole lot better." *female age 21*

Healthcare providers often tell women that less than 5% of women have sexual side effects when taking the pill. That's because most studies that have asked women about the sexual side effects of taking the pill have only included women who had been taking it for five years or more. But women who experience a drop in sexual desire often stop taking the pill within the first year. So sexual side effects are greatly under-represented. Also, these studies are easy to manipulate, and most of the studies have been funded by the drug companies who have a vested interested in the outcome.

Are Women Too Suggestible to Deserve Adequate Warnings?

"My doctor never told me that I could have any of those side effects. Sure, I was expecting weight gain and such, but not depression and NO sex drive." *female age 21*

"This is the third brand of pill I have been on. The first was a three-month kind, which left me spotting for weeks, made me frustrated and took away my sex drive. The second made me very depressed with a sex drive that rose and fell like crazy. This third one has leveled out my emotions and might be making my sex drive a little stronger than before." *female age 20*

Healthcare providers don't always warn women about the sexual side effects of hormonal birth control. Some feel that to warn women about sexual side effects would plant the idea in a woman's mind. Fortunately, there are different pill formulations and types of estrogen and progestin that a woman can take. With the help of an astute healthcare provider, a woman who is not doing well with one type of pill might try a different one or a different delivery system such as the NuvaRing or IUD. (The copper IUD known as Paragard does not release hormones, while the Mirena, Kyleena, Liletta and Skyla IUDs release from 13.5 mg to 52 mg of the progestin levonorgestrel which is a hormone.)

So What's Going On?

"No change whatsoever... Still horny as a dog." *female age 21*

"The pill has totally suppressed my sex drive. I have hardly any desire." *female age 22*

"I definitely enjoy sex way more knowing that I won't get pregnant if the condom breaks or slips off." *female age 24*

While testosterone tends to be associated with men's bodies, having a certain amount of it is necessary for most women to have a healthy sex drive. Unfortunately, birth-control pills lower the amount of testosterone in most women's bodies. This can sometimes reduce or totally kill the sex drives of some women. Exactly how much testosterone a woman needs can vary: one woman might handle a drop in testosterone with no adverse effects, while another will want to curl up with a book instead of a lover.

There is also another factor: some women's sex drives are more testosterone dependent, while for other women, it's the kind of relationship they are in that's the bigger issue. Researchers have also found that women who live in a country where they don't expect to enjoy sex report fewer sexual side effects from the pill than women who live in countries where they do expect to enjoy sex.

The Importance of Smell

For some women, their partner's smell or scent registers in a sexual way. They might cherish wearing a lover's shirt that has his scent on it. (This would be his scent, as opposed to his smelly BO. There's a big difference!) Unfortunately, a woman's ability to smell a man's scent is inversely impacted by hormonal methods of birth control like the pill. So if smell is an important turn-on for a woman, the pill might be impacting her in ways that people usually don't think about.

The Pill and Pelvic Pain

Women who use hormonal birth control are six times more likely to experience pelvic pain than women who don't use hormonal birth control. This could be due to a thinning of the skin on the genitals that occurs when the level of testosterone in a woman's body falls too low, which is a side effect of use hormonal birth control. When women who are using hormonal birth control have chronic pain during sex or the skin on their genitals is frequently irritated, one of the first things pelvic pain specialists often recommend is they stop using the hormonal birth control.

Pill-Related Benefits

A woman who is using a highly effective method of birth control is more likely to want sex than a woman who has to worry about becoming pregnant. Also, pills can help women who have premenstrual mood issues, as well as helping to decrease period flow and cramping. This might explain why some women prefer pills with a higher dose of estrogen than low-dose pills, because the extra estrogen might help decrease the bleeding, cramping, and premenstrual mood fluctuation.

Some formulations of the pill decrease acne. This might help a woman to feel more sexually attractive. But these pills zap zits because they excel at reducing testosterone which can cause acne, so the cost of clearer skin could be a lower sex drive.

Gauging Your Sex Drive Before You Start Taking The Pill

You might find it's helpful to jot down the answers to the following questions before you start taking the pill. Then you'll have something to refer back to in six months or a year to make sure there haven't been changes in your mood and sex drive that could be related to the pill.

😎 If you've been having sex, write down how many times a month and how satisfying it is or isn't.

😎 Are there times of the month when you feel especially horny? See if it changes after you start taking the pill.

😎 If you have a partner, are you aware of his scent? Is it a turn-on, toss-up, or a turn-off?

👓 How many times a month are you masturbating? It can be helpful to compare the frequency before and a few moths after you start taking the pill.

👓 Jot down a few things about how your life is going in general. How are things at school, at work, with your friends and roommates? How do you feel about yourself? Do you like yourself?

👓 Do a screen capture of your social media posts. In a few months, this might help you to better recall your mood before you started taking the pill.

👓 Relationship quality: if you are in a relationship, take a pre-pill inventory of what's going right and what's not.

Keep in mind that it's perfectly normal for couples to feel less horny over time, which has nothing to do with the pill. If that's been happening, you'll need to decide if some of it is related to using hormonal birth control or not.

More Reader Comments

"I was on the shot, the ring and the pill. The shot made me bleed for 6 months straight, the ring gave me headaches so bad that I threw up, and the pill made me cry all the time. My next adventure in birth control will be the diaphragm."

female age 26

"I use the NuvaRing, and I love it. I haven't noticed a change in sex drive, but I have noticed that I seem to be constantly wet."

female age 19

"On the pill, it's harder to maintain your weight and tone even when you are eating right and exercising regularly. It fluctuates your water weight and feeling of attractiveness which can affect your desire for sex." *female age 22*

"I'm on the combined pill. My sex drive has dipped a bit, but that may be because the initial lust-driven 'we must have sex every night' has died down a little. Of course, staying at his parents house for two months didn't help." *female age 21*

"I think my sex drive is lower. But it is something that happens gradually, so it is hard to be sure. It definitely makes my discharge thicker, which sometimes makes it a little harder to have sex. I am not as wet and we have to use lube sometimes. I used to be on Ortho Tri-Cyclin Lo, and that had a huge effect on my sex drive. I was extremely depressed and did not want sex at all." *female age 26*

"I was on Mirena for 3 years, and I sunk into a period of low sexual drive. Also, in my 3rd year, it made me have my period every week for 3 weeks at a time. Now that I am on Ortho Tri-Cyclin Lo, I have increased sexual energy, and less problems."
female age 28

"These days I am so horny, that I don't think it's affected me!"
female age 33

"I hate the pill. Makes me a total bitch." *female age 25*

"I used the pill in college—went through three different brands and had so many side effects and very little desire for sex. Now I just use condoms and feel like my horny self again.
female age 25

"When I was on the pill, both combined and pop, I found that my desire definitely waned." *female age 40*

"The pill has totally suppressed my sex drive. I have hardly any desire." *female age 22*

"I use the NuvaRing. I absolutely love it! I no longer forget to take pills, it is more reliable, and my partner doesn't feel it."
female age 21

With Gratitude to Cynthia Graham and John Bancroft for being among the few who are trying to do this kind of research in spite of a pharmaceutical industry has not wanted these questions to be asked.

Rape & Abuse: Good Sex after Bad

Some sexual acts are uninvited and forced, leaving confusion in their wake, especially when the person involved is an otherwise kind and important figure in your life. This chapter looks at the aftermath of abuse and rape with an eye on learning to have good sex after bad. The information it provides is a small drop in a large and sometimes difficult bucket.

While sexual assault is not unique, you are. What works for someone else might not work for you. Be diligent in finding information that is helpful and be cautious when self-described experts tell you what you should do instead of giving you a wide platter to choose from.

The first part of this chapter assumes that the person who experienced the assault or abuse is female and that the perpetrator is male. That's how it usually is, but not always. The last part of the chapter is for straight guys who have been raped by other men, although gay men get raped as well.

Rape Versus Abuse

Rape and abuse are often lumped together, as if the experiences are the same because they are both sex crimes. Depending on who you are and what happened, this may or may not be true. Let's consider two women whose only similarity in life is that both had sex forced on them.

The first woman grew up in a safe and loving home. Her parents were always there for her. The men she chose for lovers were respectful and decent. In times of stress and tumult, her family was a resource she could fall back on. When she was raped at age 24, her family and friends circled the wagons and stood by her. When she was trying to rebuild her sex life after the assault, she had the memory of many satisfying nights with loving men to help her recall that sex could be wonderful as well as wicked.

The second woman had a very different family. The man her mom remarried had sex with her from the time she was 8. When her grades began to drop and she started to become isolated at school, her mom chalked it up to "growing pains." Troublesome signs that a less-chaotic parent would have picked up on went ignored. While the house was well-maintained and she was fed, clothed and clean, home was not a safe place. As she grew into a young woman, her choice of sexual partners reflected the chaos she grew up in.

These two very different women provide a sense that the challenges sexual-assault victims face are not the same. The second woman has no memories to fall back on of sex being wonderful and loving. There was constant emotional abandonment that has become part of the mortar that binds her entire psyche. This is very different from the first woman's challenge regarding her rape, which is to deal with the kinds of issues that one might address after a terrorist attack.

There is also no way of predicting which victims of abuse or rape will have sexual and relationship issues. Some of it has to do with a person's temperament and constitution. It might also have to do with whether there was something good that she could hold onto in her mind.

Sexual Confusion in a House of Abuse

For some women who experienced childhood abuse, the times they were abused might have been the only times they were treated with tenderness. Think of how confusing this must have been. For other women who experienced childhood abuse, the family member might have otherwise been an important and loving part of her life. This can make sorting things out incredibly difficult and confusing.

Equally difficult are situations in which the girl's own mother was jealous of her, as if she were competition for the woman's husband or boyfriend. Non-abused sons who grow up in situations where a girl is being abused can also find it difficult to process what is unfolding around them. Some are isolated and depressed. Others grow up finding it a challenge to respect the sexual rights and emotions of others.

Learning to Have Good Sex After Bad

Women who have been raped or abused sometimes report that their bodies are betraying them. Perhaps it's just that their bodies are trying to protect them, and the nerves and muscles beneath their skin have no way of knowing that the danger has passed.

Think of what happens in your body when a loving partner is tenderly kissing the sides of your neck. As you are becoming sexually aroused, your heart beats faster, you breathe more quickly, and your skin starts to perspire. You might not be consciously aware of it, but your hearing and vision also become more acute.

A woman who has never been abused might experience these body sensations as a sign of the good things to come. But for a woman who has been abused or assaulted, her body is apt to confuse these signs with danger. Far from trying to betray her, her body might be trying to protect her. Her nerves and muscles are still preparing for combat rather than for relaxation and pleasure. So one of the first things a woman might do is to become aware of sexually-charged situations that cause her body tone to go from "Oh boy!" to "Yikes!" or those that make her feel numb or disassociated.

For one woman, the trigger might be a quick, admiring glance from a man in a restaurant. Another woman's body might be totally into having sex until she feels her lover's penis enter her vagina.

As a woman begins to recognize these triggers, she can become more proactive. One woman might find it helpful to stay with the bad feeling and observe how it unfolds within her. Another might remind herself the situation isn't the dangerous one that her body is confusing it with. If it happens during lovemaking, she and her partner might have a signal so they change positions or stop. Maybe her lover can say something reassuring to her, or perhaps they switch on a light so she can physically see his face in addition to hearing the sound of his voice. It might also be helpful if there were comforting environmental cues at the start of their lovemaking, such as certain music or a particular light, or having a special object that she can feel or grasp that helps her feel safe enough to stay in the here and now.

"Initially, my now-husband had to learn how to stop and comfort me when I had flashbacks during sex. Thankfully those no longer occur. I really need to have music on, or something to concentrate on that adds to the sex. If it is silent, or we have relaxing sex without music or awesome satin sheets or something that provides other sensations, then I will have a lot of trouble not disassociating." *female age 27*

Masturbation to the Rescue

For some women who have been sexually abused or assaulted, masturbation can provide an important bridge to healthy sexual enjoyment. When she masturbates, she can retrain her body to anticipate a good sexual outcome. For a woman who has never had a good sexual experience, masturbation can be the first step in learning how good sex can feel. And for a woman who has had good sex in the past, it can be a safe way for her to remember how good sex used to feel.

If she has a trusting, loving relationship with a partner, it might be a huge step for a woman to pleasure herself while he holds her. Hopefully, he can understand how big of a step this can be, and not to feel like she's rejecting him because the sight of his hard penis throws her into a panic. All things in good time.

Her partner will also need to be comfortable with masturbation himself, as there may be times when she suddenly needs to put the brakes on during lovemaking. He needs to have the option of getting himself off by hand. Hopefully they can talk about this, and she can appreciate and respect his need to get off, and he can appreciate and respect her sudden need for space.

"Masturbation had lost a lot of its fun. Isn't that terribly sad? I'm finding it again now, and it makes me proud of myself.
female age 27

"I was a frequent masturbator before the rape, but for a while after I didn't really want any sexual things at all. Masturbating helped me to start enjoying my body again." *female age 19*

[After being raped at age 12] "I was 14 and my older friend was telling me about how she could have orgasms in the shower. I tried it, and the experience was so amazing and so all-my-own that I began to feel a lot better about what sex and sexuality should be." *female age 18*

"Fantasy men were always nice to me—patient, kind, concerned about me, etc. Not like in real life. In a weird way, it taught me what and who to look for in real life." *female age 30*

What Some Women Have Found Helpful

There isn't a right or wrong way to have sex after you have been raped. There are different options, and only you can decide what's right for you. Here are some things other women have found to be helpful:

Setting Limits & Feeling Safe: If the places and situations where you used to date and have sex no longer feel safe, see if it helps to treat yourself like the nervous parents of 16-year-old. Set the kind of limits for yourself that they would for her. Should you be home by 10 or midnight? What about only double-dating with a trusted friend? Don't go to a party without a friend. If you are in a social situation and start to feel unsafe, don't stick around. Go home. If a guy you like asks you to have a beer, there's no reason why you can't say, "Not now, but coffee on Sunday would be really nice." Decide ahead of time how much physical contact you are going to allow—a handshake, a kiss, a feel above the waist, a feel below...

But as the women of the Seattle Institute for Sex Therapy so aptly note, if you discover that you are exclusively selecting men to date who you feel safe with, but who you don't feel sexually attracted to, or it's been a long time and you're still not able to get as sexually excited as you used to, it might be a good idea to seek some counseling.

Re-Virginization: OK, it was bad enough being a virgin the first time! If you are planning on having sex with a guy and you think you might need to stop groping each other midway, or will be needing special reassurance, then it's best to tell him that you had been sexually assaulted. Most guys will be very understanding and will try to help in any way they can once they know what's going on. It's perfectly fine to say, "The old me might have been pulling your pants off by now, but with the new me, it could be a couple of months before you even get to feel under my bra. I have no idea how it's going to go, but I need to be able to totally trust that if I say stop, you'll stop at that very moment."

You should also warn him that you might have days when you can't get enough of him sexually and other days when you have the sexual sensibilities of a 90-year-old nun.

On the days when you need to send him off to the bathroom to masturbate, let him know that it still might be really important that the two of you do something romantic together, like taking a walk, or going to the bookstore or to a movie, or flying a kite, or doing any number of things together that couples like to do. And on those days when you need physical contact but want him to keep his penis in his pants, talk to him about cuddling together, holding hands, or exchanging back or foot rubs. If it's not too much for him or you, a warm bath together or dip in a hot tub might feel great.

If You Have a Partner: Your partner isn't the man who raped you, but he can be almost as affected by the rape as you are. One of the first challenges is that he might try to seriously hurt the rapist. That's to be expected when someone intentionally harms a loved one. And even though you know he wasn't the one who harmed you nor would he ever want to, guys might not be at the top of your most-favored-sex list right now. He will need to be aware that it might take months before sex returns to normal. For other women, things will return to normal much sooner. You can't predict, and you can't tell. Hopefully, he will read all he can and educate himself about the reactions that victims of sexual assault can have, and learn how to be an ally of the healing process. Patience will have its rewards.

Flashbacks: Some women who have been sexually assaulted have flashbacks; others don't. You and your partner need to be aware that flashbacks sometimes happen when you are at the peak of sexual excitement and are orgasming left and right. Your partner needs to understand that flashbacks are not because he is doing anything that's wrong. Learn about the things that trigger flashbacks and come up with a strategy for dealing with them. Have faith that they will decrease with time.

Don't Confuse the Female Body's Protective Mechanism with Being Turned On

Researchers have discovered that there is a difference between what makes a vagina lubricate and what turns a woman on mentally. It is not unusual for a woman's vagina to lubricate in situations where she is frightened or terrified. This will protect her vagina from tearing if intercourse is forced upon her.

This primitive reflex can be very confusing for a woman who has had sex forced on her. For instance, if she had an orgasm while being raped, she might wonder if she has a secret thing for violence and somehow invited the rape. She should understand that other women who have been raped have had orgasms, and those orgasms are the product of a body in terror that's spewing out a flood of adrenalin while physical pressure is being placed on her genitals. This kind of reaction is not limited to women. Erections are no stranger to the gallows. It's been known for many centuries that men who are executed by hanging often die with erections, and some even ejaculate. While this may have something to do with the body's response to asphyxiation, terror also plays a role. These men were no more sexually turned-on by being in the gallows than is a woman in a violent situation in which sex is being forced on her.

Ways to Help Prevent Rape

Before you read about ways to prevent rape, keep in mind that women who have been raped sometimes go overboard in trying to avoid situations that cause them anxiety. The extreme avoidance can reinforce anxiety and stress disorders. So it is important for those who have been raped to conquer the temptation to avoid too much. The key is in using common sense. Do a browser search for practical ways to help prevent rape. Also, never get drunk or stoned outside of the safety of your own home or that of your sexual partner's.

Strategy

According to interviews with incarcerated rapists, they do not pick a victim based on how she looks or how she is dressed. Their first criteria is not getting caught. So what a rapist is looking for is a highly vulnerable victim. He want to be able to easily isolate her from others and to commit his crime without drawing the attention of others.

The sex offender's goal is to find ways to control a victim. He is good at getting women to engage in light forms of romance or sex play, not so much at their invitation, but in a way that she doesn't think to scream "STOP IT!" He manages to take her off-guard, doing things that feel good enough so she gets confused. He will try to physically isolate her and emotionally confuse her. She is suddenly wondering, "Did I invite this?" If she didn't put a stop to it immediately, he will have invaded her personal space and personal boundaries, and then there's no stopping him. After committing his crime, his next goal is to not get caught.

If You Have Been Raped—The First Hours After

The thing you don't want to do is to disturb any of the evidence, and unfortunately, the evidence is on you and in you. Do not shower, douche, wash your hands, change your clothes, drink anything or even brush your teeth. Saliva can be used to identify a rapist as well as his semen. If you think you might have been drugged and you have to urinate, do so in a bottle and take it with you to the hospital. Be sure to tell the doctor about any suspicions of being drugged. The way they find out if you have been drugged is through testing your urine, and some drugs pass through your system quickly. (In some states, the threshold of evidence is lower if it is discovered that the victim was drugged.)

If you are a minor, you don't need to have a parent's permission to have a "rape kit" done at the hospital. So there's no reason to fear going to the hospital if you've been doing something that would make your parents angry.

You should take extra clothing that you can change into after they have collected all the evidence at the hospital. If you can, ask a friend to go with you or to meet you at the hospital. If you live in a dorm, ask a resident advisor to go with you as well. It's OK if the friend stays with you during the exam and during your entire hospital visit. Your friend can be your ears, eyes, and brain. If you or your friend are able, call RAINN (800-656-HOPE). See if there is a victim advocate who can meet you at the hospital.

As a victim of a sexual assault, you have priority over just about everything other than life-threatening illnesses. So unless you see people being wheeled in with panicked-looking doctors hovering around them, you should get in sooner than later. If a long time has gone by, ask your friend to remind the person at the desk that you are a rape victim and haven't been seen. If you prefer a doctor of your same sex, let them know. If they can, they will get you one.

Going to the hospital doesn't mean you need to speak to the police or press charges. But it's essential to go to the hospital for a couple of reasons. If at some point you do decide to press charges, they will have the necessary evidence. It will be much harder otherwise. The people in the ER can give you the morning-after pill to help prevent pregnancy, and they can treat any physical trauma. Going to the hospital right away greatly increases your chances to receive victim's services if you should need them, and in a lot of states, the state will pay for your expenses. The people in the ER should be able to explain your options and connect you with counseling and other help. It is a very, very good idea to visit a hospital emergency room right away. There are virtually no downsides. As with a car accident, you have no idea of the kinds of emotional or physical trauma that might present itself in a couple of days or weeks. Having everything on record at the ER will make it easier for you to get free services if you should need them in the future.

How People Act after Being Raped

There is no manual for how to act after a sexual assault. Some people will be hysterical while others will be unusually calm. Some will be agitated, others will be numb. It is unwise to judge a person's emotional experience of a sexual assault based on their behavior following it.

Rape in Marriage

People assume that rape in a marriage isn't really rape, and it's less serious than sexual assault that is caused by a stranger. But spousal rape might be even more devastating than stranger rape. The stranger never said, "To have and to hold, to love and to cherish, till death do us part." Women who are raped by their husbands are likely to be raped a number of times before finally leaving. The rape can be oral, anal and vaginal. Dealing with it can be a particular challenge when the victim lives with the rapist.

Further Humiliation

Some rapists will force their victims to pretend they are enjoying the rape. Rape experts indicate that it's a good idea to go along with the rapist on this one if he is so inclined. It seems that if the rapist is unable to complete the act, he is more apt to further injure his victim. Think of how seriously imbalanced he is mentally if he wants you to pretend you are enjoying the experience.

Whether to Report—If It's Child Abuse

While it is important that a child who is being abused can find a trusting teacher, counselor, minister or parent to tell, reporting doesn't always improve the situation. For some girls, it makes it worse, as dysfunctional families will often try to make her the problem. There is also the reality that while some state protective services agencies are top-notch, others are as dysfunctional as the families they are supposed to be protecting children from. Between failures of the criminal-justice system and an overwhelmed social-services system, good outcomes are sometimes the exception rather than the rule.

Complicating matters further is the fact that some children make false accusations. Equally disturbing are the number of divorces where one angry parent accuses the other parent of abuse out of revenge. If they are so sure the other parent was abusing the child, why didn't they say something about it before the divorce? This shouldn't be confused with situations where the divorce came as a result of learning that a child was being abused.

Whether to Report—If You Are an Adult and It's Rape

It's no secret that few rapes are actually reported. The percentage of reports is even lower in rapes where the victim knew the offender prior to the sexual assault. There are reasons why women don't report. A common one is if the rapist is a member of your social circle or your mother's favorite cousin. Or if he's your sister's husband or a popular guy at work or school.

Other reasons for not reporting include fears that you won't be believed, fears that you will be blamed, and fears that the accused will retaliate. Some women believe that if they didn't put up a fight, the state won't consider it rape. This is not true. Not fighting may have been the best way to prevent further injury or death. The fact that you are still alive indicates that you did the smartest thing possible. While fighting may have stopped the rape, it could have just as easily ended up in you being killed or seriously injured beyond any sexual trauma.

So why should you report? There are three very good reasons:

1. Rapists tend to be bullies who may see your failure to report as an indication that you liked what they did, or that you are an easy mark for a repeat offense. Reporting a rapist can protect you from re-assault rather than putting you in harm's way.

2. One of the greatest regrets among women who don't report is knowing that their lack of action may have made it possible for the rapist to sexually assault other women. This fact, even more than the rape itself, is what haunts some women the most.

3. Even if the man is not convicted, your report puts him on law-enforcement radar. It makes it less likely that he will get away with it the next time. Even if he is not convicted, your reporting is what might save his potential victims.

Reporting—If He's In Your Social Circle

Reporting is socially easier if the rapist isn't part of your social circle. If he is, be prepared for people taking sides, and not necessarily yours. On the other hand, if you don't report, he will know you are an easy target, and you will have to live with knowing he will most likely be victimizing others. Don't waste time trying to warn him or threaten him. Your actions in not reporting him are all he will hear.

If you have reported someone from your social circle, it's probably best not to discuss it. Don't try to defend yourself or to say anything negative about him. The only people you should be speaking to about it are the police, the DA and your healthcare provider or counselor if you have one. Keeping these boundaries will hopefully make it easier for you in the long run.

Reporting—If You Are in a Sorority

Hopefully, things in the Greek system have evolved and justice is more important than keeping quiet to maintain the social order. But understand that if you were raped and report a fraternity member to the police, his house brothers will likely feel that you have reported all of them as well. And your sorority sister who had a secret crush on the guy? Get ready to meet your new worst enemy.

You won't read this advice in the "Welcome To Our Wonderful College!" booklets, but if you've been raped by a fraternity bro and decide to report him, get thee to the psych library and read about what happens in dysfunctional families when a child reports that she's been abused. Knowing how strange it can get will help you maintain a sense of irony and perspective that could be necessary if a psychodrama were to unfold around you. People join fraternal organizations with the hope of being a part of something that's bigger and better than they are. In accusing a fraternity man of rape, you are not only threatening the relationship between your sorority and his fraternity, you are taking to task the very system that has been the spawning ground of presidents, senators and supreme-court justices.

Does this mean you shouldn't report? Heck no. But it does mean that you will be standing out as an individual in an organization that is not exactly the Walden Pond of free thinking. The priority of some sorority with is to party with boys with pedigrees. They are likely to see you, rather than a fraternity man who takes uninvited liberties with his penis, as the problem.

If you are in a sorority and you report a fraternity man for rape, or if you are in any tightly-knit organization and report a fellow member, be prepared to move out and move on. But think about it: in a world where people are tortured and killed for speaking the truth, is having to find new friends such a huge price to pay for doing the right thing? Is it such a huge price to pay for helping to protect other women this person might victimize throughout his life, because that's who will suffer if there is no price to pay for sex that is forced. In the long run, wouldn't you rather be known as a woman not to mess with?

If you are raped by a fraternity member and your sorority sisters stand by you, understand you have found something truly precious.

When Straight Men are Raped by other Men

Most of us believe that rape happens to only women and gay or imprisoned men. We assume that any man who doesn't want to be sexually assaulted should be able to defend himself and fend off the attacker. But just because you are a guy doesn't mean you should be able to beat up a mugger or fend off a rapist. Rape is first and foremost about violence, power, sadism and hatred. The rapist didn't choose you because he thought you had a cute butt. He chose you because he thought he could dominate you.

When you've got a gun to your head or a knife to your throat, you suddenly have other priorities than to say, "Excuse me, Mr. Rapist, you've got it all wrong. I like girls!" Your job is to survive, and even if that means having to go down on the guy, you should do it and not think twice. Think of how many women have given you oral sex and didn't pass out!

In addition to being blind-sided with a lethal weapon, a man can be sexually assaulted by a group of men he doesn't stand a chance against. Sometimes the rape can be the result of blackmail or of being drunk or stoned. The last thing a guy who is drunk is going to be able to protect is his rear end.

Male rape can happen in other ways, as well. Not too long ago, a former National Hockey League Player revealed that he was sexually assaulted by one of his coaches when he was a teen.

Unfortunately, a man who has been raped has fewer options than a woman who has been raped. Think about it: how many guys are going to find it cathartic to tell their friends they were raped? The chances are his drinking buds will assume it's a joke.

If you are a guy who has been raped, call a rape-crisis center or even if you are the epitome of straightness, call a gay-men's health center. They tend to be understanding and helpful about sexual violence against men.

It can be really confusing if you became hard or came when you were being raped. But it's not unusual to have an erection and orgasm when the body is under extreme stress or panic. As mentioned earlier in this chapter, plenty of guys who go to the gallows meet their maker with an erection and semen in their pants.

Some rapists are aware that you might get an erection. They will intentionally stroke you to orgasm just to mess with your mind even more. So what's the big deal if you did get hard and came? The important thing is in understanding that you were violently assaulted. We should all have erections and orgasms in such situations. At least you lived to think about it, which is a very good thing.

Men who are bisexual or gay sometimes worry that being raped or abused is what gave them their same-sex orientation. And straight guys who are sexually assaulted by other males might wonder if this will impact their sexual orientation. Studies have never shown that sexual abuse or rape influences a person's sexual orientation, yet this is a myth that persists.

While you might want to keep it all inside, it could be the rape has been causing you to deal with intimate relationships in strange ways. What do you have to lose by speaking to a counselor about it for a session or two? As for reporting, the big issue is how strongly you feel about the guy being able to do this to other men, because it is likely that he will if he can.

Thanks to Stephen Braveman specializes in the sex abuse of men, including sexual abuse of men in the military.

Resources (Your state or county may have resources as well):

National Center for Victims of Crime
(855) 484-2846 or 855-4-VICTIM

Rape, Abuse, and Incest National Network
(800) 656-4673 or (800) 656-HOPE

National Domestic Violence Hotline
(800) 799-7233 or (800) 799-SAFE

Recommended Reading:

Evicting the Perpetrator by Ken Singer.

Principles of Trauma Therapy: A Guide to Symptoms, Evaluation, and Treatment by John Briere and Catherine Scott.

Child Trauma Handbook: A Guide For Helping Trauma-exposed Children And Adolescents by Ricky Greenwald.

Treating Nonoffending Parents in Child Sexual Abuse Cases: Connections for Family Safety by Jill Levenson and John Morin.

Just Before Dawn: Trauma Assessment and Treatment of Sexual Victimization by Jan Hindman

Victims No Longer: The Classic Guide for Men Recovering from Sexual Child Abuse by Mike Lew.

Readers Speak

"I was dating one guy for four years (I was 16 when it started). Over time he became more and more thoughtless during sex until the point where it had crossed the line into violence. If sex was painful he would not stop, and there was emotional violence. We started out using porn to enhance our sex lives, but after a while he would position us so he could ignore me during sex and just watch the screen. I did two years of being single without sex after that to pull myself together. When I began having sex again I had flashbacks and would panic. I used to be so sexually outgoing and playful. I would enjoy oral sex. Now I don't do that anymore. For a long time I could not joyfully give my partners oral sex because of the negative associations with it, and sometimes I still have trouble not choking, even when it is barely in my mouth. Things are slowly improving, but I am worried it will never have that carefree way about it. It is hard to relax and not over protect myself. I've been married for a year now to a wonderful and gentle man that I've been intimate with for five years.... That's how long it's taken." *female age 27*

"I have been raped twice in my life by two separate men. The first was during my 16th birthday. After the party I went to my friend's spare bedroom to sleep. My then-boyfriend came in and lay next to me. We started fooling around but things started going too far. I asked him to stop but he didn't. He kept pressuring me, saying he wouldn't do anything serious. It ended with him just shoving himself in me while I was sobbing. That was how I lost my virginity. The saddest part is that I stayed with him for two more months. The second time I was at a friend's house. Drinking and playing Dungeons and Dragons. (Yes, girls are nerds too.) I drank far too much and lay down on a mattress that was sitting in the middle of the living room. All my friends went into the den to watch TV while this guy lay next to me. I should have figured it out then, but I was really drunk. I asked him to leave me because I was too drunk to be near anyone, let alone a guy with 'intentions.' He didn't leave. He started with the foreplay. I alternated between liking it and asking him to go away. It ended with him on top of me while I told him to stop. I suppose this one was partially my fault. Needless to say, the friendship ended there. Sex since then? I've never orgasmed. That may be due to the fact that I can't trust men. I'm never comfortable being naked around anyone. And to be completely honest, I don't really like sex. I think I'm just expecting men to mistreat me after having it. To just use me. Recently I have been in a relationship with a man who was a virgin before we had sex. His love and trust have gone a long way toward helping me believe that a guy might like me for more than just sex. It's helping me to enjoy myself more." *female age 20*

"I was continually abused growing up (emotionally, spiritually, verbally, mentally, sexually), so much so I don't remember much of it. I continued the abuse voluntarily by getting involved with men who abused me. For instance, I have two kids as a result of 3-a.m. encounters when I was three-quarters asleep. I'm still pretty badly messed up and have a hard time seeing when someone is trying to be decent. I have never had normal sex. I discovered recently (in the past two years) that what I thought was normal was far from normal. I never knew that you were supposed to have feeling inside. I thought it was normal to be numb inside. My former partner could stick any number of fingers up inside me, and I could never tell him how many there were. He could even put a whole fist inside, and I didn't know. He could scratch and wiggle–nothing, nada, zip, zero, zilch. Still have that problem. Maybe I'll figure it out someday." *female age 31*

"When I was in middle school, and my body was just starting to mature, my step-dad was going through a rough time with work. He was pretty stressed. My mom was around, but she had a job so I was left alone with a man who I wasn't exactly fond of. He started getting a little too close and intimate for comfort. I told him I didn't like it. When he didn't stop, I told my mom. She didn't want to believe me. One night while she was out with her friends, I woke up and he was on top of me. I tried to scream. He stifled me. 'It'll feel good, I promise,' he told me. It didn't feel good. I screamed and flailed my body until I could get away. I ran and tried to hide. He found me and hit me so hard that I don't remember any more of that night. I was 12." I was ashamed of my body for a long time after that. But at the same time, I still really wanted the fellas who were my own age to take notice of me. I think I was looking for someone who would try to protect me. Eventually, I found myself in a good relationship that was much more about the emotional connection than a physical one. When we finally did get to that point, I felt so at ease with him that it was completely natural, pure and honest [and way good!]." *female age 18*

"I was 9 years old. My karate instructor gave me a lesson in oral sex and other such matters. This was 32 years ago. I was not in a huge hurry to lose my *official virginity.* But then I had a great boyfriend for my *first time,* so it worked out. Get someone to talk to—a professional—and don't stop until you find one that helps you to release the pain or anger. It's possible to have good sex after bad IF you take it slow and find the right person. I think about sex not as something that is being done to me, but as something that I am giving to someone else." *female age 41*

"I was molested by my dad & younger brother. It took years of therapy to overcome self-destructive behavior. The abuse took a seemingly wholesome, enjoyable act, and made it ugly. I became psychotically self-destructive with sex, alternating between frigidity and promiscuity. I was able to find good therapist and a good man who loves me. I can finally breathe and trust, relax, have fun, and enjoy sex. (We're getting married later this year.)" *female age 30*

"It was seven years ago. In my room. My cousin's husband attacked me while I was sleeping. I never had sex before then. I look at sex as something that I don't need. Sometimes it just brings back the night of the bad. My advice? Take control next time. You'd be surprised at how much better it can be the next time that way! If it's happened to you, don't hesitate to tell someone else. I didn't, and I'm still paying for it. It took me four years to come to the reality of it. Don't hide anything. If you've been raped, don't think of sex as bad. Think of it as a way to better yourself." *female age 20*

"Report it right away. My biggest regret is that I never did. The man who raped me raped others. Maybe if I had said something, they would never had to experience that. And get counseling. Don't just sit there and blame yourself. Always remember it wasn't your fault, and it doesn't make YOU a bad person." *female age 20*

"When I was about 7 or 8 years old, I was masturbated by an uncle. He gave me a dollar to 'not tell.' I never did. I began having sex at age 13 and was quite promiscuous. I believe I've had about 50 sexual partners, but only 6 or 7 of those in the past 10 or 12 years. I now realize that my behavior probably has something to do with the experience. I've learned to forgive, and to realize that people are better than their worst moments." *female age 33*

"I can't imagine a single situation in which rushing out and boning the first willing, semi-attractive person with a pulse is a good idea to help you overcome an unfortunate sexual encounter." *female age 18*

"Relax and take your time. My fiancee and I weren't exactly rockin' the first few times. I needed to build trust and security, and then I could relax and truly enjoy myself." *female age 30*

"When I was 6- to 8-years-old, my best friend's dad molested me. He would make me give him oral sex, and touch him, and he'd touch me.... I try not to make too big of a deal about it. I have good relationships with women and like to think I am a relatively emotionally stable person. However, I still have frequent dreams about him abusing me, and sometimes I have sex fantasies about him as well. These disturb me because he abused me. I was so young that I think I repressed most of the negative thoughts. All I can remember are the way things felt." *male age 21*

A Very Special Thanks to Robin J. Wilson, David S. Prescott, and to Alessandra Rellini at the University of Vermont and Cindy Meston for making the introduction! These are some of the most thoughtful, intelligent and caring people I have ever had the pleasure of working with.

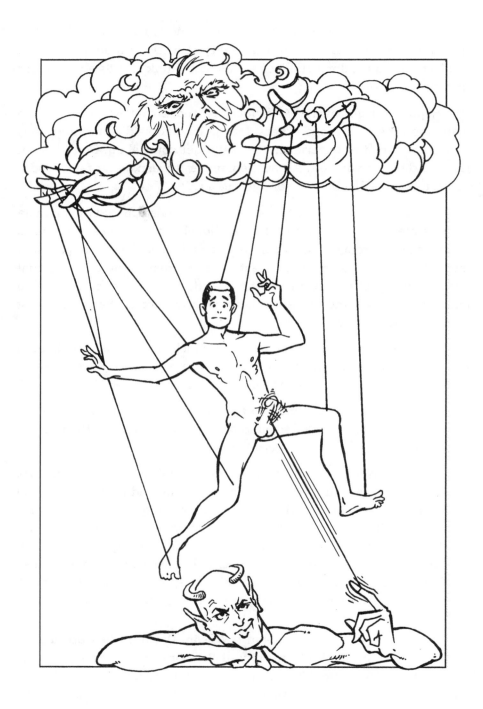

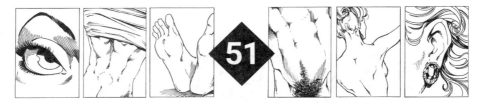

God, Sex and Goodbye!

When people ask why I wrote this book on sex, I usually say it was revenge for eight years in Catholic school. But even before I went to school, I had started to appreciate the influence of religion on people's lives—both good and bad.

One of my earliest memories as a child was being at a holy-roller revival in a big tent with people waving their arms in the air and begging the Lord to save their souls. (Our family wasn't evangelical, but the baby-sitter was.)

Later, as a teenager, I would revisit the revivals out of curiosity. Revivals were like the circus. They rolled into town for a couple of days, and then rolled out in the dark of night. The county where we lived was poor, so it was interesting to see the Evangelists arrive in shiny new Cadillacs.

At what seemed like a pre-arranged moment during the revival, one of the women who had arrived in the new Caddys would start screaming that she'd had inoperable cancer and had been saved by Jesus. She would then crawl up the aisle to the collection basket, waving serious amounts of cash as she wept and wailed. Sometimes the preacher would lay his hands on her and she would faint, other times not.

On the second night of the revival, at the very same moment, this same woman would be wearing a different colored wig and would scream that the Lord had saved her from the ravages of alcoholism and sexual excess. Again, with big bills in each hand. Many in the audience followed, admitting to their own transgressions of the flesh, and asking that Satan be cast from their souls.

The most important thing I learned at the revivals wasn't that they were well-planned and highly orchestrated. Rather, it was their impact on the people who went to them. Even to my young self, I could see how

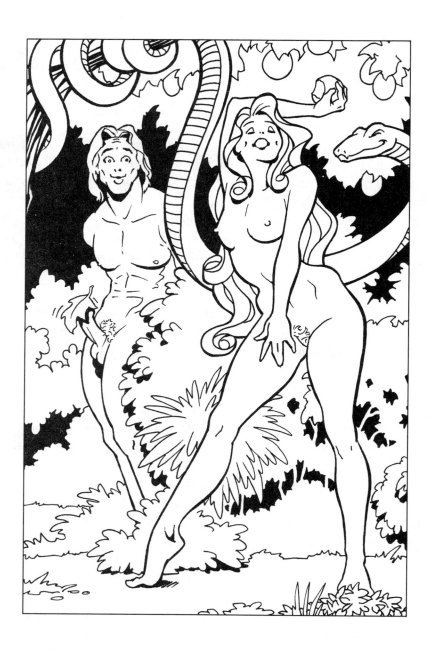

these events put hope into the lives of people who didn't have much. It's where they went to confess and be saved, until the next time.

Maybe that's why people would show up at those revival tents and wave their arms in the air and not notice that the woman who started the parade of bill-waving sinners was a ringer from the bank of the preacher. I didn't know then, and I still don't know, if that was such a bad thing. It's hard for any of us to live our lives without hope.

As for my own personal experience with religion and hope, there was a radio evangelist by the name of Brother Popoff who I sometimes listened to on the all-night radio station that beamed up from Mexico. He was on after The Wolfman. If you sent him money, he promised to send you a special prayer cloth. So I taped some dimes and quarters to a card, and sent him what I had.

A few weeks later, a piece of red cloth arrived in the mail. It was about one-foot square, with no seams on the sides. The accompanying note said for me to lay it over anything that was troubling me. So I went to bed every night with that red prayer cloth tucked inside the front of my briefs.

I never did see much of a dividend, but then again, not too many people go on to write books on sex that sell a million copies.

Vaya Con Dios!

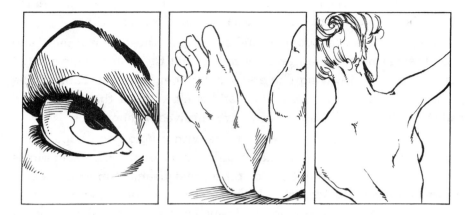

Free Chapters at Guide2Getting.com

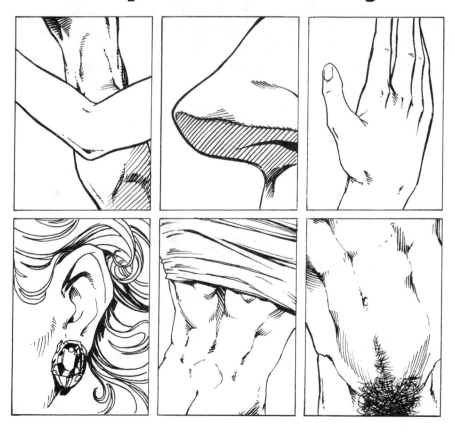

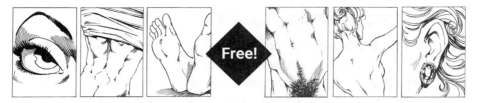

Why I Put The Next 16 Chapters And the Glossary On The Website

I originally wrote this book for people who wanted to have better sex. But then it started winning awards and being used in college sex-ed courses. So I tried to make the book all things to all people, and it started to grow, and grow, and grow. It grew to 1,200 pages and cost nearly $30 US dollars.

People started to feel overwhelmed by its size. They weren't reading it like they did earlier editions that weren't so huge. So with this new edition, I've worked hard to take the *Guide To Getting It On* back to its roots. It is more than 500 pages shorter, which allows it to be less than $20 US dollars. It is also the most up-to-date book on sex you will find and the most fun to read.

To accomplish these changes, there were some chapters that were near and dear to my heart that I needed to leave out. They were chapters in the second half of the book that a lot of people didn't read, but they were some of my favorites. For instance, I had spent more than a year writing the chapter on *Sex in the 1800s*. If you think that today's surge in nationalism and blaming immigrants for all that ails us is new, this would be the chapter to read. It also explains how modern dating came to be.

I have made these chapters available as free downloads on the book's website at www.Guide2Getting.com/free. As an added benefit, the book's illustrator colorized the illustrations from these chapters by hand. I've included a brief description of what the chapters cover in the pages that follow, and I've included the illustrations from them. I hope you'll have fun comparing these illustrations in black and white with the color versions in the free chapters you can download.

I also moved the book's extensive 50-page glossary of sex terms and sex slang to the website as well. You'll find every word there!

Chapter: **Explaining Sex to Kids**

This chapter doesn't pretend to have all the answers about children and sex; it's simply a way of getting you to think about the subject before most parents do, which is sometimes too late for an effective response. Topics range from talking about genitals and masturbation to periods, sex play and porn. *Read the entire chapter for free at Guide2Getting. com/kids.*

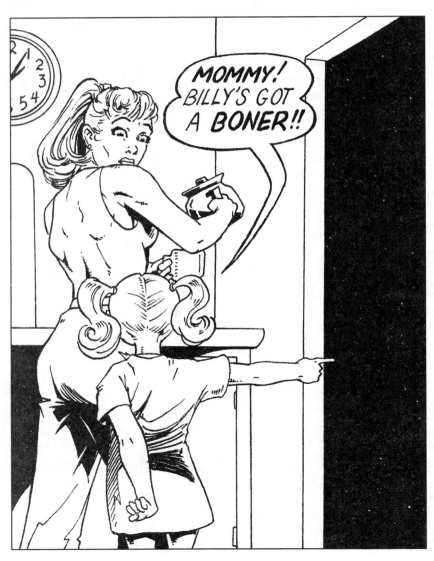

Chapter: **The Historical Breast & Bra**

Before the 1920s, women were skeptical about bras. They preferred to wear corsets. Yet today, there's hardly a woman in Western culture who doesn't have bras, including a favorite one or two. She can also make a sexual statement by not wearing a bra. And there are plenty of straight teenage boys who equate success in dating with whether a girl let him take her bra off (or took it off for him).

This chapter looks at breasts and the bras that hold them up. It begins with a peek at breasts in different times and different places. It then focuses on the fascinating evolution of the bra: how it came to be in 1860, and why bras didn't become "sexy" until more than 70 years later. *Get the chapter at Guide2Getting. com/breasts.*

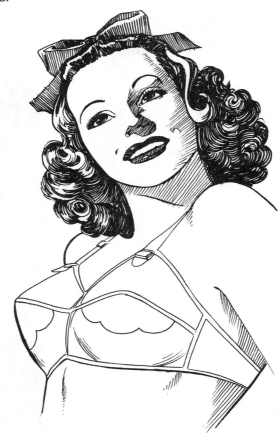

Chapter: Sex during Pregnancy

Some pregnant women will want more intimacy than ever before, while others will want space—sometimes huge amounts of space. This can be confusing for a dad-to-be, as he is never quite sure if the love of his life wants to snuggle or pluck his eyes out. Also, don't think that the dad-to-be isn't experiencing his own set of pregnancy-related emotions. These may cause him to hesitate sexually while his child-to-be is turning somersaults half a penis-length away. The mom-to-be might be wanting to rip his clothes off, and he's suddenly prim and proper.

This chapter is about sex during pregnancy, from orgasm-related uterine contractions to swelling vulvas and fetal brain development. *Read the entire chapter at www.Guide2Getting.com/pregnancy.*

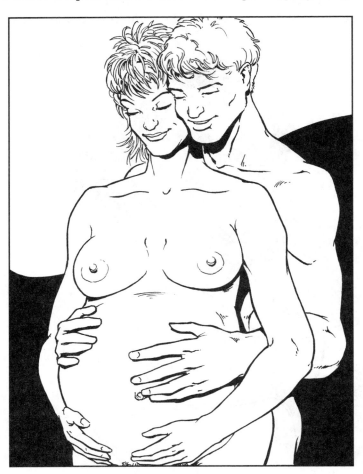

Chapter: On Needles and Pins
Piercings, Tattoos & Sex

Who knew that "tramp stamps" would show up on the butts of more women than tear drops in prison-yard tattoos? At least 24% of people ages 18 to 50 have tattoos and 14% have body piercings. For young adults between 18 and 25, the number of body piercings increases to between 35% and 50%, and this doesn't include pierced ears. If you want to know how any of that impacts sex, this is a chapter to read! *Get it for free at Guide-2Getting.com/piercings.*

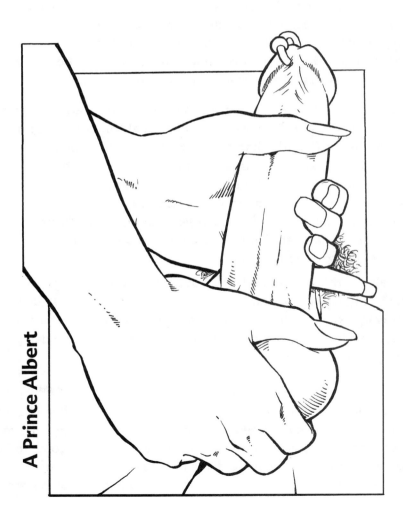

A Prince Albert

Chapter: Sex & Breast, Brain & Ball Cancer

After seeing the title of this chapter, you are probably thinking, "Just the uplifting chapter I've been wanting to read!" Actually, you might be surprised.

If you are wondering about the subject of sex and cancer, the following account of a 37-year-old reader with breast cancer might be helpful. The readers' experiences that fill this chapter contain tips and suggestions that are better than what's in much of the professional literature.

"I hate cancer, hate having lost a breast. I went through a horrid jealous phase, envying other women their whole breasts, their health, their fertility (treatments put me into early menopause). But that's a draining response, so I don't dwell on it. Now, I just try to appreciate beauty when I see it."

"Treatments for cancer can cause discomfort, fatigue and intense pain. Still, it's possible to be sexual throughout treatment, just differently than before. Self-pleasure through masturbation is easiest because you set the pace. Try masturbating even if you have a partner because then you can guide them as to what feels best. I started with self-pleasure for sleep and pain relief a few days after surgery. Later, masturbating in front of my partner also helped be a turn-on at times when I didn't feel up to active sex."

"I talked with my best friend about sex and body image. She said, 'You know, no man has ever pursued us for our fabulous cleavage. We both have small breasts, so we are beautiful and desirable for other reasons,' and then she gave this wonderful dirty chuckle..." *female age 37*

This is from a reader whose 20-year-old boyfriend has brain cancer:

"Sometimes we have sex just to feel closer in a hard time like after we heard he was going to need a second surgery. It's comforting to be that close to the person you love and know that nothing is going to happen to them right then, even if outside of those moments you are living in constant fear." *Get the chapter at www.Guide2Getting.com/cancer.*

Chapter: **Men's Underwear**

It used to be that men's underwear was anything but sexy. Then, manufacturers like Calvin Klein teamed up with homoerotic photographers to make men look hot in their white briefs. Mind you, the men they used in their photo shoots would have looked sexy wearing a loincloth made of cornhusks. The real emphasis of these ads boiled down to the bulge in the crotch—with all visual roads drawing your eye to the package behind the fly. The ads had two primary targets: gay men and straight women who buy underwear for their husbands and boyfriends. Nail these two groups, and straight men are putty in the corporate hand.

Read the chapter at www.Guide2Getting.com/briefs.

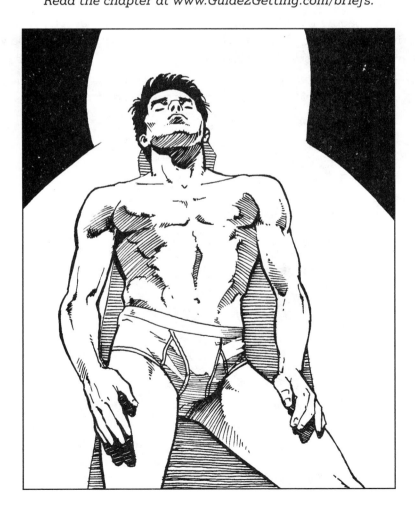

Chapter: **Sex When You Are Horny & Disabled**

A 22-year-old man with cerebral palsy who has virtually no control over his body's movements started using his wheelchair as an antisocial ramming device. He eventually wrote on his word-board that he was so horny he couldn't stand it anymore. Although his body has the same sexual urges and desires as an able-bodied 22-year-old, he has no ability to walk, talk, access porn, or masturbate like other young adults.

As quickly as they began, this young man's wheelchair tantrums stopped. The reason? A nurse's aide mercifully began giving him handjobs. But then she was caught and fired instantly. The board-and-care home threatened to file a complaint against her for sexual abuse.

Many people not only disapprove of sex for the severely disabled, but find the concept offensive. They feel we need to protect people who are disabled from sex. This chapter does not agree. *www.Guide2Getting.com/disabled.*

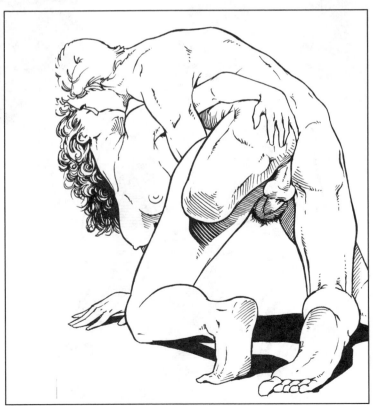

Chapter: Shaving Down Below

"I'm more aware of myself and my sexuality when I'm shaved. It feels sensual, like the first time you wear silk underwear. It's too much trouble to keep up, though. If there was an easy way, I think I'd do it more often." *female age 36*

"Shaving is painful and I look about 12 years old, it grosses me out. Trimming works! Borrow a beard trimmer and go for it! One crew cut coming up!" *female age 29*

We have managed to put golf carts on Mars and we've engineered cows with genes that nature never intended. But we have yet to find a particularly good way to remove unwanted body hair. In this chapter, we look at temporary methods for removing unwanted body hair like shaving and waxing, then at permanent methods

Read the entire chapter at www.Guide2Getting.com/shaving.

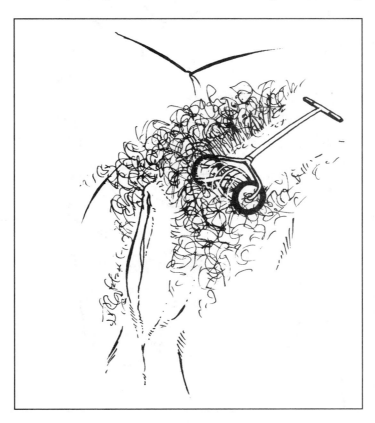

Chapter: **Sex & Hysterectomy**

Does this illustration make you feel uncomfortable? Many women have their ovaries and uteruses removed, which is the equivalent of a man having his testicles taken off. The chapter looks at whether having a uterus removed impacts a woman's experience of sex. *Read the entire chapter at www.Guide2Getting.com/hysterectomy.*

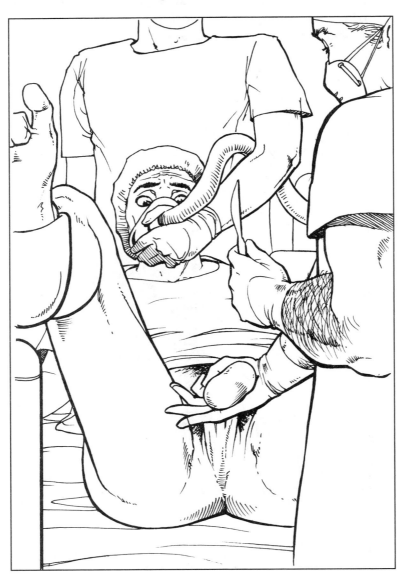

Chapter: Talking To Your Partner about Sex

"Students will often say, 'Okay, so I know communication and feedback are so important, but I just don't know what to say or how to bring it up. So I end up not saying anything because I don't want to upset my partner or ruin the moment.'"

> — *from a college instructor who uses*
> *'The Guide' in his sex ed courses*

This chapter offers tips and suggestions to hopefully make it easier for you to talk to your partner about sex.

Read the entire chapter at www.Guide2Getting.com/talking.

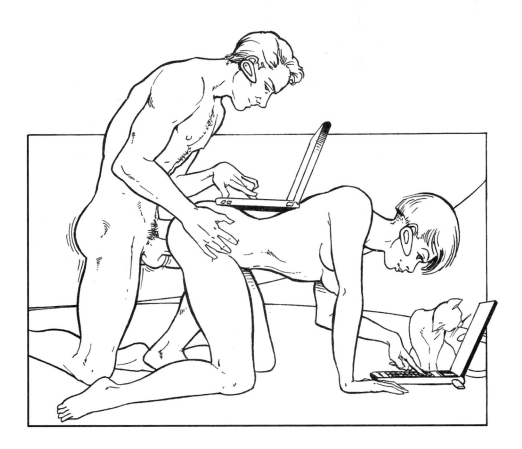

Chapter: Intersex

When we talk about a person's sex or gender, we're usually talking about whether they are male or female. This is generally based on what's between their legs and what is in their chromosomes. We think of a person's sex or gender as an either-or thing—pull down their pants, and either a penis or vagina will be staring back at you. While this is true for the vast majority of people, it's a distinction humans make, not nature. Nature is not constricted by pink or blue.

Nature made the sexes on a continuum, with most of our bodies falling toward one end or the other. However, there are a number of people born with an intersex condition, where their genitals don't shout "Boy!" or "Girl!" Many people with intersex conditions look typically male or female on the outside, but inside there may be some blending of the parts we call male and female. An example is the girl who is a high-school cheerleader and who feels 100% female. A lot of straight guys get a stirring in their pants when she walks by. But she has what's called androgen insensitivity syndrome or AIS. She has XY chromosomes like most men do but her androgen receptors did not work like those of a typical male. So she has a woman's brain and a woman's body, and her genitals like those of most other girls', but her vagina isn't quite as deep as that of a woman who is XX and she doesn't have ovaries. Chances are, she won't learn about her AIS until she goes to see a gynecologist to find out why her friends have started their periods but she hasn't. To say that she's in for a bit of a surprise is to put it mildly, but this doesn't change the fact that she's every bit as much a girl as any other female at her school.

Read the entire chapter at www.Guide2Getting.com/intersex.

Chapter: Barbie The Icon

You might be wondering why Barbie received her own chapter, and why it was one of my most favorite chapters. Perhaps the following comments from readers will explain:

"I had lots of Barbies. She and my giant panda bear got naked and 'did it,' and my sister and I dressed her up in Ken's clothes." *female age 18*

"My Barbie had Ken on her ALL the time. If I knew then what I know now, Barbie would have been on top more often." *female age 44*

"She had kinky fantasies and a lot of BDSM. Barbie was a fun girl." *fem 18*

"Yes, my Barbies had sex. And since I also had a twelve-inch Luke Sky-walker doll, they did it A LOT." *female age 34*

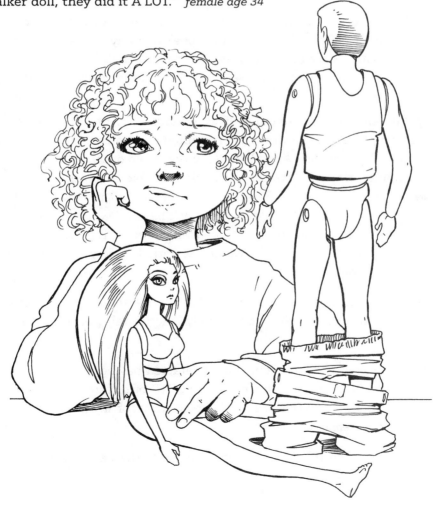

"My friend had a Ken and we used to make them have sex by making their little plastic bodies rub against each other when they were lying in Barbie's little nylon bed. We were about ten and were disappointed that Ken's underwear was glued on." *female age 22*

"My basement was a temple to Barbie and all her relatives. Barbie lived in a soap opera complete with abortions, sex changes, and adultery. She and Ken frequently got naked in their Laura Ashley canopy bed." *fem 24*

"Barbie and Ken had a very active relationship and 'sex' life. It's hard to say it was a sex life without any genitalia. I guess I used them to emulate the adults around me. Barbie and Ken often went skinny dipping at the ocean, and slept nude most times." *female age 35*

"You know those parts in movies that parents were always trying to hide from younger children? I got a slight peek one day, but all I saw were sheets moving. After I saw that, Barbie and Ken made those sounds and simulated those actions. But I wasn't sure what they were really doing."
female age 22

"My Barbies had intimate family lives, detailed jobs, etc. There was a lot of adultery in Barbie's world which resulted in divorces, private investigators, and alcoholism. All the adultery was acted out in full detail, from Ken coming on to his secretary at work to Barbie throwing all of Ken's clothes out the window... Barbie helped me act out my own questions about being an adult. I'm a feminist now, I have a healthy relationship, earn more than my spouse, don't wear make-up or high-heeled shoes, and my husband helps with all the housework. It's okay to let little girls play with Barbie." *female age 24*

"There was one summer when I was fairly obsessed with the fact that Ken had no dick. Beach Ken had a totally inaccurately placed suggestion of one, but no balls." *female age 21*

"I think I was 7 or 8 when our Barbies started having all sorts of high-drama romances, and there were ALL SORTS of different sexual experiences going on. My Barbies were a big outlet for my sexual curiosity growing up." *female age 22*

See the entire chapter at www.Guide2Getting.com/barbie

Chapter: Kink in the Animal Kingdom

"Humans are the only animals who have sex for pleasure in addition to reproduction." "Non human animals only have sex for reproduction and dominance." Until recently, this is what many biologists had told us. Fortunately, they have been reconsidering the idea that humans are the only animals who like to have sex for more than just dominance and reproduction. *Read the entire chapter at www.Guide2Getting.com/ kingdom.*

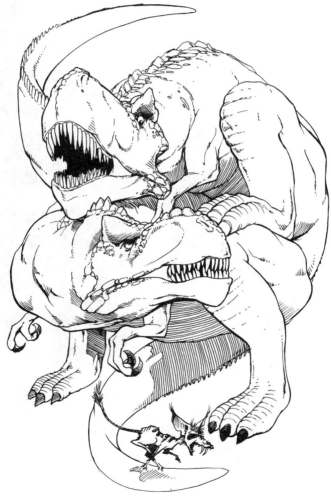

An artist's conception of how the tyrannosaurus had sex, eg "I got some tail last night." (Thanks to dinosaur artist Luis Rey for inspiration.)

Chapter: What's Masculine, Feminine & Erotic?

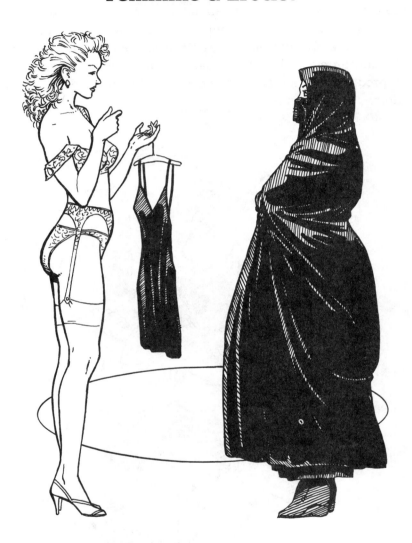

Who is the sexual prisoner:

    a. The Western Woman

    b. The Moslem Woman

    c. Neither

    d. Both

Once you start chipping away at what's masculine and feminine in different cultures, you can't help but notice that these are concepts that are often constructed by society. But there are also fascinating layers and nuances that we look at in this chapter. *Read the entire chapter at www.Guide2Getting.com/roles*

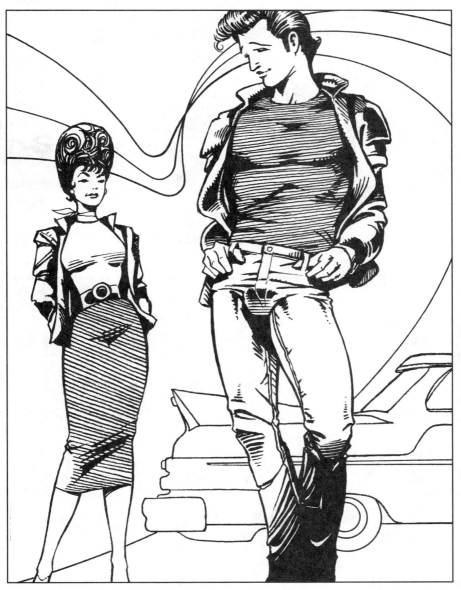

Sex roles, anyone?

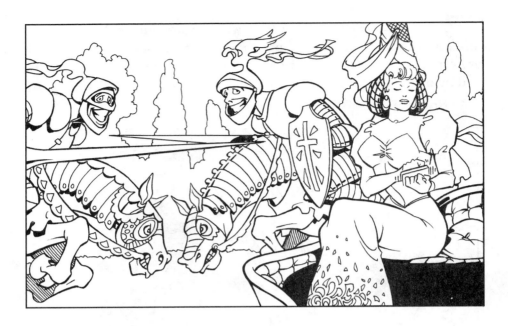

*Are these sex-role differences
due to biology, culture, custom or some of each?*

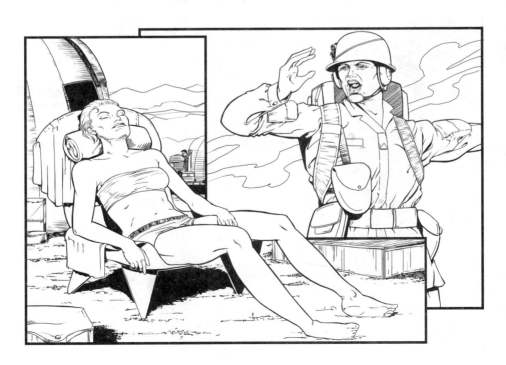

Chapter: Sex in the Military

"Things the military could do to help sex be better? Make the damn uniforms easier to get out of!" *female, age 19*

"My sister, who is also in the service is married to a serviceman. She recently returned from a TDY (temporary duty) assignment, and while there, engaged in an extramarital affair with another married serviceman. These things happen a lot." *female age 25*

It's not like soldiers leave their sex drives in their home towns. But providing helpful information about sex for new recruits is not a priority of the military. So we have put this information together based on clandestine reports from the field. Hopefully, this book's intelligence is better than that of some governmental agencies. Here's from an interview with a member of Special Services who was on leave from Afghanistan:

Some soldiers say they are too exhausted or traumatized to want very much sex when they're in combat. What's it been like for you?

"I enjoy sex and have it whenever I can. I have a much higher sex drive now than when I was in high school. My body is on hyper alert when I'm out on patrol and I can't shut it off just because I'm back at base. After what I see and do out there, the sex helps me reconnect with a sense of humanity."

Where do you find sex in Afghanistan?
There's a lot of sex on base!!!

What about prostitution?
I've been with prostitutes in Iraq and in Afghanistan. They're not out in the open, but you can find them if you ask around. Some that I've been with speak English. I've spent entire nights just talking with them. The women are exotic, and I find that very appealing. It's different than being with a woman here at home.

What about the female soldiers on base? Are they up for sex?
This isn't going to sound so good, but there's a lot of people having a lot of sex on base and I don't see relationships back home being a detriment. If you work hard to please a woman on base sexually, and you do a good job, the women will talk about you to other women. Word gets around if you're good and who you are, so it's not at all unusual for a woman to come around in the afternoon or night and ask if you're available to have sex. It's real straightforward, nobody gets embarrassed, none of the games like when you're back home. If you're available and

she's someone you'd like to have sex with, then you say yes. Or maybe you'll say I'm really sorry, but there's already someone I'll be with tonight.' And yes, the women have sex with each other. Most of the women aren't gay, it just happens. And maybe it's nice having sex with other women when you're surrounded by so many guys.

Is there much relationship drama on base?

Good God yes. Guys aren't used to women being trained soldiers, and some of these women won't hesitate to hurt you physically, and I mean hit you, pull a knife on you, and even shoot you. Everything is turned up on a base in a war zone, including the drama.

How are women treated on the bases?

Terribly. A woman who is in the military needs to have seriously thick skin. Guys are going to be talking trash to her from morning to night, 'Bend over and let's see what you've got...' kind of stuff. A woman needs to be tough and able to ignore it. Guys will behave when a commanding officer is around, but the minute he or she is gone...

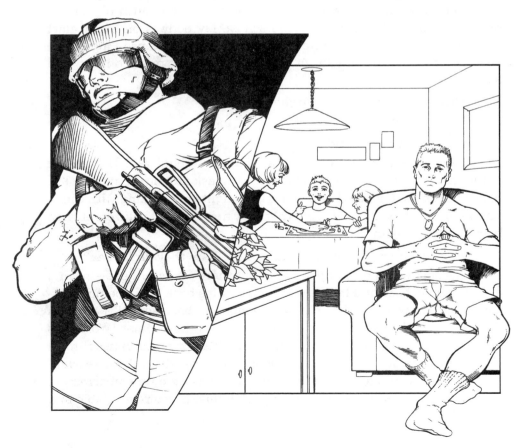

Chapter: "I Knew the Bride"
Long Term Relationships

The title of this chapter refers to a song about the singer's former lover before she was married. He knew her when she was a bit more wild than her traditional flowing white wedding dress might indicate. So what happens when you leave it all behind and enter a new phase of life? This chapter is about sex in marriage and long term relationships. *Read the entire chapter at www.Guide2Getting.com/marriage*

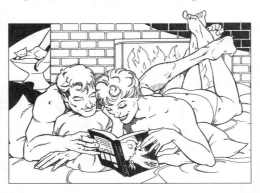

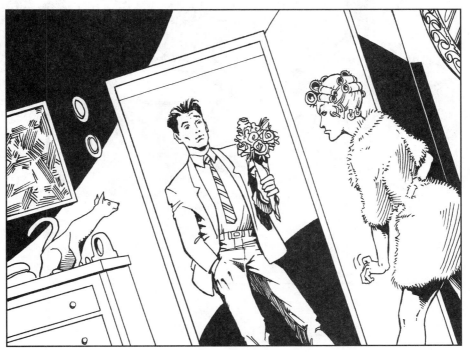

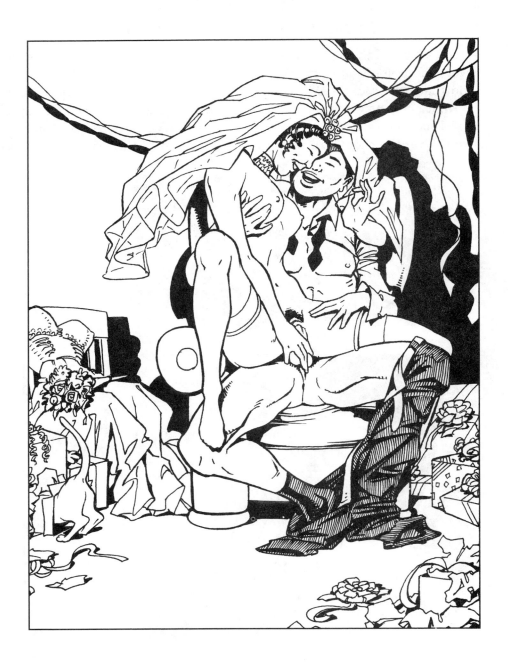

TROLL—when someone on the Internet posts messages that are designed to enrage people, such as cat-meat recipes on a pet-lover forum. To those who respond, the reply will sometimes be YHBT.YHL.HAND which means "you have been trolled, you have lost, have a nice day."

TUBAL LIGATION—female sterilization where the Fallopian tubes are sealed.

TUBES—free websites that are aggregators of porn content. Some of the better known tubes are Pornotube, Xtube, Pornhub, Redtube, Xhamster and Spankwire. Many of the videos are pirated, but some are from genuine amateurs who get off from posting and having fans. Porn tubes have drastically changed the way porn sites operate. It used to be porn viewers expected to take a sh[...] then have to subscribe with a monthly fee. Now, it's [...] porn for free, with the price they pay subs[...]am of pop-ups, and countless viruses[...]

TURKEY DUMP—[...] Thanksgiving and breaks u[...] breakup that happens soo[...]

TWINK—a yo[...]at helpless or is not th[...]to be white and withou[...]. Twink and twinking ar[...]o with sex.

UHSE, BEATE—[...]ded and run by Beate Rote[...]ith her young son, stole a plan[...]ey were pulling into Germany at t[...]one of the finest museums of sexuality[...]

> The Guide's incredible Dictionary of Sex Terms and Sex Slang now resides at Guide2Getting.com/glossary It's the most unusual and amazing glossary you will ever find.

UM-FRIEND—according to the [...] Poly, this is a person no one else knows you are having sex with: "This is Dan, my–um–friend."

UNDERWEAR SWAPPING or TRADING—in Japan, there is such a large market for unlaundered teenage girls' underwear that the legislature outlawed the sale of used underwear by teenagers. Japanese teenage girls could go to small stores called burusera and sell their soiled knickers for $20, $30 or more per pair (the more fragrant or soiled, the higher the price). In other parts of the world, some gay men are into *briefs swapping*, and some college women have learned that if they create the right online presence, they can sell their soiled panties to horny straight guys.

UNDESCENDED TESTICLE—testicles are not formed in the scrotum, but in the abdomen. Before birth, they usually descend into the scrotum. About 3.5% of the time, a testicle doesn't descend into the scrotum, so the boy is born with an undescended testicle. The majority of undescended testi

W

X-Y-Z

For a great glossary of sex terms and slang, and for posts on sports, nature, sex, and our mostly wonderful videos, visit **www.Guide2Getting.com**